Rare Diseases of the Immune System

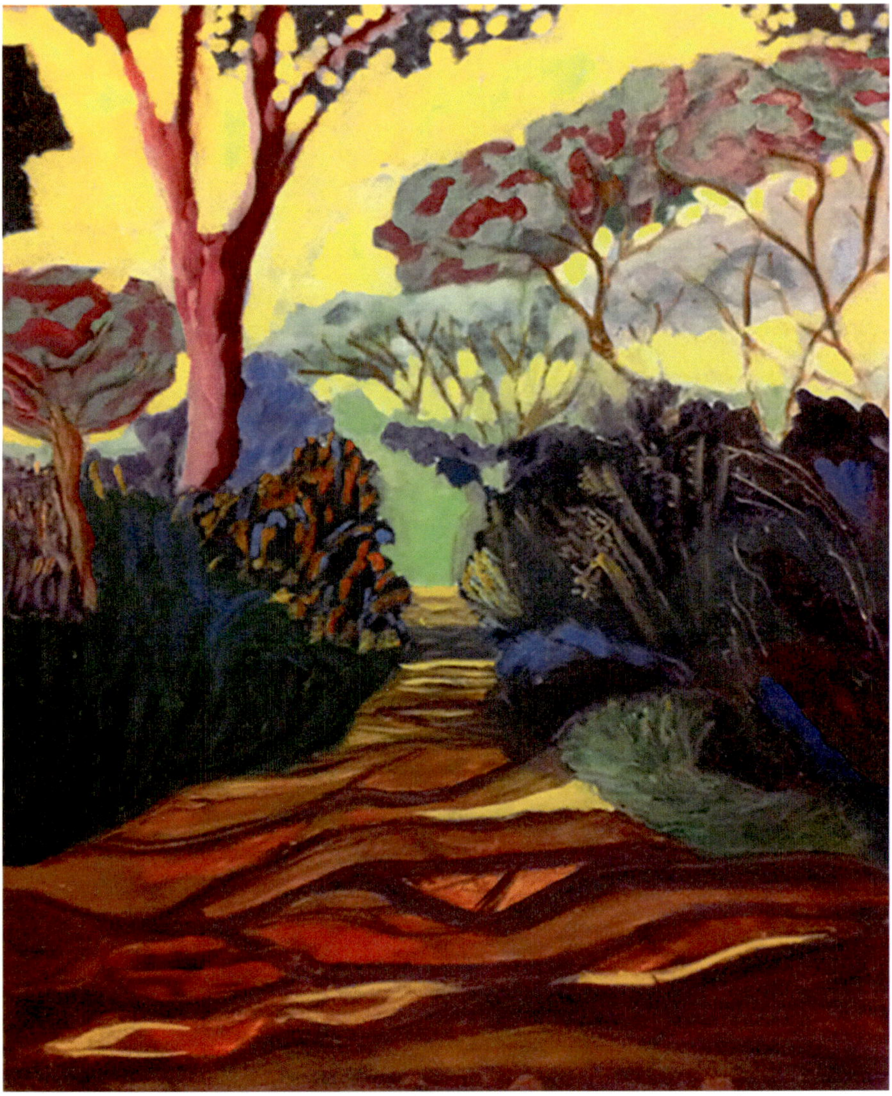

Pineta, Laura Maddii Emmi (Private collection)

Javier Martín • Francisco David Carmona
Editors

Genetics of Rare Autoimmune Diseases

Springer

Editors
Javier Martín
Institute of Parasitology and Biomedicine
Lopez-Neyra
CSIC
Granada
Spain

Francisco David Carmona
Department of Genetics
University of Granada
Armilla
Granada
Spain

ISSN 2282-6505 ISSN 2283-6403 (electronic)
Rare Diseases of the Immune System
ISBN 978-3-030-03933-2 ISBN 978-3-030-03934-9 (eBook)
https://doi.org/10.1007/978-3-030-03934-9

This Springer imprint is published by the registered company Springer Nature Switzerland AG
The registered company address is: Gewerbestrasse 11, 6330 Cham, Switzerland

Preface

Autoimmunity is characterized by progressive tissue damage due to pathogenic processes whose primary cause is the loss of tolerance of the immune system against self-peptides of the organism. The clinical manifestations of such abnormal immune responses depend on the affected cells or tissues, resulting in a heterogeneous group of severe immune-mediated conditions known as autoimmune diseases.

Autoimmune diseases have a relatively low prevalence individually, and, because of that, they are considered rare in most cases. Besides, most of them have a multifactorial etiology, in which a complex interaction between environmental and polygenic factors is responsible for their development and progression. As a consequence, these conditions received little attention during the last century in comparison with other more common diseases. However, the overall prevalence of autoimmunity has been estimated around 5–8% in Western countries which, together with their chronic and disabling nature in most cases, implies a considerable socioeconomic burden for both the patients and the healthcare systems.

The increase in the sample size of the study cohorts and the use of novel technologies for genome-level data analysis during the last decade have substantially increased our knowledge of the molecular mechanisms involved in the susceptibility and expression of autoimmune diseases. It is currently known that common human genetic variation and epigenetics are directly involved in their pathophysiology. The elucidation of the genetic basis of autoimmunity is definitively helping in the identification of accurate diagnostic and prognostic markers as well as in the implementation of more effective personalized therapies.

This volume is aimed at providing an updated overview of the recent progress gained on the molecular mechanisms that underlie the most relevant rare autoimmune diseases, providing a critical point of view about the possible future directions by basic and clinical researchers of worldwide renown. The two main reasons that motivated us to coordinate this fascinating initiative were the growing interest in this topic and the reduced number of documents related to it available in the literature.

We would like to sincerely thank the authors that made possible the publication of this book, as we are confident that a broad range of students, practicing physicians, and scientists of related disciplines will benefit from their valuable knowledge on this field, which was acquired during many years of high effort, passion, and dedication.

Granada, Spain Javier Martín
Granada, Spain Francisco David Carmona

Contents

Systemic Lupus Erythematosus

1

Susan K. Vester and Timothy J. Vyse

Contents

1.1 Introduction

Systemic lupus erythematosus (SLE) is a chronic autoimmune inflammatory disease. It is clinically very heterogeneous, and multiple organ systems can be affected including the skin, kidneys, nervous system, heart, lungs, and the musculoskeletal system, with severity of disease ranging from mild to life-threatening. SLE is characterized by the production of autoantibodies against cell nuclear components such as DNA, histones, and ribonucleoproteins [1]. The prevalence of

S. K. Vester
Department of Medical and Molecular Genetics, King's College London, London, UK
e-mail: susan.vester@kcl.ac.uk

T. J. Vyse (✉)
Department of Medical and Molecular Genetics, King's College London, Guy's Hospital, London, UK
e-mail: timothy.vyse@kcl.ac.uk

J. Martín, F. D. Carmona (eds.), *Genetics of Rare Autoimmune Diseases*,
Rare Diseases of the Immune System, https://doi.org/10.1007/978-3-030-03934-9_1

SLE is ancestry-dependent, being more prevalent in non-European populations such as Afro-Caribbean, African American, and Asian. Ninety percent of patients are female, and in a majority of cases, onset of disease occurs during or after childbearing years [2, 3]. Juvenile onset makes up 15–20% of lupus cases, is less biased toward females, and is characterized with a more severe outcome and higher disease activity [4]. SLE is typically a genetically complex disease that has a strong genetic component, with an estimated heritability of 44–66% [5, 6]. Studies have shown that twin concordance rates are much higher in monozygotic twins (24–57%) than dizygotic twins (2%) [7, 8]. While siblings, parents, and offspring of affected patients have a higher than average risk of developing SLE (sibling risk λs of over 20), heredity is complex and in most cases does not follow a Mendelian pattern of inheritance [5, 9]. Earlier onset of disease and severe disease presentation are thought to correlate with higher genetic burden [10]. Environmental factors such as smoking; exposure to UV light; medication; viral infections, for instance, Epstein-Barr virus; and hormonal factors (estrogen, prolactin) contribute to the development of SLE, making this a multifactorial disease [11]. Pathways that have been implicated in the pathogenesis of SLE through genetic advances include impaired apoptosis and autophagy leading to clearance defects and thus increased exposure to nuclear autoantigens, type I interferon signaling including nucleic acid sensing and interferon (IFN) response, B lymphocyte hyperactivity, and altered immune cell signaling. Gaining a better understanding of the underlying pathways resulting in the development of SLE through genetic studies will lead the way in the development of targeted therapies. The clinically heterogeneous spectrum of SLE may represent several distinct, but related diseases that may respond differently to treatment [12].

1.2 Rare Monogenic Causes of SLE

While SLE is in most cases a complex genetic disease with polygenic inheritance, familial forms of lupus have been described as early as the 1950s [13–16]. Monogenic causes of lupus are rare, especially in adult cohorts, and disease phenotype can vary from classic manifestation. However, they provide clear genotype-phenotype relationships that give insight into the underlying biological pathways involved. Suggestive of a monogenic cause of lupus or lupus-like disease can be early age of onset; severe, atypical, or refractory manifestation; a family history of the disease (with Mendelian inheritance); parental consanguinity; or male gender [17]. Deficiencies in classical complement components were among the first to be described. Mutations have mainly been observed in early pathway components *C1Q*, *C1R*, *C1S*, *C4*, and *C2*, but some rarer are known in terminal pathway components *C3* and *C5–C9* [18]. While penetrance of these autosomal recessive complete complement deficiencies is high, not every individual will develop SLE as a result: 93% of *C1Q* deficiencies, 75% of *C4* deficiencies, 57% of *C1R*/*C1S* deficiencies, 32–33% of *C2* deficiencies, and 10% of *C3* deficiencies develop SLE [19]. Of note, both *C2* and C4's C4A and C4B genes are clustered on the class III major histocompatibility complex (MHC) on chromosome 6 [20]. Complement deficiencies lead to an impaired uptake of apoptotic material, and both C1 and C4 deficiencies (which cause SLE in more than 75% of cases) are thought to additionally compromise self-tolerance [21]. While complement deficiencies have long been recognized as a cause of monogenic SLE, mutations in components of nucleic acid sensing, type I IFN, immune clearance, and lymphocyte signaling pathways have been discovered. This includes impaired clearance through an autosomal dominant inherited mutation in *DNASE1* [22] or a *DNASE1L3* null mutation, which leads to an autosomal recessive form of SLE characterized by pediatric onset of disease and kidney involvement [23]. A mutation in *PRKCD* (protein kinase Cδ) leading to dysregulated apoptosis and B cell proliferation was further found in a family with an autosomal recessive form of SLE [24]. Lupus-like diseases such as autosomal dominant familial chilblain lupus and autosomal recessive Aicardi-Goutières syndrome have shed further light on monogenic causal variants including *TREX1*, *SAMHD1*, *RNASEH2A*, *RNASEH2B*, *RNASEH2C*, *ADAR*, and *IFIH1* involved in the nucleic acid sensing and the type I IFN pathway [25]. Other monogenic causes of lupus-like diseases have implicated over 16 further genes [26, 27].

1.3 The MHC

HLA antigens are extremely polymorphic due to selective pressure to present a wide variety of antigens. Associations between the MHC and SLE were first described in humans as early as 1971 [28, 29]. Classical MHC class II alleles HLA-DR3 (DRB1*0301) and HLA-DR2 (DRB1*1501), along with their haplotypes, have been consistently associated with SLE in European populations [30]. Indeed, in female-dominated European cohorts, the MHC region accounts for the greatest genetic risk of SLE [31–33]. Assessing causality of variants within the MHC is challenging due to the high linkage disequilibrium observed; however, it has become apparent that the MHC harbors multiple, distinct association signals [34–37].

1.4 Polygenic Causes of SLE

Up until the early 2000s, associations with the MHC, antibody receptor genes (e.g., *FCGR2A*), as well as monogenic complement deficiencies were some of the few known genetic factors of SLE [38]. Linkage analysis and candidate gene studies in subsequent years yielded further associations, including nine independently identified and replicated linkages. Meta-analysis of candidate genes confirmed association with genes such as *PTPN22*, *IL10*, *CTLA4*, and *MBL* [39]. However, it was not until the advent of new technologies such as genome-wide association studies (GWAS) and next-generation sequencing (NGS) that our knowledge of the genetics

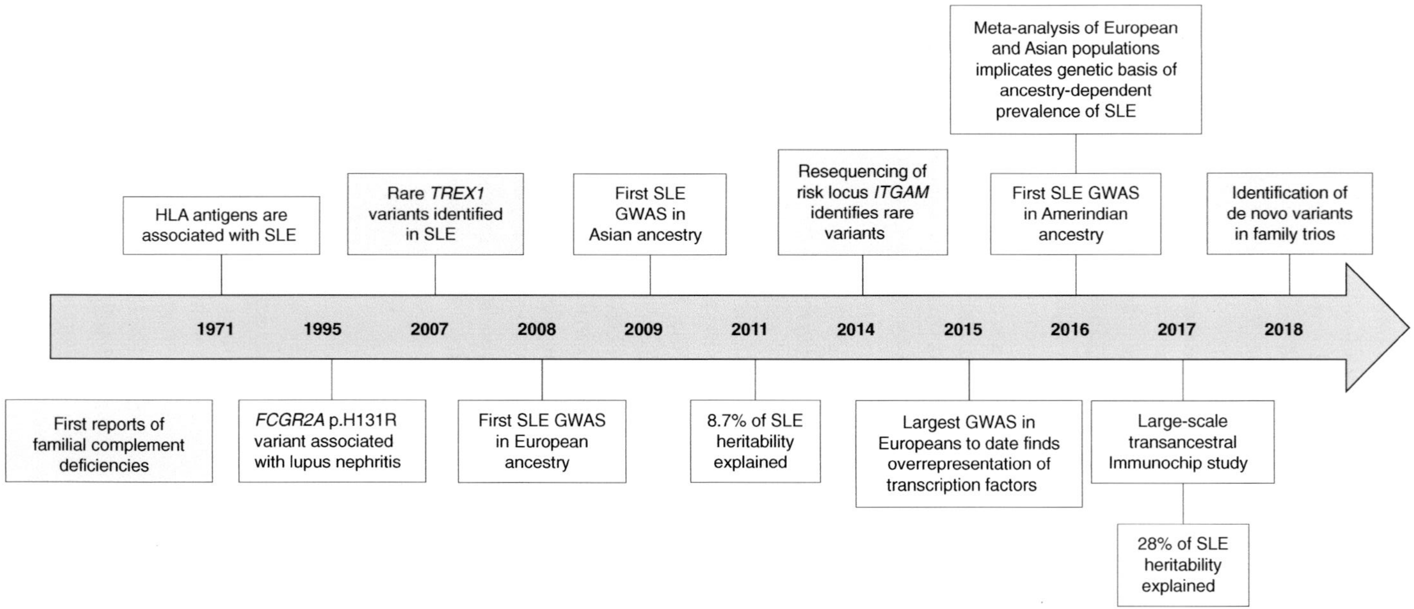

Fig. 1.1 Timeline of major advances in the discovery of common and rare variants in SLE genetics. Shaded boxes indicate discovery of rare variants. See text for details

of genetically complex diseases has enormously increased (see Fig. 1.1). A polygenic disease such as SLE will harbor contributions from both common and rare variants. Such sequence variation can take the form of single nucleotide polymorphisms (SNPs), approximately 90% of sequence variants observed, or structural variation, for instance, inversions or insertions and deletions, termed copy number variations (CNVs) [40, 41]. Common variants have a minor allele frequency (MAF) of 5% and over, while low-frequency variants have a MAF of 1–5%, and rare variants have a frequency of less than 1%. In the following, no distinction will be made between rare and low-frequency variants.

1.4.1 Common Variants

Some years ago, the "common disease, common variant" hypothesis was put forward, suggesting that common variants with modest effect size are found throughout the population and will contribute to complex disease susceptibility [42, 43]. GWAS have been extensively utilized to identify association of common variants with disease. Studying this association is hampered by the fact that common variants are found in both healthy controls and in patients, albeit to a lesser extent in the control population if a variant is associated with disease risk. Common variants have been found to confer only modest risk with 1.1–1.5-fold odds ratios [44]. Both the frequency and effect size of a variant have an impact on the sample size needed to detect significant associations [45]. The first four GWAS in SLE in European populations were published 10 years ago in 2008, after many successful discoveries had been made in other autoimmune diseases [31–33, 46]. Nine of these loci were independently replicated the following year [47]. Since then a further three GWAS have been conducted in European populations [48–50], seven GWAS in Asian populations [51–57], and one GWAS in an Amerindian population [58]. Meta-analysis and large-scale replication studies soon followed [36, 59–62]. Over half of GWAS SNPs have been found to be shared between populations. The genetic risk score of SLE is lowest in European populations and increases in Amerindian and South Asian populations, then East Asian populations, and is highest in African populations [61]. This corresponds with prevalence of SLE in different ethnic groups. In addition, a large transancestral Immunochip study including European, African, and Hispanic Amerindian ancestry identified novel loci and showed that both ancestry-dependent and ancestry-independent SLE risk alleles exist [63]. The Immunochip includes SNPs and small insertion deletions for autoimmune and inflammatory diseases [64]. While in 2011 only 8.7% of SLE disease heritability could be explained [65], over 80 risk loci are now robustly associated with SLE risk at a genome-wide significance level of $p < 5 \times 10^{-8}$, calculating the explained heritability of SLE at around 28%. Thus, over 50% of observed SLE heritability cannot be explained through common variation, a caveat being that heritability is difficult to calculate in complex diseases [66]. The results of GWAS have led to the identification and consolidation of the three major pathways involved in SLE pathogenesis: waste clearance, IFN signaling, and lymphocyte signaling [26]. Common disease-associated loci are located outside of protein-coding regions, and an overrepresentation of transcription factors has been found among SLE susceptibility genes, suggesting that common SLE-associated variants perform regulatory roles [48]. This is in accord with the proposed omnigenic model of common variation, which suggests that association signals will be located in gene regulatory networks that impact core disease-related genes in relevant cell types [67]. Studying the functional consequences of regulatory variation is challenging, as these SNPs can be located in intergenic and intragenic regions and have short- and long-range interactions [68]. Expression quantitative trait loci (eQTLs) along with colocalization methods are used to map GWAS results to find causative variants and genes, where possible [69]. Over 80% annotation and analysis of the noncoding genome has been provided by the Encyclopedia of DNA Elements, the Roadmap Epigenomics Consortium, and the Blueprint Epigenome project [70–72]. How these data can be used to further the investigation of SLE risk loci has been recently reviewed [66].

1.4.2 Missing Heritability

The identification of common variants through GWAS has increased our understanding of SLE genetics. However, there is still an observable difference in heritability estimated from familial clustering, and that can be explained by genetic variants, termed *missing heritability*. Many explanations might account for this missing heritability. This includes common variants with effect sizes below the genome-wide significance threshold in current study sizes, rare or low-frequency variants that fall below genome-wide significance due to frequency or effect size, structural variants such as inversions or CNVs, epigenetic factors, or gene-gene interactions such as regulatory haplotypes [73].

1.4.3 Rare Variants

While rare variants self-evidently are individually very uncommon in the population, they are collectively common. On average, rare variants are evolutionary "younger" than common variants, and thus differences in allele frequencies in different ancestries are more pronounced for rare variants than for common variation [74]. However, unaffected individuals will also harbor rare or private mutations that may or may not influence disease risk [75]. Rare variants can be both protein-coding and noncoding; however, non-synonymous protein-coding variants are more likely to have a greater effect size than common regulatory variants. It has been suggested that these rare variants fall into core disease genes that may make druggable targets [67]. High-penetrant rare variants, especially, have the ability to lead the way in the development of novel therapies. Designing functional studies for protein-coding variants is easier than for regulatory variants, as studying the genotype-phenotype relationship is more straightforward. Methods to identify rare variation include imputation using HapMap, 1000 Genomes, UK10K, or the

Haplotype Reference Consortium and custom genotyping arrays such as Immunochip, UK Biobank Axiom Array, or Illumina HumanExome BeadChip (although the coverage of rare and low-frequency variants is incomplete). However, the most robust and reliable method of detection is using NGS approaches such as targeted resequencing, whole-exome sequencing (WES), or whole-genome sequencing (WGS) [76].

1.4.3.1 Resequencing of Known Risk Loci

Targeted resequencing of risk loci can yield rare as well as common variants and can help to identify functional variants. However, this approach is not always very successful, as common loci do not necessarily harbor rare variants. Hunt et al. [77] reported a negligible impact on heritability from rare variants through resequencing of known GWAS loci in different autoimmune diseases and suggested that rare variants might be found in a discrete set of genes. Targeted resequencing has however been successfully performed in other diseases such as asthma, psoriasis, or inflammatory bowel disease (IBD) [78–80]. Rare variants in the DNA exonuclease *TREX1* (initially discovered in patients with monogenic forms of lupus-like disease) were found at a rate of around 2% in European SLE cohorts [81] and 0.5% in a multi-ancestral study [82]. In addition, the monogenic risk locus *DNASE1* was found to harbor further rare variants [83]. Resequencing of the common risk locus *ITGAM* yielded two novel protein-coding variants that, albeit case-specific, were shown to be functionally damaging [84]. Resequencing of the *IRF8* risk locus revealed variants including a deletion-insertion polymorphism, found to be in strong linkage disequilibrium with two genotyped and SLE-associated SNPs [85], and resequencing of *IRF5* leads to the discovery of further functional variants [86]. SLE risk-associated genes *IKBKE* and *IFIH1* were resequenced, and both rare and common variation were found [87]. Interestingly, rare variants in the nucleic acid-sensing gene *IFIH1* were identified as a cause of Aicardi-Goutières syndrome (see Sect. 1.2), and common genetic variation at this locus also appears to contribute as a risk in GWAS [48]. A similar observation has been made at the *RNASEH2C* locus [61, 62].

1.4.3.2 Identification of De Novo Mutations

Due to their low frequency, rare variants may not statistically associate with disease but, if pathogenic, will contribute to the development of SLE. A relatively high de novo mutation rate has been observed in humans, and each individual is estimated to have one de novo mutation in their genome, irrespective of disease status [88]. Thus, the simple presence of a de novo mutation is not sufficient to imply causality, and differentiation between causal and random variation will need to be made; rare variants need not be disease-causing as such [89]. WES and WGS can be used as hypothesis-free approaches to study the underlying genetics of disease. WES is currently less cost-prohibitive than WGS, but only captures 1–2% of the human genome, and WGS may perform better at calling exonic variants [90]. Large-scale exome-wide case control studies in diseases such as type 2 diabetes or IBD have had limited success at detecting rare variant associations [91, 92]. Approaches to overcome this limitation include studying extreme phenotypes [93] or looking for de novo mutations in extended families or family trios. A first example of using WES in polygenic cases of SLE to discover new candidate genes through de novo mutations has recently been published [94]. WES was performed in a cohort of 30 unrelated patients and their unaffected parents (family trios) with extreme phenotype, i.e., severe disease comprising young age of onset and clinical features associated with poorer outcome. Fourteen novel de novo missense mutations were discovered in 11 patients that were absent in the parents and unaffected siblings, none of which were among any of the >80 known SLE-associated genes. Some of these de novo mutations may be random background variation, which is why it is important to further study the variants and genes implicated. Five of the discovered variants, all CpG transitions, were observed at very low frequencies in ExAC, and five variants were predicted to be possibly damaging (CADD Phred score > 5). For one of these genes, *C1QTNF4*, found to be harboring a p.His198Gln de novo mutation, gene-level metrics support a potential role in SLE, although no further rare variant associations were discovered for this gene. *C1QTNF4* is constrained against missense variants and has a modest CADD score of 12.3. The function of C1QTNF4 is currently poorly understood; however, it has structural homology with both C1q and tumor necrosis factor (TNF) superfamily members, important pathways in the pathogenesis of SLE. Mutant p.His198Gln-C1QTNF4 appears to inhibit some TNF-mediated cellular responses in vitro, including NF-κB activation and TNF-induced cell death, suggesting a causal role of this mutation [94]. Another gene discovered to harbor a de novo mutation, *PRKCB*, has previously been reported in a consanguineous family with monogenic SLE [24] (see Sect. 1.2). While different pathogenicity-predictive tools for protein-coding variation are available [95], examining the role of rare, noncoding variants in WGS data is challenging. It is difficult to predict and test the functional significance of noncoding mutations, many of which will have no impact on pathogenesis.

1.4.3.3 Rare Variant Association Analysis

Statistical methods to study association of rare variation comprise genomic region-based tests. These include burden tests, variance-component tests, combined tests, and others. Burden tests collapse causal genetic variants of the same effect size and direction into a single score, e.g., by gene, exon, or family of genes, and a regression analysis with the disease can then be performed [76]. Burden of rare variants might implicate genes in SLE pathogenesis that have so far not been identified as contributing to risk. Pullabhatla et al. [94] performed a burden test of rare exonic variants on imputed data and found association of rare variants in *PRKCD* with SLE. Furthermore, they observed association of collective rare exonic variants in the DNA methyltransferase *DNMT3A* with anti-dsDNA and renal involvement with hypocomplementemia in a subphenotype analysis. Variance-component tests examine the distribution of genetic effects within a set of variants, independently of the direction of the effect, which can be weighted [76]. Wang et al. [87] performed a sequence kernel association test to examine association of SLE with rare variants, discovered by resequencing of risk loci *IKBKE* and *IFIH1*. The publication was not able to show any significant association with these rare variants; however, they could be pathogenic in the individual. These association tests have limitations such as power, replication, and confounding effects, and using family-based designs can be beneficial [76].

1.4.4 Structural Variants

Although structural variants can be both common and rare, GWAS prioritize SNPs which make up most of the sequence variation observed. Structural variants such as inversions or CNVs will also contribute to lupus susceptibility. CNVs often span whole or multiple genes and are likely to have a functional impact [73, 96]. While it is not easy to detect CNVs, new analysis tools for NGS data are making studying this structural variation easier. In particular interesting for a female-biased disease such as SLE, a disease-unrelated autosomal burden of rare CNVs has been reported in females [97]. Low copy number of the IgG Fc receptor FCGR3B gene is associated with SLE susceptibility [98–100]. Additionally, it has been suggested that complement *C4* with CNV is a risk factor for SLE; however, extensive LD at the MHC makes this contentious [101].

1.5 Epigenetic Mechanisms

Epigenetic alterations such as DNA methylation, histone modification, DNA hydroxymethylation, or noncoding RNA are known to contribute to the development of SLE. For instance, DNA hypomethylation and thus overexpression of inflammatory genes have been observed in SLE [102, 103]. Furthermore, DNA hypomethylation of apoptotic DNA appears to be involved in triggering autoantibody production [104]. Interestingly, rare variants in the DNA methyltransferase *DNMT3A* have been associated with SLE subphenotypes (see Sect. 1.4.3.2). SLE is predominantly observed in females, suggesting a direct or indirect effect of the sex chromosomes. Further insight into the role of the X chromosome in SLE has been gained from patients with X chromosomal abnormalities. The prevalence of patients with Klinefelter syndrome (47,XXY karyotype) in SLE is much higher than in the general population, with the risk of Klinefelter patients developing SLE much closer to female (46,XX), than male (46,XY) risk [105]. A higher prevalence of SLE was also reported in 47,XXX women than 46,XX women [106], and in addition, Turner's syndrome (45,XO) may be underrepresented in SLE [107]. Together these findings suggest an X chromosome gene dosage effect [105–107], for which genes that escape X inactivation are potential candidates. Six loci harboring common variants associated with SLE have been identified on the X chromosome, including *PRPS2*, *TLR7*, *CXorf21*, *LINC01420*, *NAA10-HCFC1-TMEM187*, and *IRAK1-MECP2*, in different populations [48, 108–111].

1.6 Modified Penetrance Through Regulatory Haplotypes

Both common regulatory and rare protein-coding variants, whether sequence variation such as SNPs or structural variation, make up the inter-individual variation that can lead to the development of disease. While variation is often studied on an individual variant level, variation should be viewed in context and not as independent entities, as there will, naturally, be interaction between a variant and its allelic setting. Coding variants especially, both in monogenic and polygenic inheritance, show a strong genotype-phenotype correlation; however, penetrance is often incomplete. While HLA variation has been viewed in terms of haplotypes for many years, it makes sense to think of other variation in the context of their regulatory haplotype. Noncoding variation has the ability to influence the expression of proteins, while pathogenic coding variation will have an impact on a gene's function. Thus, *cis*-regulatory variation will have an impact on the expression of the pathogenic gene product and hence will contribute to the penetrance of directly disease-causing variants through dosage effects (see Fig. 1.2). Indeed, there appears to be a negative selection of haplotypes that leads to higher penetrance of pathogenic coding variants through expression or splicing [112]. In a disease such as SLE with high clinical variability, the interplay between regulatory and coding variation may well contribute to the clinical heterogeneity observed. Thinking about the complete genetic makeup makes sense, especially when considering population differences based on ethnicity and thus underlying genetic differences. An example of modified penetrance by the interplay of rare and coding variation has been reported in monogenic SLE. Demirkaya et al. [113] described a novel, high-penetrant mutation in *C1R* as a cause of familial SLE in a consanguineous Turkish family with four affected patients homozygous for a 1 base pair deletion. One of the more severely affected patients had more additional SLE risk alleles than the other three affected family members (no classic SLE-associated HLA alleles were identified in this family), while one young family member with the deletion was not yet affected. Other rare monogenic complement deficiencies leading to SLE (see Sect. 1.2) have high,

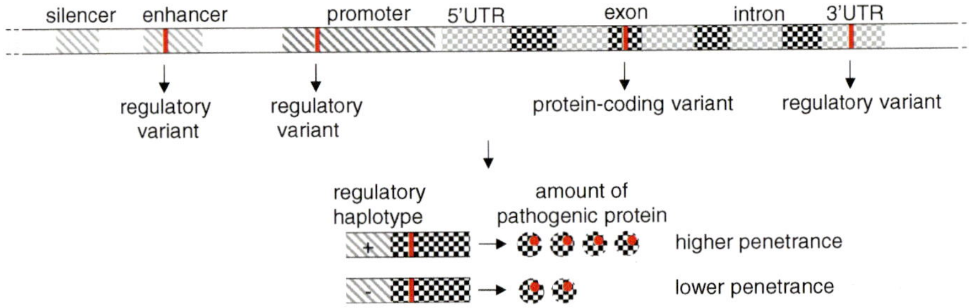

Fig. 1.2 Modified penetrance of protein-coding variation through regulatory haplotypes. Penetrance of protein-coding variation is dependent on the allelic regulatory haplotype made up of common or rare noncoding variants. The amount of mutated, here pathogenic, protein produced is dependent on how regulatory variation influences expressivity of this protein. *UTR* untranslated region

but incomplete penetrance. This implicates a role of modifying alleles in disease expressivity, as rare and common gene variants will collectively contribute to disease severity. Non-HLA haplotypes that influence risk of developing SLE have been described. *IRF5* haplotypes, consisting of a splice site variant, an exonic variant, and a variant in the 3′ untranslated region (3′UTR), are either protective or confer risk, demonstrating that multiple, in this case common, variants can jointly influence disease risk [86]. Furthermore, a *TREX1* risk haplotype made up of common variants was relatively common in European ancestry and had a higher frequency of neurological involvement [82]. Thus, both risk of developing SLE and severity of disease manifestation may be influenced by rare and common variant haplotypes.

1.7 Conclusions

In the last decade, much progress has been made in identifying the underlying genetic causes of SLE. Both common and rare variants have been identified; however, missing heritability is still observed. Initially, high-penetrant rare monogenic forms of SLE were described in family-based studies. Common variants have mainly been identified through population-based studies, especially since the advent of GWAS in 2008. However, identifying functionally causative variants from GWAS hits is not trivial, and thus the underlying pathogenic pathways remain poorly understood. While the interplay between variants remains understudied, observing them in terms of their haplotype is going to find increasing application. Elucidating the causal impact of risk variants and their underlying pathogenic pathways is of pivotal importance for exploring new therapeutic approaches. Family-based studies, especially of extreme phenotypes, yielding high-penetrant rare variants can inform new core genes and pathways. These are of particular importance for improving care of SLE patients, as these rare variants have the potential to be targeted therapeutically.

References

1. Kaul A, Gordon C, Crow MK, Touma Z, Urowitz MB, van Vollenhoven R, et al. Systemic lupus erythematosus. Nat Rev Dis Primers. 2016;2:16039.
2. Pons-Estel GJ, Alarcón GS, Scofield L, Reinlib L, Cooper GS. Understanding the epidemiology and progression of systemic lupus erythematosus. Semin Arthritis Rheum. 2010;39(4):257–68.
3. Rees F, Doherty M, Grainge MJ, Lanyon P, Zhang W. The worldwide incidence and prevalence of systemic lupus erythematosus: a systematic review of epidemiological studies. Rheumatology. 2017;56(11):1945–61.
4. Brunner HI, Gladman DD, Ibanez D, Urowitz MD, Silverman ED. Difference in disease features between childhood-onset and adult-onset systemic lupus erythematosus. Arthritis Rheum. 2008;58(2):556–62.
5. Kuo C-F, Grainge MJ, Valdes AM, See L-C, Luo S-F, Yu K-H, et al. Familial aggregation of systemic lupus erythematosus and coaggregation of autoimmune diseases in affected families. JAMA Intern Med. 2015;175(9):1518–26.

6. Lawrence JS, Martins CL, Drake GL. A family survey of lupus erythematosus. 1. Heritability. J Rheumatol. 1987;14(5):913–21.
7. Deapen D, Escalante A, Weinrib L, Horwitz D, Bachman B, Roy-Burman P, et al. A revised estimate of twin concordance in systemic lupus erythematosus. Arthritis Rheum. 1982;35(3):311–8.
8. Block SR, Winfield JB, Lockshin MD, D'Angelo WA, Christian CL. Studies of twins with systemic lupus erythematosus. A review of the literature and presentation of 12 additional sets. Am J Med. 1975;59(4):533–52.
9. Alarcon-Segovia ME, Cardiel MH, Caeiro F, Massardo L, Villa AR, Pons-Estel BA. Familial aggregation of systemic lupus erythematosus, rheumatoid arthritis, and other autoimmune diseases in 1,177 lupus patients from the GLADEL cohort. Arthritis Rheum. 2005;52(4):1138–47.
10. Webb R, Kelly JA, Somers EC, Hughes T, Kaufman KM, Sanchez E, et al. Early disease onset is predicted by a higher genetic risk for lupus and is associated with a more severe phenotype in lupus patients. Ann Rheum Dis. 2011;70(1):151–6.
11. Parks CG, de Souza Espindola Santos A, Barbhaiya M, Costenbader KH. Understanding the role of environmental factors in the development of systemic lupus erythematosus. Best Pract Res Clin Rheumatol. 2017;31(3):306–20.
12. Crow YJ. Lupus: how much "complexity" is really (just) genetic heterogeneity? Arthritis Rheum. 2011;63(12):3661–4.
13. Glagov S, Gechman E. Familial occurence of disseminated lupus erythematosus. N Engl J Med. 1956;255(20):936–40.
14. Marlow AA, Peabody HD, Nickel WR. Familial occurrence of systemic lupus erythematosus. JAMA. 1960;173(15):1641–3.
15. Agnello V, De Bracco MME, Kunkel HG. Hereditary C2 deficiency with some manifestations of systemic lupus erythematosus. J Immunol. 1972;108(3):837–40.
16. Moncada B, Day NKB, Good RA, Windhorst D. Lupus-erythematosus-like syndrome with a familial defect of complement. N Engl J Med. 1972;286(13):689–93.
17. Lo MS, Tsokos GC. Monogenic lupus. Int J Clin Rheumtol. 2014;9(6):543–6.
18. Morgan BP, Walport MJ. Complement deficiency and disease. Immunol Today. 1991;12(9):301–6.
19. Arason GJ, Jorgensen GH, Ludviksson BR. Primary immunodeficiency and autoimmunity: lessons from human diseases. Scand J Immunol. 2010;71(5):317–28.
20. Atkinson JP, Yung Yu C. Genetic susceptibility and class III complement genes. In: Systemic lupus erythematosus. 5th ed. New York: Elsevier; 2011. p. 21–45.
21. Costa-Reis P, Sullivan KE. Monogenic lupus: it's all new! Curr Opin Immunol. 2017;49:87–95.
22. Yasutomo K, Horiuchi T, Kagami S, Tsukamoto H, Hashimura C, Urushihara M, et al. Mutation of DNASE1 in people with systemic lupus erythematosus. Nat Genet. 2001;28(4):313–4.
23. Al-Mayouf SM, Sunker A, Abdwani R, Abrawi SA, Almurshedi F, Alhashmi N, et al. Loss-of-function variant in DNASE1L3 causes a familial form of systemic lupus erythematosus. Nat Genet. 2011;43(12):1186–8.
24. Belot A, Kasher PR, Trotter EW, Foray AP, Debaud AL, Rice GI, et al. Protein kinase Cδ deficiency causes Mendelian systemic lupus erythematosus with B cell-defective apoptosis and hyperproliferation. Arthritis Rheum. 2013;65(8):2161–71.
25. Crow YJ, Chase DS, Schmidt JL, Szynkiewicz M, Forte GM, Gornall HL, et al. Characterization of human disease phenotypes associated with mutations in TREX1, RNASEH2A, RNASEH2B, RNASEH2C, SAMHD1, ADAR, and IFIH1. Am J Med Genet Part A. 2015;167(A):296–312.
26. Tsokos GC, Lo MS, Reis PC, Sullivan KE. New insights into the immunopathogenesis of systemic lupus erythematosus. Nat Publ Gr. 2016;12(12):716–30.
27. Lo MS. Monogenic lupus. Curr Rheumatol Rep. 2016;18:71.
28. Grumet FC, Coukell A, Bodmer JG, Bodmer WF, McDevitt HO. Histocompatibility (HL-A) antigens associated with systemic lupus erythematosus. N Engl J Med. 1971;285(4):193–6.
29. Waters H, Konrad P, Walford RL. The distribution of HL-A histocompatibility factors and genes in patients with systemic lupus erythematosus. Tissue Antigens. 1971;1(2):68–73.

30. Tsao BP. Update on human systemic lupus erythematosus genetics. Curr Opin Rheumatol. 2004;16(5):513–21.
31. Harley JB, Alarcón-Riquelme ME, Criswell LA, Jacob CO, Kimberly RP, Moser KL, et al. Genome-wide association scan in women with systemic lupus erythematosus identifies susceptibility variants in ITGAM, PXK, KIAA1542 and other loci. Nat Genet. 2008;40(2):204–10.
32. Hom G, Ph D, Graham RR, Modrek B, Taylor KE, Ortmann W, et al. Association of systemic lupus erythematosus with C8orf13-BLK and ITGAM-ITGAX. N Engl J Med. 2008;358:900–9.
33. Graham RR, Cotsapas C, Davies L, Hackett R, Lessard CJ, Leon JM, et al. Genetic variants near TNFAIP3 on 6q23 are associated with systemic lupus erythematosus. Nat Genet. 2008;40(9):1059–61.
34. Fernando MMA, Stevens CR, Sabeti PC, Walsh EC, McWhinnie AJM, Shah A, et al. Identification of two independent risk factors for lupus within the MHC in United Kingdom families. PLoS Genet. 2007;3(11):2109–21.
35. Rioux JD, Goyette P, Vyse TJ, Hammarstrom L, Fernando MMA, Green T, et al. Mapping of multiple susceptibility variants within the MHC region for 7 immune-mediated diseases. Proc Natl Acad Sci. 2009;106(44):18680–5.
36. Morris DL, Taylor KE, Fernando MMA, Nititham J, Alarcón-Riquelme ME, Barcellos LF, et al. Unraveling multiple MHC gene associations with systemic lupus erythematosus: model choice indicates a role for HLA alleles and non-HLA genes in Europeans. Am J Hum Genet. 2012;91(5):778–93.
37. Morris DL, Fernando MMA, Taylor KE, Chung SA, Nititham J, Alarcón-Riquelme ME, et al. MHC associations with clinical and autoantibody manifestations in European SLE. Genes Immun. 2014;15(4):210–7.
38. Wakeland EK, Liu K, Graham RR, Behrens TW. Delineating the genetic basis of systemic lupus erythematosus. Immunity. 2001;15(3):397–408.
39. Sestak AL, Nath SK, Sawalha AH, Harley JB. Current status of lupus genetics. Arthritis Res Ther. 2007;9(3):210.
40. Collins FS, Brooks LD, Chakravarti A. A DNA polymorphism discovery resource for research on human genetic variation. Genome Res. 1998;8(12):1229–31.
41. Zarrei M, MacDonald JR, Merico D, Scherer SW. A copy number variation map of the human genome. Nat Rev Genet. 2015;16(3):172–83.
42. Reich DE, Lander ES. On the allelic spectrum of human disease. Trends Genet. 2001;17(9):502–10.
43. Becker KG. The common variants/multiple disease hypothesis of common complex genetic disorders. Med Hypotheses. 2004;62(2):309–17.
44. Manolio TA, Brooks LD, Collins FS. A HapMap harvest of insights into the genetics of common disease. J Clin Invest. 2008;118(5):1590–605.
45. Spencer CCA, Su Z, Donnelly P, Marchini J. Designing genome-wide association studies: sample size, power, imputation, and the choice of genotyping chip. PLoS Genet. 2009;5(5):e1000477.
46. Kozyrev SV, Abelson AK, Wojcik J, Zaghlool A, Linga Reddy MVP, Sanchez E, et al. Functional variants in the B-cell gene BANK1 are associated with systemic lupus erythematosus. Nat Genet. 2008;40(2):211–6.
47. Suarez-Gestal M, Calaza M, Endreffy E, Pullmann R, Ordi-Ros J, Domenico Sebastiani G, et al. Replication of recently identified systemic lupus erythematosus genetic associations: a case-control study. Arthritis Res Ther. 2009;11(3):1–9.
48. Bentham J, Morris DL, Cunninghame Graham DS, Pinder CL, Tombleson P, Behrens TW, et al. Genetic association analyses implicate aberrant regulation of innate and adaptive immunity genes in the pathogenesis of systemic lupus erythematosus. Nat Genet. 2015;47(12):1457–64.
49. Demirci FY, Wang X, Kelly JA, Morris DL, Barmada MM, Feingold E, et al. Identification of a new susceptibility locus for systemic lupus erythematosus on chromosome 12 in individuals of European ancestry. Arthritis Rheumatol. 2016;68(1):174–83.

50. Armstrong DL, Zidovetzki R, Alarcón-Riquelme ME, Tsao BP, Criswell LA, Kimberly RP, et al. GWAS identifies novel SLE susceptibility genes and explains the association of the HLA region. Genes Immun. 2014;15(6):347–54.
51. Han J-W, Zheng H-F, Cui Y, Sun L-D, Ye D-Q, Hu Z, et al. Genome-wide association study in a Chinese Han population identifies nine new susceptibility loci for systemic lupus erythematosus. Nat Genet. 2009;41(11):1234–7.
52. Yang W, Shen N, Ye DQ, Liu Q, Zhang Y, Qian XX, et al. Genome-wide association study in Asian populations identifies variants in ETS1 and WDFY4 associated with systemic lupus erythematosus. PLoS Genet. 2010;6(2):e1000841.
53. Okada Y, Shimane K, Kochi Y, Tahira T, Suzuki A, Higasa K, et al. A genome-wide association study identified AFF1 as a susceptibility locus for systemic lupus erythematosus in Japanese. PLoS Genet. 2012;8(1):e1002455.
54. Lee H-S, Kim T, Bang SY, Na YJ, Kim I, Kim K, et al. Ethnic specificity of lupus-associated loci identified in a genome-wide association study in Korean women. Ann Rheum Dis. 2014;73(6):1240–5.
55. Lessard CJ, Sajuthi S, Zhao J, Kim K, Ice JA, Li H, et al. Identification of a systemic lupus erythematosus risk locus spanning ATG16L2, FCHSD2, and P2RY2 in Koreans. Arthritis Rheumatol. 2016;68(5):1197–209.
56. Sun C, Molineros JE, Looger LL, Zhou XJ, Kim K, Okada Y, et al. High-density genotyping of immune-related loci identifies new SLE risk variants in individuals with Asian ancestry. Nat Genet. 2016;48(3):323–30.
57. Liu L, Zuo X, Zhu Z, Wen L, Yang C, Zhu C, et al. Genome-wide association study identifies three novel susceptibility loci for systemic lupus erythematosus in Han Chinese. Br J Dermatol. 2018;179(2):506–8. https://doi.org/10.1111/bjd.16500.
58. Alarcón-Riquelme ME, Ziegler JT, Molineros J, Howard TD, Moreno-Estrada A, Sánchez-Rodríguez E, et al. Genome-wide association study in an Amerindian ancestry population reveals novel systemic lupus erythematosus risk loci and the role of European admixture. Arthritis Rheumatol. 2016;68(4):932–43.
59. Kaiser R, Taylor KE, Deng Y, Zhao J, Li Y, Nititham J, et al. Single-nucleotide polymorphisms in VKORC1 are risk factors for systemic lupus erythematosus in Asians. Arthritis Rheum. 2013;65(1):211–5.
60. Zhang J, Zhang L, Zhang Y, Yang J, Guo M, Sun L, et al. Gene-based meta-analysis of genome-wide association study data identifies independent single-nucleotide polymorphisms in ANXA6 as being associated with systemic lupus erythematosus in Asian populations. Arthritis Rheumatol. 2015;67(11):2966–77.
61. Morris DL, Sheng Y, Zhang Y, Wang Y-F, Zhu Z, Tombleson P, et al. Genome-wide association meta-analysis in Chinese and European individuals identifies ten new loci associated with systemic lupus erythematosus. Nat Genet. 2016;48(8):940–6.
62. Molineros JE, Yang W, jie ZX, Sun C, Okada Y, Zhang H, et al. Confirmation of five novel susceptibility loci for systemic lupus erythematosus (SLE) and integrated network analysis of 82 SLE susceptibility loci. Hum Mol Genet. 2017;26(6):1205–16.
63. Langefeld CD, Ainsworth HC, Cunninghame Graham DS, Kelly JA, Comeau ME, Harley JB, et al. Transancestral mapping and genetic load in systemic lupus erythematosus. Nat Commun. 2017;8:16021.
64. Cortes A, Brown MA. Promise and pitfalls of the immunochip. Arthritis Res Ther. 2011;13(1):101.
65. So HC, Gui AHS, Cherny SS, Sham PC. Evaluating the heritability explained by known susceptibility variants: a survey of ten complex diseases. Genet Epidemiol. 2011;35(5):310–7.
66. Chen L, Morris DL, Vyse TJ. Genetic advances in systemic lupus erythematosus: an update. Curr Opin Rheumatol. 2017;29(5):423–33.
67. Boyle EA, Li YI, Pritchard JK. Perspective an expanded view of complex traits: From polygenic to omnigenic. Cell. 2017;169(7):1177–86.
68. Martin P, McGovern A, Orozco G, Duffus K, Yarwood A, Schoenfelder S, et al. Capture Hi-C reveals novel candidate genes and complex long-range interactions with related autoimmune risk loci. Nat Commun. 2015;6:1–7.

69. Odhams CA, Cortini A, Chen L, Roberts AL, Buil A, Small KS, et al. Mapping eQTLs with RNA-seq reveals novel susceptibility genes, non-coding RNAs and alternative-splicing events in systemic lupus erythematosus. Hum Mol Genet. 2017;26(5):1003–17.
70. Chen L, Ge B, Casale FP, Vasquez L, Kwan T, Garrido-Martín D, et al. Genetic drivers of epigenetic and transcriptional variation in human immune cells. Cell. 2016;167(5):1398–414.
71. Dunham I, Kundaje A, Aldred SF, Collins PJ, Davis CA, Doyle F, et al. An integrated encyclopedia of DNA elements in the human genome. Nature. 2012;489(7414):57–74.
72. Roadmap Epigenomics Consortium, Kundaje A, Meuleman W, Ernst J, Bilenky M, Yen A, et al. Integrative analysis of 111 reference human epigenomes. Nature. 2015;518(7539):317–29.
73. Manolio TA, Collins FS, Cox NJ, Goldstein DB, Hindorff LA, Hunter DJ, et al. Finding the missing heritability of complex diseases. Nature. 2009;461(7265):747–53.
74. Altshuler DM, Durbin RM, Abecasis GR, Bentley DR, Chakravarti A, Clark AG, et al. An integrated map of genetic variation from 1,092 human genomes. Nature. 2012;491(7422):56–65.
75. Keinan A, Clark AG. Recent explosive human population growth has resulted in an excess of rare genetic variants. Science. 2012;740:740–4.
76. Bomba L, Walter K, Soranzo N. The impact of rare and low-frequency genetic variants in common disease. Genome Biol. 2017;18(1):1–17.
77. Hunt KA, Mistry V, Bockett NA, Ahmad T, Ban M, Barker JN, et al. Negligible impact of rare autoimmune-locus coding-region variants on missing heritability. Nature. 2013;498(7453):232–5.
78. Torgerson DG, Capurso D, Mathias RA, Graves PE, Hernandez RD, Beaty TH, et al. Resequencing candidate genes implicates rare variants in asthma susceptibility. Am J Hum Genet. 2012;90(2):273–81.
79. Jordan CT, Cao L, Roberson EDO, Duan S, Helms CA, Nair RP, et al. Rare and common variants in CARD14, encoding an epidermal regulator of NF-kappaB, in psoriasis. Am J Hum Genet. 2012;90(5):796–808.
80. Rivas MA, Beaudoin M, Gardet A, Stevens C, Sharma Y, Zhang CK, et al. Deep resequencing of GWAS loci identifies independent rare variants associated with inflammatory bowel disease. Nat Genet. 2011;43(11):1066–73.
81. Lee-Kirsch MA, Gong M, Chowdhury D, Senenko L, Engel K, Lee YA, et al. Mutations in the gene encoding the 3′-5′ DNA exonuclease TREX1 are associated with systemic lupus erythematosus. Nat Genet. 2007;39(9):1065–7.
82. Namjou B, Kothari PH, Kelly JA, Glenn SB, Ojwang JO, Adler A, et al. Evaluation of the TREX1 gene in a large multi-ancestral lupus cohort. Genes Immun. 2011;12(4):270–9.
83. Bodaño A, Amarelo J, González A, Gómez-Reino JJ, Conde C. Novel DNASE I mutations related to systemic lupus erythematosus. Arthritis Rheum. 2004;50(12):4070–1.
84. Roberts AL, Thomas ERA, Bhosle S, Game L, Obraztsova O, Aitman TJ, et al. Resequencing the susceptibility gene, ITGAM, identifies two functionally deleterious rare variants in systemic lupus erythematosus cases. Arthritis Res Ther. 2014;16(3):R114.
85. Lessard CJ, Adrianto I, Ice JA, Wiley GB, Kelly JA, Glenn SB, et al. Identification of IRF8, TMEM39A, and IKZF3-ZPBP2 as susceptibility loci for systemic lupus erythematosus in a large-scale multiracial replication study. Am J Hum Genet. 2012;90(4):648–60.
86. Graham RR, Kyogoku C, Sigurdsson S, Vlasova IA, Davies LRL, Baechler EC, et al. Three functional variants of IFN regulatory factor 5 (IRF5) define risk and protective haplotypes for human lupus. Proc Natl Acad Sci. 2007;104(16):6758–63.
87. Wang C, Ahlford A, Laxman N, Nordmark G, Eloranta ML, Gunnarsson I, et al. Contribution of IKBKE and IFIH1 gene variants to SLE susceptibility. Genes Immun. 2013;14(4):217–22.
88. Veltman JA, Brunner HG. De novo mutations in human genetic disease. Nat Rev Genet. 2012;13(8):565–75.
89. Cooper GM, Shendure J. Needles in stacks of needles: finding disease-causal variants in a wealth of genomic data. Nat Rev Genet. 2011;12(9):628–40.
90. Belkadi A, Bolze A, Itan Y, Cobat A, Vincent QB, Antipenko A, et al. Whole-genome sequencing is more powerful than whole-exome sequencing for detecting exome variants. Proc Natl Acad Sci. 2015;112(17):5473–8.

91. Fuchsberger C, Flannick J, Teslovich TM, Mahajan A, Agarwala V, Gaulton KJ, et al. The genetic architecture of type 2 diabetes. Nature. 2016;536(7614):41–7.
92. Luo Y, De Lange KM, Jostins L, Moutsianas L, Randall J, Kennedy NA, et al. Exploring the genetic architecture of inflammatory bowel disease by whole-genome sequencing identifies association at ADCY7. Nat Genet. 2017;49(2):186–92.
93. Chakravarti A, Turner TN. Revealing rate-limiting steps in complex disease biology: the crucial importance of studying rare, extreme-phenotype families. Bioessays. 2016; 38(6):578–86.
94. Pullabhatla V, Roberts AL, Lewis MJ, Mauro D, Morris DL, Odhams CA, et al. De novo mutations implicate novel genes in systemic lupus erythematosus. Hum Mol Genet. 2018;27(3):421–9.
95. Lek M, Karczewski KJ, Minikel EV, Samocha KE, Banks E, Fennell T, et al. Analysis of protein-coding genetic variation in 60,706 humans. Nature. 2016;536(7616):285–91.
96. Ruderfer DM, Hamamsy T, Lek M, Karczewski KJ, Kavanagh D, Samocha KE, et al. Patterns of genic intolerance of rare copy number variation in 59,898 human exomes. Nat Genet. 2016;48(10):1107–11.
97. Desachy G, Croen LA, Torres AR, Kharrazi M, Delorenze GN, Windham GC, et al. Increased female autosomal burden of rare copy number variants in human populations and in autism families. Mol Psychiatry. 2015;20(2):170–5.
98. Fanciulli M, Norsworthy PJ, Petretto E, Dong R, Harper L, Kamesh L, et al. FCGR3B copy number variation is associated with susceptibility to systemic, but not organ-specific, autoimmunity. Nat Genet. 2007;39(6):721–3.
99. Morris DL, Roberts AL, Witherden AS, Tarzi R, Barros P, Whittaker JC, et al. Evidence for both copy number and allelic (NA1/NA2) risk at the FCGR3B locus in systemic lupus erythematosus. Eur J Hum Genet. 2010;18(9):1027–31.
100. Mueller M, Barros P, Witherden AS, Roberts AL, Zhang Z, Schaschl H, et al. Genomic pathology of SLE-associated copy-number variation at the FCGR2C/FCGR3B/FCGR2B locus. Am J Hum Genet. 2013;92(1):28–40.
101. Boteva L, Morris DL, Cortés-Hernández J, Martin J, Vyse TJ, Fernando MMA. Genetically determined partial complement C4 deficiency states are not independent risk factors for SLE in UK and Spanish populations. Am J Hum Genet. 2012;90(3):445–56.
102. Hedrich CM. Epigenetics in SLE. Curr Rheumatol Rep. 2017;19(9):58.
103. Long H, Yin H, Wang L, Gershwin ME, Lu Q. The critical role of epigenetics in systemic lupus erythematosus and autoimmunity. J Autoimmun. 2016;74:118–38.
104. Wen ZK, Xu W, Xu L, Cao QH, Wang Y, Chu YW, et al. DNA hypomethylation is crucial for apoptotic DNA to induce systemic lupus erythematosus-like autoimmune disease in SLE-non-susceptible mice. Rheumatology. 2007;46(12):1796–803.
105. Scofield RH, Bruner GR, Namjou B, Kimberly RP, Ramsey-Goldman R, Petri M, et al. Klinefelter's syndrome (47,XXY) in male systemic lupus erythematosus patients: support for the notion of a gene-dose effect from the X chromosome. Arthritis Rheum. 2008;58(8):2511–7.
106. Liu K, Kurien BT, Zimmerman SL, Kaufman KM, Taft DH, Kottyan LC, et al. X chromosome dose and sex bias in autoimmune diseases: increased prevalence of 47,XXX in systemic lupus erythematosus and Sjögren's syndrome. Arthritis Rheumatol. 2016;68(5):1290–300.
107. Cooney CM, Bruner GR, Aberle T, Namjou-Khales B, Myers LK, Feo L, et al. 46,X,del(X)(q13) Turner's syndrome women with systemic lupus erythematosus in a pedigree multiplex for SLE. Genes Immun. 2009;10(5):478–81.
108. Zhang Y, Zhang J, Yang J, Wang Y, Zhang L, Zuo X, et al. Meta-analysis of GWAS on two Chinese populations followed by replication identifies novel genetic variants on the X chromosome associated with systemic lupus erythematosus. Hum Mol Genet. 2015;24(1):274–84.
109. Shen N, Fu Q, Deng Y, Qian X, Zhao J, Kaufman KM, et al. Sex-specific association of X-linked Toll-like receptor 7 (TLR7) with male systemic lupus erythematosus. Proc Natl Acad Sci. 2010;107(36):15838–43.

110. Zhu Z, Liang Z, Liany H, Yang C, Wen L, Lin Z, et al. Discovery of a novel genetic susceptibility locus on X chromosome for systemic lupus erythematosus. Arthritis Res Ther. 2015;17(1):349.
111. Jacob CO, Zhu J, Armstrong DL, Yan M, Han J, Zhou XJ, et al. Identification of IRAK1 as a risk gene with critical role in the pathogenesis of systemic lupus erythematosus. Proc Natl Acad Sci. 2009;106(15):6256–61.
112. Castel SE, Cervera A, Mohammadi P, Aguet F, Reverter F, Wolman A, et al. Modified penetrance of coding variants by cis-regulatory variation shapes human traits. bioRxiv. 2018;190397.
113. Demirkaya E, Zhou Q, Smith CK, Ombrello MJ, Deuitch N, Tsai WL, et al. Brief report: deficiency of complement 1r subcomponent in early-onset systemic lupus erythematosus: the role of disease-modifying alleles in a monogenic disease. Arthritis Rheumatol. 2017;69(9):1832–9.

Systemic Sclerosis

2

Elena López-Isac, Marialbert Acosta-Herrera, and Javier Martín

Contents

2.1 Introduction

Systemic sclerosis or scleroderma (SSc) is a rare and complex autoimmune disease (AD) of the connective tissue with heterogeneous clinical manifestations. It involves deregulation of the immune system, vascular damage, and extensive collagen deposition leading to fibrosis in the skin and different internal organs [1–3]. The main vascular abnormalities include Raynaud's phenomenon, renal crisis, and pulmonary arterial hypertension (PAH). The lungs, heart, kidneys, and esophagus are the principal internal organs affected by fibrosis, although this complex disease can cause severe dysfunction and failure of almost any internal organ. Esophageal dysfunction is the most common visceral complication; however lung involvement (both pulmonary hypertension and pulmonary fibrosis) is the leading cause of

E. López-Isac (✉) · M. Acosta-Herrera · J. Martín
Institute of Parasitology and Biomedicine López-Neyra (IPBLN), CSIC, PTS Granada, Granada, Spain
e-mail: elenalopezisac@ipb.csic.es; m.acostaherrera@ipb.csic.es; javiermartin@ipb.csic.es

J. Martín, F. D. Carmona (eds.), *Genetics of Rare Autoimmune Diseases*,
Rare Diseases of the Immune System, https://doi.org/10.1007/978-3-030-03934-9_2

death [4]. Immune imbalance includes altered lymphocyte activation that leads to autoantibody production, aberrant cytokine release, and deregulation of the innate immune system. The most frequent autoantibodies are anticentromere (ACA), antitopoisomerase (ATA), and anti-RNA polymerase III autoantibodies (ARA) [1, 2]. Patients with SSc are usually classified into two main subgroups according to the extent of skin involvement, limited cutaneous SSc (lcSSc) and diffuse cutaneous SSc (dcSSc), with a prevalence of approximately 65% and 35%, respectively. In lcSSc, fibrosis is mainly restricted to the skin of the hands, arms, and face. Raynaud's phenomenon appears several years before fibrosis, and pulmonary arterial hypertension (PAH) is frequent. dcSSc is characterized by a more aggressive, generalized, and rapidly progressing fibrosis that affects the skin of all body and one or more visceral organs [1–3].

The occurrence of this disease is more frequent among females, with a woman-to-man ratio ranging from 3:1 to 12:1 [5]. However, a recent study has reported a correlation between male sex and a worse outcome of the disease [6]. Large discrepancies exist regarding SSc prevalence, ranging from 7 to 700 cases per million inhabitants. These differences may be the result of substantial variation across geographic regions, ethnic differences, and the lack of consensus on disease diagnosis and classification due, mainly, to the disease rarity and to the large spectrum of clinical manifestations and severity [6, 7]. The estimated prevalence is higher among African descent population than in European descent, and the lowest prevalence has been reported in Asian population [7, 8]. Furthermore, it has been observed an increasing north to south gradient in SSc incidence across Europe. Interestingly, the presence of autoantibodies is also differential across ethnicities being the ACA more frequent in European descent population and the anti-U1-ribonucleoprotein (RNP) and anti-U3-RNP (fibrillarin) in African descent population [9].

Despite the progress in understanding the pathophysiology of SSc, the pathogenic mechanisms underlying the disease are still far from its complete knowledge. The conventional proposed model suggests that microvascular injury and endothelial cell (EC) activation are the primary events in SSc [10–12]. The hypothesis arises from the observation that vascular damage (Raynaud's phenomenon and edema) is the earliest feature that takes place in the disease. However, recent studies have strengthened the idea of autoimmunity as a central player in the onset and progression of the disease [13, 14]. The vascular inflammatory phase is more prominent in the earlier stages of SSc. This inflammatory environment and the altered immune reaction ultimately give rise to fibroblast activation, excessive deposition of collagen and other components of the extracellular matrix (ECM), and fibrosis [11]. In addition, several studies have also implicated reactive oxygen species (ROS) in the pathogenesis of SSc [15]. Tissue ischemia and activated fibroblast can lead to the generation of these chemical species. In fact, high levels of ROS have been observed in SSc, and several in vitro and mouse model studies further support the profibrogenic effect of these chemical species in fibroblast [15–17].

SSc shows a complex etiology where environmental and genetic factors seem to play a major role in the disease [2]. Several environmental factors have been linked to SSc susceptibility, such as the exposure to chemical compounds (e.g., silica, organic solvents, welding fumes, or asbestos), infectious agents (e.g., parvovirus B19, cytomegalovirus, and Epstein-Barr virus), and pregnancy-related events [2]. The current knowledge of the SSc genetic component will be addressed in the following sections of the chapter.

2.2 Genetic Component

The most compelling evidence supporting the existence of a genetic component in SSc comes from family co-occurrence. In fact, a positive familial history of SSc is the major risk factor reported to date [18]. A study comprising 703 families, first-degree relatives and siblings of patients with SSc, showed relative risk ranging from 10- to 27-fold higher than in the general population [18]. Moreover, familial and twin studies have described a high concordance of autoantibody production [19, 20]. In addition, there is interesting evidence pointing out to this genetic component, given the aforementioned differential prevalence among different populations.

The starting point for understanding the genetic bases of complex diseases is the identification of genetic markers associated with them. Single nucleotide polymorphisms (SNPs) are variations at a single position in the DNA sequence. The association of these variants with a phenotype is determined by genetic association studies, and the most commonly used are bi-allelic SNPs. Case-control studies compare the allele frequencies of one or more SNPs between cases (individuals affected by the disease) and controls (unaffected individuals). If the difference between these frequencies is statistically significant, that is, the p-value for association is below the significance threshold, then the SNP is considered as associated with the disease [21].

Nowadays, and thanks to advances in the genotyping technology and large sequencing projects, the assessment of genetic associations is directed to the entire genome in genome-wide association studies (GWASs). They have the main advantage of exploring the genome without the need of having a previous hypothesis about the biological processes involved. Besides, they are hypothesis generating, since the novel discovered *loci* may pinpoint to unexpected pathways in the pathogenesis of the disease. With the help of public information from the HapMap project [22] and The 1000 Genomes project [23] through statistical inferences, the determination of millions of SNPs provides an excellent power to infer common genetic variation in European population.

Despite the success provided by GWAS, the majority of associated SNPs have modest effect sizes, and they explain a relatively small proportion of the heritability of many complex diseases [24]. Therefore, it has been proposed that part of this "missing heritability" may lie on non-well covered region from arrays or on rare variants with large effect sizes. This issue has led to the design of a genotyping array called Immunochip, with the aim to perform a fine-mapping of *loci* associated with immune-mediated diseases in a cost-effective manner [25]. This custom genotyping platform contains 196,524 variants (including SNPs and small insertions-deletions) for fine-mapping 186 autoimmunity loci and a dense coverage of the HLA region.

The study of the genetic basis underlying SSc started with candidate gene studies, using relatively small sample sizes. In spite of this, some of them were able to identify susceptibility genes that are currently considered as firmly associated genes with the disease, such as *STAT4*, *IRF5*, and the HLA region [26]. In 2010, the first GWAS in SSc in European population was published [27]. Our group was involved in the study, which identified *CD247* as a novel gene associated with SSc risk, and confirmed the previously reported associations in the HLA region, *STAT4* and *IRF5*. Interestingly, these findings were independently replicated by Dieudé et al. [28]. One year later, a second GWAS in SSc was published by Allanore et al., which identified the genes *TNIP1*, *RHOB*, and *PSORS1C1* as novel susceptibility *loci* [29]. Our group was involved in the independent replication of the findings from this second GWAS; however, we could only confirm *TNIP1* signal as a genetic risk factor for SSc [30]. This fact highlights the relevance of a high statistical power in GWAS, since GWAS results tend to present inflated effect sizes—also called the winner's curse. Additionally, two other SSc GWAS have been performed in Korean population and a trans-ethnic meta-GWAS involving European and Japanese patients, respectively [31, 32].

Another distinctive trait of GWASs is the so-called gray zone, where SNPs with tier 2 associations (*p*-values between 5×10^{-8} and 5×10^{-3}) are located. Follow-up studies focusing on this gray zone constitute one of the most useful GWAS data mining methods, since possible real association signals could be masked in that area due to a lack of statistical power. In SSc, these types of studies have been successful in the identification of new risk *loci*. Bossini-Castillo et al. performed a follow-up focused on *IL12RB2*, a *locus* that showed suggestive signal of association in the first SSc GWAS [33]. Additionally, Martin et al. carried out a large follow-up of the GWAS that included 768 polymorphisms selected from the gray zone, and they could identify *CSK* as a genetic risk factor for SSc and confirmed previously reported associations [34]. Taking advantage of our GWAS data, we also performed a follow-up of the gray zone from the French GWAS [35] confirming *PPARG* as a susceptibility locus.

The Immunochip has gathered important achievement on the genetic component of ADs [36]. Applying this fine-mapping approach, our group identified several new SSc susceptibility *loci* (*DNASE1IL3*, *IL12A*, and *ATG5*) that implicated new biological pathways into the pathogenesis of the disease, such as apoptosis and autophagy [37]. In addition, an extensive analysis of the HLA region was performed. Later on, a second SSc Immunochip performed in an Australian cohort with relatively small sample size confirmed some of the reported associations [38].

2.2.1 Systemic Sclerosis Heritability

The large numbers of SNPs provided by GWAS and Immunochip have offered great opportunities to develop new methodologies for predicting genetic risk of complex diseases in a more accurate way [39–41]. In the case of SSc, efforts in the estimation of disease heritability have not provided conclusive reports, mainly due to limited sample sizes [26]. The significant SNPs described to date for SSc only account for

~20% of the estimated heritability [26]. Thus, it is expected that additional SSc risk *loci* remain to be discovered. Moreover, the number of well-established susceptibility *loci* is relatively low in comparison with other ADs, such as rheumatoid arthritis (RA) and systemic lupus erythematosus (SLE), for which 101 and 43 *loci* have been validated, respectively [42]. The low prevalence of SSc makes difficult the recruitment of large sample sizes required to reach a high statistical power and to effectively detect association signals. Therefore, the estimation of the heritability of SSc is a challenging task.

2.2.2 The HLA Class II in Systemic Sclerosis

The major histocompatibility complex (*MHC*) is the genetic region that represents the strongest genetic association reported to date for SSc [37], as well as for other ADs [36]. This implies that disease-associated *MHC* alleles must be responsible for an important portion of the susceptibility to autoimmune processes. In human, the *MHC* is the most polymorphic region of the genome, and its gene products are called human leukocyte antigen (HLA).

Several HLA associations with SSc have been previously described, and all of them were found in HLA class II genes [36].The analyses according to the autoantibody status showed differential associations in the HLA genes [37, 43, 44]. Moreover ancestry has been proven to influence the association of classical HLA alleles associated with SSc [43, 45].This was clearly observed in the study by Arnett et al., which included 961 European descent, 178 African descent, and 161 Hispanic descent SSc patients and 1000 healthy controls (539 Caucasian, 263 African-American, and 198 Hispanic subjects) [43]. For the overall disease, the strongest associations were found for the DRB1*1104, DQA1*0501, and DQB1*0301 haplotype and DQB1 alleles encoding a non-leucine residue at position 26 (DQB1 26 epi) in the white and Hispanic subjects, while DRB1*0804, DQA1*0501, and DQB1*0301 alleles showed the strongest signals for the black cohort. Regarding ATA-positive subgroup, HLA-DPB1*1301 was the allele most strongly associated in European descent subjects (OR = 14), in accordance with previous results [46]. However, HLA-DRB1*1104 was the allele that showed the most significant association and the highest OR for this autoantibody in the Hispanic populations, while HLA-DRB1*1104, HLA-DQB1 26 epitope, HLA-DRB1*08, and HLA-DRB1*0804 alleles were those that explained the association with ATA in the African descent. ACA-positive status was best explained by DQB1*0501 and DQB1*26 epi alleles in white and Hispanic subjects. The association analysis in ARA-positive patients revealed significant results for HLA-DRB1*0404, HLA-DRB1*11, and HLA-DQB1*03 in European and Hispanic populations but for DRB1*08 in African descent population [43].

The most comprehensive analysis of the HLA alleles in SSc reported to date was carried out in the first SSc Immunochip study published by Mayes et al. [37]. As stated above, this custom genotyping array includes a dense coverage of this genomic region, along with novel imputation methods that enable the inference of classical HLA alleles, and even polymorphic amino acid positions from genetic data allowed the authors to describe a comprehensive model that explained all the observed associations in the region in European descent population. The model includes six polymorphic amino acid positions in HLA-DRB1, HLA-DQA1, and HLA-DPB1 and seven SNPs independently associated. The analysis also confirmed the divergent HLA allele associations between ACA-positive and ATA-positive serological subgroups [37]. In the ACA-positive subgroup, the model includes 2 amino acid associations, the 13th HLA-DRB1 amino acid and the 69th HLA-DQA1 amino acid, along with 5 single-nucleotide polymorphisms (SNPs). The model provided for ATA-positive subgroup comprises 4 amino acid associations, the 67th and 86th positions in HLA-DRB1 and the positions 76th and 96th in HLA-DPB1, along with 2 SNPs [37]. Mayes et al. also reported that some of the associated protein residues cause different amino acid binding preferences in the corresponding peptide binding grooves of the HLA molecules. Moreover, the authors functionally characterized the associated SNPs and found cis-expression quantitative trait *loci* (eQTLs) for most of them [37].

2.2.3 Overview of the Genetic Component of Systemic Sclerosis Outside the HLA Region: Functional Implication of Associated Loci

In this section we would like to revisit and update the firmest genetic associations with SSc and their potential functional role in the disease pathophysiology. The genetic variants associated with the disease are mainly located in genes related to the immune response, either in the innate or in the adaptive immune system. However, well-powered high-throughput studies have contributed to highlight novel *loci* with different roles on the disease presentation. In total, there are 20 *loci* outside the HLA region firmly associated to SSc (Table 2.1). Most of them point out to genes that are closely related according to their function and that form complex interaction networks, as can be observed in a protein-protein interaction (PPI) analysis performed by means of STRING V10.0 (Fig. 2.1) [47]. These molecular networks point toward biological pathways involved in SSc onset and progression.

2.2.3.1 Innate Immunity, Interferon Signature, and Systemic Sclerosis

As it was stated in the introduction section, the inflammatory phase is an important feature of SSc pathophysiology [2, 11, 48–50]; therefore, it is not surprising that several *loci* directly involved in the regulation of the inflammatory response represent SSc susceptibility genes [29, 30, 34, 37, 51] (Table 2.1). This is the case of the genes *TNFAIP3* and *TNIP1*, which are involved in the TNF-induced NF-κB proinflammatory signaling pathway and participate in the TNF-mediated apoptosis [52].

Type I interferon (IFN) signaling, which is a master regulator of the innate immune system, stimulates natural killer and cytotoxic T-cell activity and the maturation of antigen-presenting cells (APCs). The deregulation of this pathway has

Table 2.1 Firm susceptibility *loci* for systemic sclerosis outside the HLA region

Locus	Chr	Gene name	Index SNP	SNP function	Reference
Innate immunity, interferon signature, and inflammation					
IRF5	7	IFN regulatory factor 5	rs36073657	Intronic	[27, 37, 53–58]
IRF8	16	IFN regulatory factor 8	rs11117420	Intergenic	[44, 59]
IRF7	11	IFN regulatory factor 7	rs1131665	Exonic	[60]
IRF4	6	IFN regulatory factor 4	rs9328192	Intergenic	[61]
PRDM1	6	PR/SET domain 1	rs4134466	Intergenic	[32]
TNFAIP3	6	Tumor necrosis factor alpha-induced protein	rs2230926	Exonic	[34, 37, 51]
TNIP1	5	TNFAIP3-interacting protein	rs3792783	Intronic	[29, 30]
Adaptive immune response: B- and T-cell proliferation, survival, and cytokine production					
TNFSF4	1	Tumor necrosis factor ligand superfamily member 4	rs11576547	ncRNA_ intronic	[69–71]
CD247	1	T-cell receptor zeta chain	rs2056626	Intronic	[27–29]
CSK	15	C-Src	rs1378942	Intronic	[34]
STAT4	2	Signal transducer and activator of transcription 4	rs3821236	Intronic	[27, 29]
TYK2	19	Tyrosine kinase 2	rs34536443	Exonic	[80]
IL12A	3	Interleukin 12A	rs589446, rs77583790	ncRNA_ intronic	[37]
IL12RB2	1	Interleukin 12 receptor, beta 2	rs3790566	Intronic	[33]
IL12RB1	19	Interleukin 12 receptor, beta 1	rs436857	UTR5	[79]
BLK	8	BLK proto-oncogene, Src family tyrosine kinase	rs2736340	Intergenic	[74–76]
Apoptosis, autophagy, fibrosis, and others					
DNASE1L3	3	Deoxyribonuclease I-like 3	rs35677470	Exonic	[37, 38]
ATG5	6	Autophagy related 5	rs9373839	Intronic	[37]
PPARG	3	Peroxisome proliferator-activated receptor gamma	rs310746	Intergenic	[35, 81]
GSDMA	17	Gasdermin A	rs3894194	Exonic	[32]

Chr chromosome, *SNP* single-nucleotide polymorphism

been observed in the pathogenesis of SSc, where an increased expression and activation of IFN-inducible genes have been detected in the peripheral blood and skin of patients [53]. This evidence, known as "IFN signature," is similar to the one observed in other ADs. It is noteworthy that four IFN regulatory factor (*IRF*) genes have been associated with SSc susceptibility: *IRF4*, *IRF5*, *IRF7*, and *IRF8* [27, 37, 44, 53–61]. These IRFs belong to a family of transcription factors that are activated after type I IFN induction [53, 62]. In the first GWAS in Caucasian population performed by Radstake et al. [27], the lead association outside the HLA region was in a promoter SNP of *IRF5*. Moreover, this SNP is associated with lower transcriptional activity of the gene, a longer survival, and less severity of interstitial lung

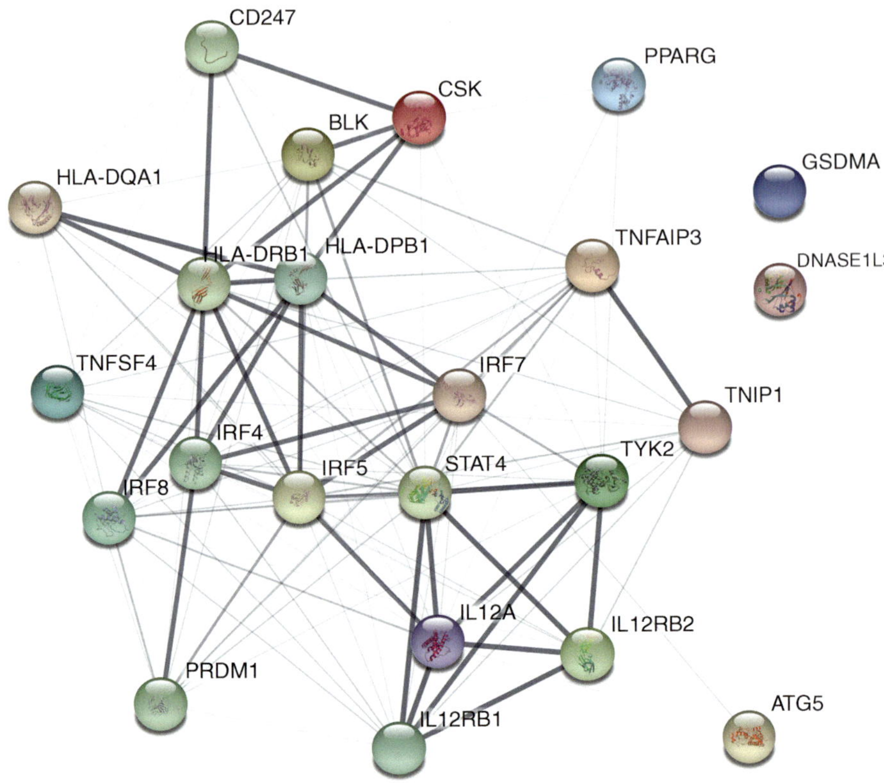

Fig. 2.1 Protein-protein interaction network of systemic sclerosis risk *loci* performed by means of STRING V10.0. The thickness of the lines depicts the confidence of data supporting the interaction. Proteins related to the immune system are highly connected. Additional associated *loci* highlight new biological processes also relevant in the disease pathogenesis

disease (ILD) in SSc patients [63]. Confirming the connection of SSc with the "IFN signature," the gene *PRDM1* has been recently associated with the disease in a trans-ethnic meta-GWAS [32]. The protein encoded by this gene acts as a repressor of the β-interferon gene expression.

2.2.3.2 Adaptive Immune Response: B- and T-Cell Proliferation, Survival, and Cytokine Production

Several components of the adaptive immune response are also involved in the disease pathophysiology, and this is reflected, as well, in the genes that have been associated with the disease. T cells show an activated phenotype and signatures of antigen-driven cell expansion [64–66]. Specifically, most of the cells observed in SSc infiltrates are T helper 2 (Th2) cells, characterized by secretion of profibrotic mediators. Moreover, a Th1-Th2 cytokine imbalance with higher levels of Th2 cytokines has been described in patients with SSc [67]. B cells, on the other hand, show dysregulated homeostasis and are also detected in skin and lung infiltrate of patients with SSc [68]. Their role is not only restricted to autoantibodies secretion but also the production of IL-6, which directly stimulates fibroblasts.

T- and B-cell biology, including cell proliferation, differentiation, survival, and activation, are represented in SSc risk factors [69–71]. For instance, *TNFSF4* is involved in T- and B-cell proliferation and survival [72]; the gene *CD247* encodes the T-cell receptor subunit that forms the T-cell receptor-CD3 complex (TCR-CD3 complex), which is negatively regulated by CSK and LYP [27, 73].The gene *BLK*, also associated with SSc genetic predisposition [74–76], is a tyrosine kinase involved in B-lymphocyte development, differentiation, and BCR signaling [77]. The gene *PRDM1*, also known as B-lymphocyte-induced maturation protein 1, is very important for epithelial and B-cell differentiation [78]. Additionally, IL12/23 and Jak/STAT signaling pathways are also overrepresented by the genetic background of SSc with associated genes such as *IL12A*, *IL12RB1*, *IL12RB2*, *STAT4*, and *TYK2* [27, 33, 37, 79, 80] (Table 2.1).

2.2.3.3 Apoptosis, Autophagy, and Fibrosis

Different *loci* in pathways belonging to the immune system are the main source of genetic risk factors in SSc. However, additional associated genes highlight new biological processes also relevant in the disease pathogenesis [32, 35, 37, 38, 81]. The gene *DNASE1L3* is a member of the deoxyribonuclease I family and is involved in DNA fragmentation, DNA breakdown during apoptosis, and the generation of the resected double-strand DNA breaks in immunoglobulin genes [82–84]. Another gene recently associated with SSc susceptibility is the *GSDMA* [32]. GSDM family proteins have a role in the regulation of cellular differentiation, likely through programmed cell death [85]. Consequently, the impaired clearance of degraded DNA and apoptosis emerges as a new process related to the disease.

Moreover, autophagy is a central player in the immune system. It is involved in B- and T-cell development, survival, cytokine production, and pathogen clearance [86]. In this sense, the gene product of *ATG5*, a gene associated with SSc [37], is involved in autophagosome elongation.

Finally, excessive collagen deposition and fibrosis is one of the hallmarks of SSc. Therefore, it can be expected that genes related to this process are also associated with the disease [35]. This is the case of the *locus PPARG*, which encodes the peroxisome proliferator-activated receptor gamma. Recent studies have shown the antifibrotic role of this molecule in vitro and in vivo [87–90] and the impairment on its expression and function in SSc patients [91].

2.2.3.4 Functional Characterization of Disease-Associated Variants

In order to provide insights into the pathological mechanisms leading to a complex disease, it becomes necessary to assign the functional consequences of the statistical associated variants. The first challenge is to identify the causal variants that are responsible for the genetic associations, as not always correspond to the lead SNP. Once the variants are identified, the next step is to connect the genetic markers to likely target genes. The development of ambitious projects focused on improving the functional characterization of human genome and epigenome, including the

ENCODE, the NIH Roadmap Epigenomics, and GTEx, has offered a valuable source of data for SNP functional annotation and prioritization [92–94].

In the case of SSc, several associated SNPs constitute missense variants, and their functional effect has been previously addressed. For instance, in vitro studies have shown that rs35677470 minor allele at *DNASE1L3* leads to an inactive form of the protein that lacks its DNase activity [95]. Similarly, *TYK2* rs34536443 minor allele leads to a near-complete loss of TYK2 catalytic function, and consequently it impairs cytokine signaling [96]. Another example is the non-synonymous SNP at *TNFAIP3* that results in a phenylalanine-to-cysteine change that reduces the inhibitory activity of TNFAIP3 at the NF-κB signaling pathway [97]. However, the vast majority of associated SNPs lie in noncoding regions of the genome, as is the case for other complex traits [98]. These SNPs might be linked to regulatory functions, rather than affecting the encoded protein themselves. In this sense, the different alleles might correlate with changes on gene expression, also known as eQTL, or overlap with chromatin marks of active enhancers (H3K4me1, H3K27ac), active promoters (H3K4me3, H3K9ac) [99], DNase hypersensitivity sites, or TF-binding sites.

Most of SSc-index SNPs overlap with promoter and enhancer histone marks in relevant cell types for the disease, such as primary T helper cells, primary B cells, primary CD8+ cells, monocytes, and fibroblasts. This fact confirms that most of the genetic variations involved in the susceptibility to SSc modulate transcriptional regulatory mechanisms. Additionally, many of the associated variants correlate with eQTLs, thus altering gene expression for the a priori candidate gene. Nonetheless, we also found genetic variants affecting additional genes. As an example, *DNASE1L3* rs35677470 missense variant—that leads to an inactive enzyme—correlates with eQTL for the neighbor genes *PXK* and *RP11-802O23.3*. These observations highlight that assigning association signals to the "nearest gene" is not a suitable strategy for some SNPs and that the functional role of certain signals may spread out to different target genes.

In addition to variants mapping in introns and intergenic regions, there are a number of SNPs located in noncoding RNAs (ncRNAs), in UTR3′ or UTR5′ regions, upstream or downstream the genes, and in splicing sites. This suggests that variants affecting mRNA processing or stability may provide additional insights into the regulatory mechanisms affecting expression of disease-implicated *loci*. Emerging evidence suggests a role of ncRNAs in autoimmunity [100], and there are also increasing evidence for the role of genetic variants underlying transcript splicing (splicing quantitative trait *loci* or sQTLs) in common diseases [101].

The establishment of the regulatory mechanisms underlying a genetic association is not always straightforward [102]. Interestingly, due to the LD patterns, the functional annotation of the index SNP might be linked to a different "SNP category." For instance, the index SNP at *IL12RB1* is a promoter variant, and its minor allele showed to decrease IL12RB1 mRNA levels [103]. This SNP is in high LD with other exonic non-synonymous, intronic, UTR3′, and splicing variants. For example, the variant rs393548 that leads to an alternative 3′ acceptor splice site results in a different transcript for the gene.

The functional characterization on epigenetic marks and relevant cell types or tissues for the disease adds valuable information to accurately design functional studies that will help us to move from genetic associations to disease genes and mechanisms [104].

2.3 Conclusions and Future Directions

Genetic association studies have been successful in determining genetic regions containing variants associated with SSc risk; however, assigning them a functional effect and uncovering the disease-causing genes is still a challenging task [26]. Until now, GWAS findings are assigned to the closest or most compelling local gene; however, the majority of associated variants lie in noncoding regions of the genome and are known to be enriched in enhancer regions, which are cell-type specific [26, 93]. Enhancers can regulate gene transcription by physical interactions with their target genes, and these can operate over large genetic distances [105]. Therefore, to fully translate these findings into mechanisms of disease and potential therapeutic targets, one of the next fundamental steps is to confidently link the associated genomic regions to genes and cell types on which they have their disease-causing effect.

Recent advances in molecular biology techniques, including nuclear dynamic technologies, have enabled the design of functional experiments to address these questions. Chromosome conformation capture technology (Capture Hi-C) has been successfully used to detect patterns of long-range interactions at the genome-wide level at high resolution between chromosomal regions in several types of cancer [106–108] and in four autoimmune diseases: RA, type 1 diabetes (T1D), psoriatic arthritis (PsA), and juvenile idiopathic arthritis (JIA) [109]. Therefore, Capture Hi-C (CHi-C) has been shown to be an effective approach to link noncoding variation to target genes, which is an important challenge for genetics and genomics of complex diseases such as SSc [108, 110].

References

1. Gabrielli A, Avvedimento EV, Krieg T. Scleroderma. N Engl J Med. 2009; 360(19):1989–2003.
2. Katsumoto TR, Whitfield ML, Connolly MK. The pathogenesis of systemic sclerosis. Annu Rev Pathol. 2011;6:509–37.
3. Denton CP, Khanna D. Systemic sclerosis. Lancet. 2017;390(10103):1685–99.
4. Steen VD, Medsger TA. Changes in causes of death in systemic sclerosis, 1972-2002. Ann Rheum Dis. 2007;66(7):940–4.
5. Amur S, Parekh A, Mummaneni P. Sex differences and genomics in autoimmune diseases. J Autoimmun. 2012;38(2–3):J254–65.
6. Elhai M, Avouac J, Walker UA, Matucci-Cerinic M, Riemekasten G, Airo P, et al. A gender gap in primary and secondary heart dysfunctions in systemic sclerosis: a EUSTAR prospective study. Ann Rheum Dis. 2016;75(1):163–9.

7. Ranque B, Mouthon L. Geoepidemiology of systemic sclerosis. Autoimmun Rev. 2010;9(5):A311–8.
8. Reveille JD. Ethnicity and race and systemic sclerosis: how it affects susceptibility, severity, antibody genetics, and clinical manifestations. Curr Rheumatol Rep. 2003;5(2):160–7.
9. Reveille JD, Fischbach M, McNearney T, Friedman AW, Aguilar MB, Lisse J, et al. Systemic sclerosis in 3 US ethnic groups: a comparison of clinical, sociodemographic, serologic, and immunogenetic determinants. Semin Arthritis Rheum. 2001;30(5):332–46.
10. Trojanowska M. Cellular and molecular aspects of vascular dysfunction in systemic sclerosis. Nat Rev Rheumatol. 2010;6(8):453–60.
11. Varga J, Abraham D. Systemic sclerosis: a prototypic multisystem fibrotic disorder. J Clin Invest. 2007;117(3):557–67.
12. Allanore Y, Simms R, Distler O, Trojanowska M, Pope J, Denton CP, et al. Systemic sclerosis. Nat Rev Dis Primers. 2015;1:15002.
13. Shah AA, Rosen A, Hummers L, Wigley F, Casciola-Rosen L. Close temporal relationship between onset of cancer and scleroderma in patients with RNA polymerase I/III antibodies. Arthritis Rheum. 2010;62(9):2787–95.
14. Airo P, Ceribelli A, Cavazzana I, Taraborelli M, Zingarelli S, Franceschini F. Malignancies in Italian patients with systemic sclerosis positive for anti-RNA polymerase III antibodies. J Rheumatol. 2011;38(7):1329–34.
15. Gabrielli A, Svegliati S, Moroncini G, Pomponio G, Santillo M, Avvedimento EV. Oxidative stress and the pathogenesis of scleroderma: the Murrell's hypothesis revisited. Semin Immunopathol. 2008;30(3):329–37.
16. Servettaz A, Goulvestre C, Kavian N, Nicco C, Guilpain P, Chereau C, et al. Selective oxidation of DNA topoisomerase 1 induces systemic sclerosis in the mouse. J Immunol. 2009;182(9):5855–64.
17. Sambo P, Baroni SS, Luchetti M, Paroncini P, Dusi S, Orlandini G, et al. Oxidative stress in scleroderma: maintenance of scleroderma fibroblast phenotype by the constitutive up-regulation of reactive oxygen species generation through the NADPH oxidase complex pathway. Arthritis Rheum. 2001;44(11):2653–64.
18. Arnett FC, Cho M, Chatterjee S, Aguilar MB, Reveille JD, Mayes MD. Familial occurrence frequencies and relative risks for systemic sclerosis (scleroderma) in three United States cohorts. Arthritis Rheum. 2001;44(6):1359–62.
19. Feghali-Bostwick C, Medsger TA Jr, Wright TM. Analysis of systemic sclerosis in twins reveals low concordance for disease and high concordance for the presence of antinuclear antibodies. Arthritis Rheum. 2003;48(7):1956–63.
20. Assassi S, Arnett FC, Reveille JD, Gourh P, Mayes MD. Clinical, immunologic, and genetic features of familial systemic sclerosis. Arthritis Rheum. 2007;56(6):2031–7.
21. Lewis CM. Genetic association studies: design, analysis and interpretation. Brief Bioinform. 2002;3(2):146–53.
22. Frazer KA, Ballinger DG, Cox DR, Hinds DA, Stuve LL, Gibbs RA, et al. A second generation human haplotype map of over 3.1 million SNPs. Nature. 2007;449(7164):851–61.
23. Abecasis GR, Auton A, Brooks LD, DePristo MA, Durbin RM, Handsaker RE, et al. An integrated map of genetic variation from 1,092 human genomes. Nature. 2012;491(7422):56–65.
24. Eichler EE, Flint J, Gibson G, Kong A, Leal SM, Moore JH, et al. Missing heritability and strategies for finding the underlying causes of complex disease. Nat Rev Genet. 2010;11(6):446–50.
25. de Bakker PI, Ferreira MA, Jia X, Neale BM, Raychaudhuri S, Voight BF. Practical aspects of imputation-driven meta-analysis of genome-wide association studies. Hum Mol Genet. 2008;17(R2):R122–8.
26. Bossini-Castillo L, Lopez-Isac E, Martin J. Immunogenetics of systemic sclerosis: defining heritability, functional variants and shared-autoimmunity pathways. J Autoimmun. 2015;64:53–65.
27. Radstake TR, Gorlova O, Rueda B, Martin JE, Alizadeh BZ, Palomino-Morales R, et al. Genome-wide association study of systemic sclerosis identifies CD247 as a new susceptibility locus. Nat Genet. 2010;42(5):426–9.

28. Dieude P, Boileau C, Guedj M, Avouac J, Ruiz B, Hachulla E, et al. Independent replication establishes the CD247 gene as a genetic systemic sclerosis susceptibility factor. Ann Rheum Dis. 2011;70(9):1695–6.
29. Allanore Y, Saad M, Dieude P, Avouac J, Distler JH, Amouyel P, et al. Genome-wide scan identifies TNIP1, PSORS1C1, and RHOB as novel risk loci for systemic sclerosis. PLoS Genet. 2011;7(7):e1002091.
30. Bossini-Castillo L, Martin JE, Broen J, Simeon CP, Beretta L, Gorlova OY, et al. Confirmation of TNIP1 but not RHOB and PSORS1C1 as systemic sclerosis risk factors in a large independent replication study. Ann Rheum Dis. 2013;72(4):602–7.
31. Zhou X, Lee JE, Arnett FC, Xiong M, Park MY, Yoo YK, et al. HLA-DPB1 and DPB2 are genetic loci for systemic sclerosis: a genome-wide association study in Koreans with replication in North Americans. Arthritis Rheum. 2009;60(12):3807–14.
32. Terao C, Kawaguchi T, Dieude P, Varga J, Kuwana M, Hudson M, et al. Transethnic meta-analysis identifies GSDMA and PRDM1 as susceptibility genes to systemic sclerosis. Ann Rheum Dis. 2017;76(6):1150–8.
33. Bossini-Castillo L, Martin JE, Broen J, Gorlova O, Simeon CP, Beretta L, et al. A GWAS follow-up study reveals the association of the IL12RB2 gene with systemic sclerosis in Caucasian populations. Hum Mol Genet. 2012;21(4):926–33.
34. Martin JE, Broen JC, Carmona FD, Teruel M, Simeon CP, Vonk MC, et al. Identification of CSK as a systemic sclerosis genetic risk factor through Genome Wide Association Study follow-up. Hum Mol Genet. 2012;21(12):2825–35.
35. Lopez-Isac E, Bossini-Castillo L, Simeon CP, Egurbide MV, Alegre-Sancho JJ, Callejas JL, et al. A genome-wide association study follow-up suggests a possible role for PPARG in systemic sclerosis susceptibility. Arthritis Res Ther. 2014;16(1):R6.
36. Parkes M, Cortes A, van Heel DA, Brown MA. Genetic insights into common pathways and complex relationships among immune-mediated diseases. Nat Rev Genet. 2013;14(9):661–73.
37. Mayes MD, Bossini-Castillo L, Gorlova O, Martin JE, Zhou X, Chen WV, et al. Immunochip analysis identifies multiple susceptibility loci for systemic sclerosis. Am J Hum Genet. 2014;94(1):47–61.
38. Zochling J, Newell F, Charlesworth JC, Leo P, Stankovich J, Cortes A, et al. An Immunochip-based interrogation of scleroderma susceptibility variants identifies a novel association at DNASE1L3. Arthritis Res Ther. 2014;16(5):438.
39. Lee SH, Wray NR, Goddard ME, Visscher PM. Estimating missing heritability for disease from genome-wide association studies. Am J Hum Genet. 2011;88(3):294–305.
40. Yang J, Benyamin B, McEvoy BP, Gordon S, Henders AK, Nyholt DR, et al. Common SNPs explain a large proportion of the heritability for human height. Nat Genet. 2010;42(7):565–9.
41. Yang J, Lee SH, Goddard ME, Visscher PM. GCTA: a tool for genome-wide complex trait analysis. Am J Hum Genet. 2011;88(1):76–82.
42. Okada Y, Wu D, Trynka G, Raj T, Terao C, Ikari K, et al. Genetics of rheumatoid arthritis contributes to biology and drug discovery. Nature. 2014;506(7488):376–81.
43. Arnett FC, Gourh P, Shete S, Ahn CW, Honey RE, Agarwal SK, et al. Major histocompatibility complex (MHC) class II alleles, haplotypes and epitopes which confer susceptibility or protection in systemic sclerosis: analyses in 1300 Caucasian, African-American and Hispanic cases and 1000 controls. Ann Rheum Dis. 2010;69(5):822–7.
44. Gorlova O, Martin JE, Rueda B, Koeleman BP, Ying J, Teruel M, et al. Identification of novel genetic markers associated with clinical phenotypes of systemic sclerosis through a genome-wide association strategy. PLoS Genet. 2011;7(7):e1002178.
45. Martin JE, Bossini-Castillo L, Martin J. Unraveling the genetic component of systemic sclerosis. Hum Genet. 2012;131(7):1023–37.
46. Gilchrist FC, Bunn C, Foley PJ, Lympany PA, Black CM, Welsh KI, et al. Class II HLA associations with autoantibodies in scleroderma: a highly significant role for HLA-DP. Genes Immun. 2001;2(2):76–81.
47. Szklarczyk D, Franceschini A, Wyder S, Forslund K, Heller D, Huerta-Cepas J, et al. STRING v10: protein-protein interaction networks, integrated over the tree of life. Nucleic Acids Res. 2015;43(Database issue):D447–52.

48. Abraham DJ, Krieg T, Distler J, Distler O. Overview of pathogenesis of systemic sclerosis. Rheumatology (Oxford). 2009;48(Suppl 3):iii3–7.
49. Gu YS, Kong J, Cheema GS, Keen CL, Wick G, Gershwin ME. The immunobiology of systemic sclerosis. Semin Arthritis Rheum. 2008;38(2):132–60.
50. Matucci-Cerinic M, Kahaleh B, Wigley FM. Review: evidence that systemic sclerosis is a vascular disease. Arthritis Rheum. 2013;65(8):1953–62.
51. Dieude P, Guedj M, Wipff J, Ruiz B, Riemekasten G, Matucci-Cerinic M, et al. Association of the TNFAIP3 rs5029939 variant with systemic sclerosis in the European Caucasian population. Ann Rheum Dis. 2010;69(11):1958–64.
52. Catrysse L, Vereecke L, Beyaert R, van Loo G. A20 in inflammation and autoimmunity. Trends Immunol. 2014;35(1):22–31.
53. Wu M, Assassi S. The role of type 1 interferon in systemic sclerosis. Front Immunol. 2013;4:266.
54. Ito I, Kawaguchi Y, Kawasaki A, Hasegawa M, Ohashi J, Hikami K, et al. Association of a functional polymorphism in the IRF5 region with systemic sclerosis in a Japanese population. Arthritis Rheum. 2009;60(6):1845–50.
55. Dieude P, Guedj M, Wipff J, Avouac J, Fajardy I, Diot E, et al. Association between the IRF5 rs2004640 functional polymorphism and systemic sclerosis: a new perspective for pulmonary fibrosis. Arthritis Rheum. 2009;60(1):225–33.
56. Dieude P, Dawidowicz K, Guedj M, Legrain Y, Wipff J, Hachulla E, et al. Phenotype-haplotype correlation of IRF5 in systemic sclerosis: role of 2 haplotypes in disease severity. J Rheumatol. 2010;37(5):987–92.
57. Carmona FD, Martin JE, Beretta L, Simeon CP, Carreira PE, Callejas JL, et al. The systemic lupus erythematosus IRF5 risk haplotype is associated with systemic sclerosis. PLoS One. 2013;8(1):e54419.
58. Kottyan LC, Zoller EE, Bene J, Lu X, Kelly JA, Rupert AM, et al. The IRF5-TNPO3 association with systemic lupus erythematosus has two components that other autoimmune disorders variably share. Hum Mol Genet. 2015;24(2):582–96.
59. Arismendi M, Giraud M, Ruzehaji N, Dieude P, Koumakis E, Ruiz B, et al. Identification of NF-kappaB and PLCL2 as new susceptibility genes and highlights on a potential role of IRF8 through interferon signature modulation in systemic sclerosis. Arthritis Res Ther. 2015;17:71.
60. Carmona FD, Gutala R, Simeon CP, Carreira P, Ortego-Centeno N, Vicente-Rabaneda E, et al. Novel identification of the IRF7 region as an anticentromere autoantibody propensity locus in systemic sclerosis. Ann Rheum Dis. 2012;71(1):114–9.
61. Lopez-Isac E, Martin JE, Assassi S, Simeon CP, Carreira P, Ortego-Centeno N, et al. Brief report: IRF4 newly identified as a common susceptibility locus for systemic sclerosis and rheumatoid arthritis in a cross-disease meta-analysis of genome-wide association studies. Arthritis Rheumatol. 2016;68(9):2338–44.
62. Honda K, Taniguchi T. IRFs: master regulators of signalling by Toll-like receptors and cytosolic pattern-recognition receptors. Nat Rev Immunol. 2006;6(9):644–58.
63. Sharif R, Mayes MD, Tan FK, Gorlova OY, Hummers LK, Shah AA, et al. IRF5 polymorphism predicts prognosis in patients with systemic sclerosis. Ann Rheum Dis. 2012;71(7):1197–202.
64. Yurovsky VV, Wigley FM, Wise RA, White B. Skewing of the CD8+ T-cell repertoire in the lungs of patients with systemic sclerosis. Hum Immunol. 1996;48(1–2):84–97.
65. Sakkas LI, Xu B, Artlett CM, Lu S, Jimenez SA, Platsoucas CD. Oligoclonal T cell expansion in the skin of patients with systemic sclerosis. J Immunol. 2002;168(7):3649–59.
66. Farge D, Henegar C, Carmagnat M, Daneshpouy M, Marjanovic Z, Rabian C, et al. Analysis of immune reconstitution after autologous bone marrow transplantation in systemic sclerosis. Arthritis Rheum. 2005;52(5):1555–63.
67. Wynn TA. Fibrotic disease and the T(H)1/T(H)2 paradigm. Nat Rev Immunol. 2004;4(8):583–94.
68. Bosello S, De Luca G, Tolusso B, Lama G, Angelucci C, Sica G, et al. B cells in systemic sclerosis: a possible target for therapy. Autoimmun Rev. 2011;10(10):624–30.

69. Bossini-Castillo L, Broen JC, Simeon CP, Beretta L, Vonk MC, Ortego-Centeno N, et al. A replication study confirms the association of TNFSF4 (OX40L) polymorphisms with systemic sclerosis in a large European cohort. Ann Rheum Dis. 2011;70(4):638–41.
70. Gourh P, Arnett FC, Tan FK, Assassi S, Divecha D, Paz G, et al. Association of TNFSF4 (OX40L) polymorphisms with susceptibility to systemic sclerosis. Ann Rheum Dis. 2010;69(3):550–5.
71. Coustet B, Bouaziz M, Dieude P, Guedj M, Bossini-Castillo L, Agarwal S, et al. Independent replication and meta analysis of association studies establish TNFSF4 as a susceptibility gene preferentially associated with the subset of anticentromere-positive patients with systemic sclerosis. J Rheumatol. 2012;39(5):997–1003.
72. Gourh P, Tan FK, Assassi S, Ahn CW, McNearney TA, Fischbach M, et al. Association of the PTPN22 R620W polymorphism with anti-topoisomerase I- and anticentromere antibody-positive systemic sclerosis. Arthritis Rheum. 2006;54(12):3945–53.
73. Zhong MC, Veillette A. Immunology: Csk keeps LYP on a leash. Nat Chem Biol. 2012;8(5):412–3.
74. Gourh P, Agarwal SK, Martin E, Divecha D, Rueda B, Bunting H, et al. Association of the C8orf13-BLK region with systemic sclerosis in North-American and European populations. J Autoimmun. 2010;34(2):155–62.
75. Ito I, Kawaguchi Y, Kawasaki A, Hasegawa M, Ohashi J, Kawamoto M, et al. Association of the FAM167A-BLK region with systemic sclerosis. Arthritis Rheum. 2010;62(3):890–5.
76. Coustet B, Dieude P, Guedj M, Bouaziz M, Avouac J, Ruiz B, et al. C8orf13-BLK is a genetic risk locus for systemic sclerosis and has additive effects with BANK1: results from a large French cohort and meta-analysis. Arthritis Rheum. 2011;63(7):2091–6.
77. Texido G, Su IH, Mecklenbrauker I, Saijo K, Malek SN, Desiderio S, et al. The B-cell-specific Src-family kinase Blk is dispensable for B-cell development and activation. Mol Cell Biol. 2000;20(4):1227–33.
78. Ott G, Rosenwald A, Campo E. Understanding MYC-driven aggressive B-cell lymphomas: pathogenesis and classification. Blood. 2013;122(24):3884–91.
79. Lopez-Isac E, Bossini-Castillo L, Guerra SG, Denton C, Fonseca C, Assassi S, et al. Identification of IL12RB1 as a novel systemic sclerosis susceptibility locus. Arthritis Rheumatol. 2014;66(12):3521–3.
80. Lopez-Isac E, Campillo-Davo D, Bossini-Castillo L, Guerra SG, Assassi S, Simeon CP, et al. Influence of TYK2 in systemic sclerosis susceptibility: a new locus in the IL-12 pathway. Ann Rheum Dis. 2016;75(8):1521–6.
81. Marangoni RG, Korman BD, Allanore Y, Dieude P, Armstrong LL, Rzhetskaya M, et al. A candidate gene study reveals association between a variant of the Peroxisome Proliferator-Activated Receptor Gamma (PPAR-gamma) gene and systemic sclerosis. Arthritis Res Ther. 2015;17:128.
82. Shiokawa D, Tanuma S. Characterization of human DNase I family endonucleases and activation of DNase gamma during apoptosis. Biochemistry. 2001;40(1):143–52.
83. Errami Y, Naura AS, Kim H, Ju J, Suzuki Y, El-Bahrawy AH, et al. Apoptotic DNA fragmentation may be a cooperative activity between caspase-activated deoxyribonuclease and the poly(ADP-ribose) polymerase-regulated DNAS1L3, an endoplasmic reticulum-localized endonuclease that translocates to the nucleus during apoptosis. J Biol Chem. 2013;288(5):3460–8.
84. Okamoto M, Okamoto N, Yashiro H, Shiokawa D, Sunaga S, Yoshimori A, et al. Involvement of DNase gamma in the resected double-strand DNA breaks in immunoglobulin genes. Biochem Biophys Res Commun. 2005;327(1):76–83.
85. Aglietti RA, Dueber EC. Recent insights into the molecular mechanisms underlying pyroptosis and gasdermin family functions. Trends Immunol. 2017;38(4):261–71.
86. Bhattacharya A, Eissa NT. Autophagy and autoimmunity crosstalks. Front Immunol. 2013;4:88.
87. Burgess HA, Daugherty LE, Thatcher TH, Lakatos HF, Ray DM, Redonnet M, et al. PPARgamma agonists inhibit TGF-beta induced pulmonary myofibroblast differentiation

and collagen production: implications for therapy of lung fibrosis. Am J Physiol Lung Cell Mol Physiol. 2005;288(6):L1146–53.
88. Kulkarni AA, Thatcher TH, Olsen KC, Maggirwar SB, Phipps RP, Sime PJ. PPAR-gamma ligands repress TGFbeta-induced myofibroblast differentiation by targeting the PI3K/Akt pathway: implications for therapy of fibrosis. PLoS One. 2011;6(1):e15909.
89. Wei J, Zhu H, Komura K, Lord G, Tomcik M, Wang W, et al. A synthetic PPAR-gamma agonist triterpenoid ameliorates experimental fibrosis: PPAR-gamma-independent suppression of fibrotic responses. Ann Rheum Dis. 2014;73(2):446–54.
90. Wu M, Melichian DS, Chang E, Warner-Blankenship M, Ghosh AK, Varga J. Rosiglitazone abrogates bleomycin-induced scleroderma and blocks profibrotic responses through peroxisome proliferator-activated receptor-gamma. Am J Pathol. 2009;174(2):519–33.
91. Wei J, Ghosh AK, Sargent JL, Komura K, Wu M, Huang QQ, et al. PPARgamma downregulation by TGFss in fibroblast and impaired expression and function in systemic sclerosis: a novel mechanism for progressive fibrogenesis. PLoS One. 2010;5(11):e13778.
92. Consortium EP. An integrated encyclopedia of DNA elements in the human genome. Nature. 2012;489(7414):57–74.
93. Roadmap Epigenomics C, Kundaje A, Meuleman W, Ernst J, Bilenky M, Yen A, et al. Integrative analysis of 111 reference human epigenomes. Nature. 2015;518(7539):317–30.
94. Consortium GT. Human genomics. The genotype-tissue expression (GTEx) pilot analysis: multitissue gene regulation in humans. Science. 2015;348(6235):648–60.
95. Ueki M, Takeshita H, Fujihara J, Iida R, Yuasa I, Kato H, et al. Caucasian-specific allele in non-synonymous single nucleotide polymorphisms of the gene encoding deoxyribonuclease I-like 3, potentially relevant to autoimmunity, produces an inactive enzyme. Clin Chim Acta. 2009;407(1–2):20–4.
96. Dendrou CA, Cortes A, Shipman L, Evans HG, Attfield KE, Jostins L, et al. Resolving TYK2 locus genotype-to-phenotype differences in autoimmunity. Sci Transl Med. 2016;8(363):363ra149.
97. Musone SL, Taylor KE, Lu TT, Nititham J, Ferreira RC, Ortmann W, et al. Multiple polymorphisms in the TNFAIP3 region are independently associated with systemic lupus erythematosus. Nat Genet. 2008;40(9):1062–4.
98. Zhang F, Lupski JR. Non-coding genetic variants in human disease. Hum Mol Genet. 2015;24(R1):R102–10.
99. Rivera CM, Ren B. Mapping human epigenomes. Cell. 2013;155(1):39–55.
100. Gupta B, Hawkins RD. Epigenomics of autoimmune diseases. Immunol Cell Biol. 2015;93(3):271–6.
101. Zhang X, Joehanes R, Chen BH, Huan T, Ying S, Munson PJ, et al. Identification of common genetic variants controlling transcript isoform variation in human whole blood. Nat Genet. 2015;47(4):345–52.
102. Spain SL, Barrett JC. Strategies for fine-mapping complex traits. Hum Mol Genet. 2015;24(R1):R111–9.
103. Takahashi N, Akahoshi M, Matsuda A, Ebe K, Inomata N, Obara K, et al. Association of the IL12RB1 promoter polymorphisms with increased risk of atopic dermatitis and other allergic phenotypes. Hum Mol Genet. 2005;14(21):3149–59.
104. Trynka G, Sandor C, Han B, Xu H, Stranger BE, Liu XS, et al. Chromatin marks identify critical cell types for fine mapping complex trait variants. Nat Genet. 2013;45(2):124–30.
105. Schoenfelder S, Clay I, Fraser P. The transcriptional interactome: gene expression in 3D. Curr Opin Genet Dev. 2010;20(2):127–33.
106. Dryden NH, Broome LR, Dudbridge F, Johnson N, Orr N, Schoenfelder S, et al. Unbiased analysis of potential targets of breast cancer susceptibility loci by capture Hi-C. Genome Res. 2014;24(11):1854–68.
107. Jager R, Migliorini G, Henrion M, Kandaswamy R, Speedy HE, Heindl A, et al. Capture Hi-C identifies the chromatin interactome of colorectal cancer risk loci. Nat Commun. 2015;6:6178.

108. Schoenfelder S, Furlan-Magaril M, Mifsud B, Tavares-Cadete F, Sugar R, Javierre BM, et al. The pluripotent regulatory circuitry connecting promoters to their long-range interacting elements. Genome Res. 2015;25(4):582–97.
109. Martin P, McGovern A, Orozco G, Duffus K, Yarwood A, Schoenfelder S, et al. Capture Hi-C reveals novel candidate genes and complex long-range interactions with related autoimmune risk loci. Nat Commun. 2015;6:10069.
110. Mifsud B, Tavares-Cadete F, Young AN, Sugar R, Schoenfelder S, Ferreira L, et al. Mapping long-range promoter contacts in human cells with high-resolution capture Hi-C. Nat Genet. 2015;47(6):598–606.

Behçet's Disease

3

Lourdes Ortiz-Fernández
and Maria Francisca González-Escribano

Contents

3.1 Introduction

Behçet's disease (BD) is a complex systemic syndrome characterized by inflammatory lesions of blood vessels throughout the body, being small vessels the most frequently involved. This pathology is a rare and debilitating vasculitis, which presents a wide range of clinical phenotypes. The main clinical features are genital ulceration, ocular involvement (mainly uveitis), and skin lesions, but patients also can suffer gastrointestinal involvement, arthritis, and neurological disorders, among other symptoms, which lead to significant morbidity and mortality [1]. The lack of a pathognomonic sign and the absence of specific biomarkers of the disease make difficult the diagnosis of BD which is based on criteria and classification systems

L. Ortiz-Fernández (✉)
Instituto de Parasitología y Biomedicina 'López-Neyra', IPBLN-CSIC, Parque Tecnológico Ciencias de la Salud, Granada, Spain

M. F. González-Escribano
Servicio de Inmunología, Hospital Universitario Virgen del Rocío (IBiS, CSIC, US), Sevilla, Spain
e-mail: mariaf.gonzalez.sspa@juntadeandalucia.es

J. Martín, F. D. Carmona (eds.), *Genetics of Rare Autoimmune Diseases*,
Rare Diseases of the Immune System, https://doi.org/10.1007/978-3-030-03934-9_3

being the most widely used those proposed by the International BD Study Group (ICBD) in 1990 [2]. BD is found worldwide; however, its prevalence varies along the different geographical regions. The highest prevalence is found in Turkey, followed by Japan and Iran, and it is very low in North America and in Western countries; in fact, BD is also known as "Silk Road disease" given its particular geographical distribution overlap with the ancient trading route stretching from China to the Mediterranean area [3]. Regarding the gender distribution and onset, both genders are affected equally, although with geographical differences, and the disease typically arises in the third or fourth decade of life, being uncommon in children or patients above 50s [4].

With respect to the immunological data, multiple alterations have been described in the homeostasis of the T cells in BD patients. Accordingly, activation of γ/δ T lymphocytes in both peripheral blood and mucous lesions has been described [5, 6]. Besides, imbalances in T helper (Th) cell populations have been extensively studied in BD, and Th1 infiltrates have been observed in oral and genital ulcers and cutaneous and gastrointestinal lesions. Consistently, an increase in Th1 cytokines has also been found in blood [7–9]. In addition, high levels of IL23 and IL17 have been described in peripheral blood mononuclear cells of BD patients [10]. IL23 induces the production of IL17 by T lymphocytes, and this cytokine promotes a neutrophil-mediated inflammatory response. Therefore, high levels of IL23 are consistent with the hyperactivation of neutrophils observed in the early phases of the lesion infiltration [11], which leads to the increase in the levels of reactive oxygen species, endothelial adhesion, chemotaxis, and phagocytosis [12–15]. All these data suggest that the Th17/Th1 balance plays an important role in the regulation of the inflammation in BD [16].

Despite high efforts, the etiology of BD remains unclear. However, cumulative evidences suggest that certain infectious agents and environmental factors may trigger the disease in genetically predisposed individuals. It has been proposed that different virus and bacteria could play a role in the BD development. Of special note are Herpes simplex virus I, which DNA has been isolated from genital ulcers and saliva samples of patients [17], and *Streptococcus sanguinis* that has been related with the formation of recurrent aphthous lesions [18]. Nevertheless, the present chapter focuses on the genetic component, in which great advances have been made in recent years.

3.2 Genetic Component of Behçet's Disease

The substantial genetic contribution to the pathogenesis of this disease is strongly supported by several facts. In addition to the aforementioned geographical variation in prevalence [3], familial aggregation has been extensively reported. The results of these studies revealed a higher frequency of the cases among the relatives of the patients than in the general population [19–22] with the highest sibling recurrence risk ratio, in the Turkish population (between 11.4 and 52.5) [20]. Besides, although there are few studies in BD, the disease concordance rate was higher in monozygotic twins compared with dizygotic ones [23]. Finally, specific associations of different genes with BD susceptibility have been robustly described [24]. From a genetic point of view, BD is considered as a complex disease, in which multiple genes are involved, each of them with a modest effect in the disease, being able to be related with the onset as well as with its severity and progression.

We will examine throughout this chapter the current knowledge of the BD genetic background on the basis of the recent advances in this subject. Firstly, the HLA region (which represents the main genetic contributor to the disease) will be thoroughly reviewed together with the main confirmed associated loci outside the HLA region. Besides, we summarized the results of other studies that propose new susceptibility genetic factors, and, finally, we will highlight the most important molecular pathways implicated in the disease.

3.2.1 HLA Region

The major histocompatibility complex (MHC) region includes the largest number of genetic associations for a wide range of pathological conditions, including most of the immune-mediated diseases. The earliest association of BD with the human MHC (HLA) was reported in the 1970s [25]. These initial studies, using serological typing method, revealed that HLA-B51 had a relevant relationship with the disease, so that it was detected with a relative small sample size. Decades later, with the availability of DNA-based methods and larger study cohorts, the specific association of HLA-B*51 with the disease was well established and repeatedly contrasted in different ethnic groups [24]. Multiple studies exploring other additional susceptibility loci in the HLA region have suggested the association of diverse HLA molecules with the disease. In this sense, in addition to other HLA-B molecules [26, 27], some studies have reported other classic class I HLA molecules (HLA-A and HLA-C) as associated to the disease, although in general these results were less consistent [28–30]. As we stated above, the association between HLA-B*51 and BD is well established worldwide as the strongest genetic risk factor for this condition, but the functional basis of this association in the pathogenesis of BD has not been elucidated yet. For this reason, other loci located within the HLA region have been proposed as major contributors. Specifically, a study published in 1999 in the Japanese population proposed for the first time that the causative gene of the HLA region was *MICA*, a gene located very close to *HLA-B* with strong linkage disequilibrium (LD) [31–33]. Although this idea was embraced by the scientific community at the beginning, later studies performed in different populations were inconsistent [34–38]. The problems encountered to clarify which gene is true responsible of the association are related to the complexity of the HLA region, which is particularly dense in genes related with the immune system and shows a strong LD, making difficult to clarify whether the identified risk signals are independent each other or whether they are reflections of the primary association. This problem is aggravated in the case of rare diseases, such as BD, because the sample size, relatively low compared with other pathologies with more prevalence, limits the statistical power of the individual studies.

Given the advance of the new typing approaches during the last years, new data have been raised from fine-mapping studies, thus allowing the typing of the entire region. Four independent studies performed in different populations, and following a comprehensive approach that combines high-throughput genomics with the novel algorithms of HLA imputation [39, 40], have been published [41–44]. All of these studies concluded that the *HLA-B*51* haplotype represents the strongest association factor with the disease but also discarded an association of any HLA class II molecule, something that was previously proposed using older methodologies [41–44]. However, these studies showed discrepancies regarding the independent association of other HLA class I factors. In the context of the HLA-B locus, *HLA-B*15* and *HLA-B*27* were identified as risk factors and *HLA-B*49* as a protective factor with independent effects of *HLA-B*51* in one study in the Turkish population [42]. Additionally, the allelic group *HLA-B*57* was shown to confer susceptibility to BD in two studies conducted in the Spanish and Turkish populations [42, 43]. With regard to the *HLA-A* locus, variation within the gene was also associated with disease predisposition in different studies. Specifically, three of these studies found that the *HLA-A*03* group is an independent protective factor for BD [42–44]. In addition, one of these studies reported suggested evidence that *HLA-A*26* could be also an independent risk factor for BD [42]. Only one study described an independent association of the *HLA-C* locus, specifically *HLA-C*1602* [41], which had been previously suggested by two smaller studies from Southern European [45, 46]. However, it should be noted that this independent association of the *HLA-C* haplotype was not consistent with the rest of the studies that evaluated the contribution of this locus [26, 42–44]. On the other hand, although the results of one of these studies returned the idea of the *MICA* gene as the causal susceptibility marker for BD [41], the results of the other large-scale genetic studies did not support an independent association of the *MICA* gene with BD [34–38, 42, 43].

Many of the HLA class I molecules have a dual function, and they present peptides to the CD8 T cells, but they also control the activity of the natural killer cells because they are ligands of some of their receptors (KIR). The relevant amino acid positions in one or the other function are located in different parts of the molecule. Therefore, deciphering the amino acid positions involved in BD susceptibility may definitively help to better understand the functional implications of the HLA system in the disease pathophysiology. In an effort to identify the motifs that may explain the variety of protective and risk effects conferred by HLA class I molecules in BD, the possible association of polymorphic amino acid residues has been analyzed in some studies [41, 43]. One of them proposed a model comprising five amino acids located in three positions of HLA-B, 67 (glutamic acid, Glu, or phenylalanine, Phe), 97 (threonine, Thr), and 116 (leucine, Leu), as well as one position in HLA-A, 161 (Glu) [41]. According to one of those studies in which an omnibus test was performed, the most relevant amino acid position for disease risk was *HLA-B* 97. Six possible residues can be harbored at this position, with two of them conferring risk (Thr and valine, Val), another two conferring protection (arginine, Arg, and serine, Ser), and the remaining two being neutral (asparagine, Asn, and tryptophan, Trp). In addition, according to this model, the position 66 of HLA-A represented an independent association (with lysine, Lys conferring risk and Asn protection) [43]. Interestingly, the four more relevant positions (HLA-B 67, 97, 116 and HLA-A 66) are located in the binding groove of their corresponding molecules. These data brought additional evidences supporting the importance of the peptide binding by the class I HLA molecules in BD. Nevertheless, the study of the most relevant amino acid positions has to be interpreted with caution, and it is evident that each HLA-B molecule has a specific set of amino acids in its polymorphic positions, with many of them in LD with each other, thus increasing the difficulty to evaluate dependency at the amino acid level. Therefore, it should be noted that dependency does not exclude biological influence. Therefore, only by complementing the knowledge gained by this type of approaches with those provided by functional studies, it would be possible to elucidate the precise etiopathogenic role of these molecules in disease, which would be essential for a personalized medicine [43].

3.2.2 Non-HLA Region

The contribution of the HLA region to the genetic component of BD has been estimated to be approximately 20% [47], which indicates that other genes outside the region may have to be involved in this pathology. For many years, a large number of candidate gene studies tried to unravel the complex genetic architecture of BD outside of the HLA region. However, those studies yielded contradictory results that were not usually replicated in independent populations. The identification of the genetic factors involved in the susceptibility to complex diseases represents an enormous challenge, given that the effect of each gene in the development of this type of diseases is relatively low independently. To detect genes with low or medium effects, very large sample sizes are needed, and, given the condition of BD as a rare disease, most of candidate gene studies performed did not have enough statistical power. Additionally, the lack of replication among studies could be also related to specific population associations due to particular genetic architectures. Due to the above, few consistent associations with BD have been identified to date (Table 3.1).

3.2.2.1 Confirmed Risk *Loci*

Interleukin 23 receptor (IL23-R). This gene represents the most consistently associated non-HLA locus with BD, as it has been repeatedly identified as a risk factor for this disease in different populations and multiple independent studies [26, 43, 44, 48–56]. It is worth mentioning that this gene is a known risk factor for a multitude of immune-related diseases [57–59]. *IL23R* encodes a subunit of the IL-23 receptor which is expressed on the surface of Th17 cells and macrophages and binds the subunit p19 of IL-23, a pro-inflammatory cytokine composed by p19 and p40 (which is

Table 3.1 Confirmed risk loci for Behçet's disease outside the HLA region

Locus	Location	Gene name	SNP	SNP function	References
IL23-R	1p31.3	Interleukin 23 receptor	rs1495965	Intergenic	[26, 43, 44, 48–56]
			rs924080	Intergenic	
			rs10889664	Intergenic	
IL-10	1q32.1	Interleukin 10	rs1518110	Intronic	[26, 44, 48–51, 55, 61]
			rs1518111	Intronic	
			rs1800871	Intronic	
IL12A	3q25.33	Interleukin 12A	rs17810546	Intergenic	[43, 44, 55, 67, 68]
			rs1874886	Intergenic	
STAT4	2q32.2-q32.3	Signal transducer and activator of transcription-4	rs7574070	Intronic	[53, 55, 68, 71]
			rs7572482	Intronic	
			rs897200	Intergenic	
ERAP1	5q15	Endoplasmic reticulum aminopeptidase 1	rs17482078	Missense (Arg725Gln)	[55, 68, 74, 75]
			rs10050860	Missense (Asp575Asn)	
			rs2287987	Missense (Met349Val)	
			rs13154629	Intronic	
FUT2	19q13.33	Fucosyltransferase 2	rs681343	Synonymous	[44, 104]
			rs601338	Missense (Trp143Ter)	
			rs602662	Missense (Ser258Gly)	
			rs632111	3′-UTR	
KLRC4	12p13.2	Killer cell lectin-like receptor C4	rs2617170	Missense (Asn104Ser)	[55, 68]
			rs1841958	Missense (Ile129Ser)	
CCR1-CCR3	3p21.31	C-C motif chemokine receptor	rs7616215	Intergenic	[68, 90]
			rs13084057	Intergenic	
			rs13092160	Exonic	
			rs13075270	Exonic	

SNP single-nucleotide polymorphism

common with IL-12 and binds to IL12RB1). The IL-23/IL-23R complex promotes the polarization of the T cells to Th17 and increases the levels of inflammatory cytokines such as IL-1, IL-6, IL-17, and TNFα [60]. Although there are strong evidences supporting that the variants of *IL23R* influence BD susceptibility through their effects on IL-23R itself, an additional role of these variants as markers of other nearby genes, such as *IL12RB2*, cannot be discarded [49]. *IL12RB2* gene encodes the IL-12 receptor beta 2, and the complex IL-12/IL12RB2 has a crucial role in Th1 cell differentiation. Thus, although the causal mechanism of the association remains unclear, all these evidences support an important role of the IL-23/IL-17 pathway in the pathophysiology of immune-mediated diseases, including BD.

Interleukin 10 (IL10). This gene was identified together with *IL23R* as susceptibility factor for BD, and this association has been subsequently replicated in different populations [26, 44, 48–51, 55, 61, 62]. IL-10 is a potent anti-inflammatory molecule that inhibits the activation of macrophages and the synthesis of pro-inflammatory cytokines (including IL-1, IL-6, and TNFα); therefore, it suppresses Th1 cell activation [63]. Imbalances in the regulation of Th1 activation could cause deviations toward a Th1 profile, which could predispose to the disease. Interestingly, several genetic variants within this gene have been associated with the levels of expression. Specifically, the SNP reported by the Remmers group is associated with a decrease of the *IL10* expression levels in monocytes [49, 64, 65]. Besides, it has been demonstrated that a low expression of *IL10* in mouse leads to inflammation processes [66].

Interleukin 12A (IL12A). This gene encodes a subunit of IL-12, a cytokine that plays an important role in the polarization of the immune response toward Th1 and also in the production of IFNγ by both the T lymphocytes and the NK cells, so it is related to the production of pro-inflammatory cytokines [67]. Several studies reported association of this gene with BD [43, 44, 55, 68, 69], although further investigation is needed to clarify the causal variant.

The signal transducer and activator of transcription-4 (STAT4). This gene represents a shared genetic susceptibility factor for several autoimmune diseases, including rheumatoid arthritis (RA), systemic lupus erythematosus (SLE), and Sjögren's syndrome, among others [70, 71]. Regarding BD, the association with this gene has been extensively reported in different populations [53, 55, 69, 72]. STAT4 is a transcription factor that is activated by cytokines such as IL-12 and IL-23, which, as stated above, are involved in the differentiation of lymphocytes into Th1 and Th17 [73]. Two of the identified risk variants of this gene have been implicated in changes of *STAT4* mRNA expression [69, 74], although further experiments are needed to better understand the way in which this genetic variation affect the pathogenesis of BD.

The endoplasmic reticulum aminopeptidase 1 (ERAP1). The association of a missense variant of *ERAP1*, p.Arg725Gln, was described for the first time by Kirino and colleagues, whose data suggested that the associated variant contributes to disease susceptibility through a strong interaction or epistasis with HLA-B51 [69]. After that, additional studies have replicated these first results [55, 75, 76]. It is noteworthy that the association of this gene with other HLA class I-related diseases such as ankylosing spondylitis (AS) and psoriasis has been thoroughly investigated in the last years, and the implication of *ERAP1* with these diseases has been always reported through an epistatic interaction with the corresponding associated HLA allele in each case [57, 77–79]. This gene encodes an aminopeptidase with an ubiquitous distribution, which plays an important role trimming the N-terminal end of the peptides in the endoplasmic reticulum, a critical step of the processing of the peptides to optimize their length for HLA I molecule binding [80].

Fucosyltransferase 2 (FUT2). This association was firstly reported by Xavier and collaborators [81] but also in a recently published large-scale study [44]. This gene encodes the alpha [1, 2] fucosyltransferase, a molecule that produces in fluids and intestinal mucosa the secreted H antigen, which is the precursor of the ABO histo-blood group antigens [82]. It has been described that homozygosity in two missense variants (p.Trp143Ter and p.Ile129Phe) leads to an ABO nonsecretor phenotype [82]. Of note, these variants are also linked with other immune-mediated disorders such as Crohn's disease and type 1 diabetes [83–85]. The nonsecretor phenotype has also been associated with resistance to several infectious agents [86, 87] and the gut microbiome composition [88, 89]. These evidences support the hypothesis that relationship between infectious agents and the genetic component is crucial for the development of BD.

Killer cell lectin-like receptor C4 (KLRC4). This gene has been found as a susceptibility locus in two large-scale genetic studies. Two non-synonymous variants in high LD (p.Ile29Ser and p.Asn104Ser) seem to be part of the susceptibility haplotype for BD [55, 69]. The *KLRC4* gene, also known as *NKG2F*, encodes a c-type lectin receptor expressed on NK cells. Although the specific function of this molecule is unknown, the haplotype related with the disease has reported to be associated with a high natural cytotoxic activity on peripheral blood cells [90].

CCR1-CCR3. This locus harbors a cluster of chemokine receptor genes with a high LD among them [69, 91]. Through binding to its ligands, these receptors act as a key regulator in leukocyte trafficking and in the homeostasis of the immune system [92]. The risk allele reported by Hou et al. has been associated with a reduced expression of both, *CCR1* and *CCR3,* in peripheral blood mononuclear cells (PBMCs) [91] and another variant located in the same region was also related with a lower expression of *CCR1* in human primary monocytes [69].

3.2.2.2 Suggested Risk *Loci*

The number of genes identified in large-scale genetic studies is higher than that exposed in the previous section, and includes genes such as *KIAA1529, CPVL, LOC100129342, UBASH3A, UBAC2* [93], *GIMAP* [94], *JRKL-CNTN5* [43], *IL1A-IL1B, IRF8, CEBPB-PTPN1* [44]. However, the association of these *loci* with BD remains unconfirmed. In some cases, specific replication studies have been performed in other populations but the results obtained are contradictories [26, 95]. In other cases the association has recently been described in only one population [44].

New approaches such as next-generation sequencing (NGS) have being recently implemented for the investigation of the rare polymorphisms. In a recent study, 21 candidate genes were evaluated for BD association through deep exonic resequencing with the aim of identifying low-frequency non-synonymous variants [56]. The association of rare variants in four genes (*IL23R*, *NOD2*, *TLR4*, and *MEFV*) with BD is supported by the results obtained in this work. In a later study, seven genes related with immune-mediated diseases were analyzed using NGS. The findings of this second study suggested the influence of rare variants of, at least, *NOD2*, *PSTPIP1*, and *MVK* in the pathogenesis of BD [96]. More independent studies performed in other populations and/or with other approaches are necessary to confirm or discard these suggested associations.

3.3 Molecular Pathways

In the last years, large achievements have been accomplished to understand the genetic basis of BD. Although multiple studies will still be necessary for a fully comprehension of the pathophysiology underlying this disorder, given the last advances, we can outline a model that integrates the main molecular pathways involved in the development of this disease.

As it is described before, several functional studies have established that the T lymphocytes are the most important cell population involved in the immunopathogenesis of BD. These data are in concordance with the results yielded by genetic studies, because several of the BD susceptibility genes (e.g., *STAT4*, *IL12*, *IL23R*) are involved in the differentiation of naïve CD4+ T cells into mature Th1 effector cell or in the maintenance of Th17 cells [97] and others in the balance of Th1 cells (IL10). In addition, the association of the IL-23/IL-17 pathway with BD is also supported by genetic data and provides evidences of the essential role that this pathway has in the pathophysiology of multiple immune-mediated diseases, especially BD.

The genetic association of *ERAP1*, *FUT2*, and *KLRC4* supports the hypothesis that the disease would be triggered by environmental agents in which microorganisms would play a key role. On this sense, the association of *FUT2* could be related with the immune response to invasive microorganisms and the microbiota composition.

3.4 Conclusions and Future Perspectives

Despite the impressive increase in our knowledge of the genetic basis of BD during the last years, the list of the confirmed risk loci for this type of vasculitis remains significantly lower than other immune-mediated diseases [98, 99]. One of the main limitations in the genetic study of this disease is the lack of statistical power, which is conditioned by the low prevalence of this disorder and that does not permit to identify susceptibility signals with modest effects for which large sample size is required. Therefore, additional strategies are necessary to unravel the genetic component underlying BD. In this sense, one new approach which is been successfully applied is the combination of the genetic data from different diseases with similar features considering them as a single phenotype (cross-phenotype meta-analysis), and numerous shared genetic components have been described in the last years using this methodology [100–102].

On the other hand, the way in which the information of genetics variants is translated into pathogenetic mechanisms remains unclear for most of the variants associated with BD, which are located mostly in noncoding region, as occurs in many immune-mediated diseases. This fact suggests that these variants could affect different regulatory elements in the genome. Thus, further studies should be focused on the effects that the associated variants produce. In this sense, the role of epigenetics in the pathogenesis of immune-mediated diseases seems now undeniable, and the contribution of epigenetic dysregulation in vasculitis is increasingly recognized. The genetic-epigenetic relationships are taking on great importance in a field in which functional data are emerging [103]. Expanding our knowledge of how these epigenetic mechanisms interact with the polymorphisms will help to better understand the pathogenesis of this disease.

References

1. Jennette JC, Falk RJ, Bacon PA, Basu N, Cid MC, Ferrario F, et al. 2012 revised International Chapel Hill Consensus Conference Nomenclature of Vasculitides. Arthritis Rheum. 2013;65(1):1–11.
2. Criteria for diagnosis of Behçet's disease. International Study Group for Behçet's Disease. Lancet. 1990;335(8697):1078–80.
3. Sakane T, Takeno M, Suzuki N, Inaba G. Behçet's disease. N Engl J Med. 1999; 341(17):1284–91.
4. Yurdakul S, Yazici H. Behçet's syndrome. Best Pract Res Clin Rheumatol. 2008; 22(5):793–809.
5. Hamzaoui K, Hamzaoui A, Hentati F, Kahan A, Ayed K, Chabbou A, et al. Phenotype and functional profile of T cells expressing gamma delta receptor from patients with active Behçet's disease. J Rheumatol. 1994;21(12):2301–6.
6. Freysdottir J, Hussain L, Farmer I, Lau SH, Fortune F. Diversity of gammadelta T cells in patients with Behcet's disease is indicative of polyclonal activation. Oral Dis. 2006;12(3):271–7.
7. Ben Ahmed M, Houman H, Miled M, Dellagi K, Louzir H. Involvement of chemokines and Th1 cytokines in the pathogenesis of mucocutaneous lesions of Behçet's disease. Arthritis Rheum. 2004;50(7):2291–5.
8. Dalghous AM, Freysdottir J, Fortune F. Expression of cytokines, chemokines, and chemokine receptors in oral ulcers of patients with Behcet's disease (BD) and recurrent aphthous stomatitis is Th1-associated, although Th2-association is also observed in patients with BD. Scand J Rheumatol. 2006;35(6):472–5.
9. Ferrante A, Ciccia F, Principato A, Giardina AR, Impastato R, Peralta S, et al. A Th1 but not a Th17 response is present in the gastrointestinal involvement of Behçet's disease. Clin Exp Rheumatol. 2010;28(4 Suppl 60):S27–30.
10. Chi W, Zhou S, Yang P, Chen L. $CD4^+$ T cells from Behcet patients produce high levels of IL-17. Eye Sci. 2011;26(2):65–9.
11. Eksioglu-Demiralp E, Direskeneli H, Kibaroglu A, Yavuz S, Ergun T, Akoglu T. Neutrophil activation in Behçet's disease. Clin Exp Rheumatol. 2001;19(5 Suppl 24):S19–24.
12. Kobayashi M, Ito M, Nakagawa A, Matsushita M, Nishikimi N, Sakurai T, et al. Neutrophil and endothelial cell activation in the vasa vasorum in vasculo-Behçet disease. Histopathology. 2000;36(4):362–71.
13. Carletto A, Pacor ML, Biasi D, Caramaschi P, Zeminian S, Bellavite P, et al. Changes of neutrophil migration without modification of in vitro metabolism and adhesion in Behçet's disease. J Rheumatol. 1997;24(7):1332–6.
14. Efthimiou J, Addison IE, Johnson BV. In vivo leucocyte migration in Behçet's syndrome. Ann Rheum Dis. 1989;48(3):206–10.
15. Neves FS, Carrasco S, Goldenstein-Schainberg C, Gonçalves CR, de Mello SB. Neutrophil hyperchemotaxis in Behçet's disease: a possible role for monocytes orchestrating bacterial-induced innate immune responses. Clin Rheumatol. 2009;28(12):1403–10.
16. Kim J, Park JA, Lee EY, Lee YJ, Song YW, Lee EB. Imbalance of Th17 to Th1 cells in Behçet's disease. Clin Exp Rheumatol. 2010;28(4 Suppl 60):S16–9.
17. Studd M, McCance DJ, Lehner T. Detection of HSV-1 DNA in patients with Behçet's syndrome and in patients with recurrent oral ulcers by the polymerase chain reaction. J Med Microbiol. 1991;34(1):39–43.

18. Cho SB, Zheng Z, Ahn KJ, Choi MJ, Cho S, Kim DY, et al. Serum IgA reactivity against GroEL of Streptococcus sanguinis and human heterogeneous nuclear ribonucleoprotein A2/B1 in patients with Behçet disease. Br J Dermatol. 2013;168(5):977–83.
19. Koné-Paut I, Geisler I, Wechsler B, Ozen S, Ozdogan H, Rozenbaum M, et al. Familial aggregation in Behçet's disease: high frequency in siblings and parents of pediatric probands. J Pediatr. 1999;135(1):89–93.
20. Gül A, Inanç M, Ocal L, Aral O, Koniçe M. Familial aggregation of Behçet's disease in Turkey. Ann Rheum Dis. 2000;59(8):622–5.
21. Fietta P. Behçet's disease: familial clustering and immunogenetics. Clin Exp Rheumatol. 2005;23(4 Suppl 38):S96–105.
22. Yilmaz S, Cimen KA. Familial Behçet's disease. Rheumatol Int. 2010;30(8):1107–9.
23. Masatlioglu S, Seyahi E, Tahir Turanli E, Fresko I, Gogus F, Senates E, et al. A twin study in Behçet's syndrome. Clin Exp Rheumatol. 2010;28(4 Suppl 60):S62–6.
24. de Menthon M, Lavalley MP, Maldini C, Guillevin L, Mahr A. HLA-B51/B5 and the risk of Behçet's disease: a systematic review and meta-analysis of case-control genetic association studies. Arthritis Rheum. 2009;61(10):1287–96.
25. Ohno S, Aoki K, Sugiura S, Nakayama E, Itakura K, Aizawa M. Letter: HL-A5 and Behçet's disease. Lancet. 1973;2(7842):1383–4.
26. Montes-Cano MA, Conde-Jaldón M, García-Lozano JR, Ortiz-Fernández L, Ortego-Centeno N, Castillo-Palma MJ, et al. HLA and non-HLA genes in Behçet's disease: a multicentric study in the Spanish population. Arthritis Res Ther. 2013;15(5):R145.
27. Gül A, Uyar FA, Inanç M, Ocal L, Barrett JH, Aral O, et al. A weak association of HLA-B*2702 with Behçet's disease. Genes Immun. 2002;3(6):368–72.
28. Takeuchi M, Kastner DL, Remmers EF. The immunogenetics of Behçet's disease: a comprehensive review. J Autoimmun. 2015;64:137–48.
29. Meguro A, Inoko H, Ota M, Katsuyama Y, Oka A, Okada E, et al. Genetics of Behçet disease inside and outside the MHC. Ann Rheum Dis. 2010;69(4):747–54.
30. Kang EH, Kim JY, Takeuchi F, Kim JW, Shin K, Lee EY, et al. Associations between the HLA-A polymorphism and the clinical manifestations of Behcet's disease. Arthritis Res Ther. 2011;13(2):R49.
31. Yabuki K, Mizuki N, Ota M, Katsuyama Y, Palimeris G, Stavropoulos C, et al. Association of MICA gene and HLA-B*5101 with Behçet's disease in Greece. Invest Ophthalmol Vis Sci. 1999;40(9):1921–6.
32. Mizuki N, Ota M, Katsuyama Y, Yabuki K, Ando H, Goto K, et al. Association analysis between the MIC-A and HLA-B alleles in Japanese patients with Behçet's disease. Arthritis Rheum. 1999;42(9):1961–6.
33. Ota M, Mizuki N, Katsuyama Y, Tamiya G, Shiina T, Oka A, et al. The critical region for Behçet disease in the human major histocompatibility complex is reduced to a 46-kb segment centromeric of HLA-B, by association analysis using refined microsatellite mapping. Am J Hum Genet. 1999;64(5):1406–10.
34. González-Escribano MF, Rodríguez MR, Aguilar F, Alvarez A, Sanchez-Roman J, Núñez-Roldán A. Lack of association of MICA transmembrane region polymorphism and Behçet's disease in Spain. Tissue Antigens. 1999;54(3):278–81.
35. Mizuki N, Ota M, Yabuki K, Katsuyama Y, Ando H, Palimeris GD, et al. Localization of the pathogenic gene of Behçet's disease by microsatellite analysis of three different populations. Invest Ophthalmol Vis Sci. 2000;41(12):3702–8.
36. Salvarani C, Boiardi L, Mantovani V, Olivieri I, Ciancio G, Cantini F, et al. Association of MICA alleles and HLA-B51 in Italian patients with Behçet's disease. J Rheumatol. 2001;28(8):1867–70.
37. Park SH, Park KS, Seo YI, Min DJ, Kim WU, Kim TG, et al. Association of MICA polymorphism with HLA-B51 and disease severity in Korean patients with Behcet's disease. J Korean Med Sci. 2002;17(3):366–70.

38. Cohen R, Metzger S, Nahir M, Chajek-Shaul T. Association of the MIC-A gene and HLA-B51 with Behçet's disease in Arabs and non-Ashkenazi Jews in Israel. Ann Rheum Dis. 2002;61(2):157–60.
39. Browning BL, Browning SR. A unified approach to genotype imputation and haplotype-phase inference for large data sets of trios and unrelated individuals. Am J Hum Genet. 2009;84(2):210–23.
40. Jia X, Han B, Onengut-Gumuscu S, Chen WM, Concannon PJ, Rich SS, et al. Imputing amino acid polymorphisms in human leukocyte antigens. PLoS One. 2013;8(6):e64683.
41. Hughes T, Coit P, Adler A, Yilmaz V, Aksu K, Düzgün N, et al. Identification of multiple independent susceptibility loci in the HLA region in Behçet's disease. Nat Genet. 2013;45(3):319–24.
42. Ombrello MJ, Kirino Y, de Bakker PI, Gül A, Kastner DL, Remmers EF. Behçet disease-associated MHC class I residues implicate antigen binding and regulation of cell-mediated cytotoxicity. Proc Natl Acad Sci U S A. 2014;111(24):8867–72.
43. Ortiz-Fernández L, Carmona FD, Montes-Cano MA, García-Lozano JR, Conde-Jaldón M, Ortego-Centeno N, et al. Genetic analysis with the Immunochip Platform in Behçet disease. Identification of residues associated in the HLA class I region and new susceptibility loci. PLoS One. 2016;11(8):e0161305.
44. Takeuchi M, Mizuki N, Meguro A, Ombrello MJ, Kirino Y, Satorius C, et al. Dense genotyping of immune-related loci implicates host responses to microbial exposure in Behçet's disease susceptibility. Nat Genet. 2017;49(3):438–43.
45. Bettencourt A, Pereira C, Carvalho L, Carvalho C, Patto JV, Bastos M, et al. New insights of HLA class I association to Behçet's disease in Portuguese patients. Tissue Antigens. 2008;72(4):379–82.
46. Sanz L, González-Escribano F, de Pablo R, Núñez-Roldán A, Kreisler M, Vilches C. HLA-Cw*1602: a new susceptibility marker of Behçet's disease in southern Spain. Tissue Antigens. 1998;51(1):111–4.
47. Yazici H, Fresko I, Yurdakul S. Behçet's syndrome: disease manifestations, management, and advances in treatment. Nat Clin Pract Rheumatol. 2007;3(3):148–55.
48. Mizuki N, Meguro A, Ota M, Ohno S, Shiota T, Kawagoe T, et al. Genome-wide association studies identify IL23R-IL12RB2 and IL10 as Behçet's disease susceptibility loci. Nat Genet. 2010;42(8):703–6.
49. Remmers EF, Cosan F, Kirino Y, Ombrello MJ, Abaci N, Satorius C, et al. Genome-wide association study identifies variants in the MHC class I, IL10, and IL23R-IL12RB2 regions associated with Behçet's disease. Nat Genet. 2010;42(8):698–702.
50. Carapito R, Shahram F, Michel S, Le Gentil M, Radosavljevic M, Meguro A, et al. On the genetics of the Silk Route: association analysis of HLA, IL10, and IL23R-IL12RB2 regions with Behçet's disease in an Iranian population. Immunogenetics. 2015;67(5–6):289–93.
51. Xavier JM, Shahram F, Davatchi F, Rosa A, Crespo J, Abdollahi BS, et al. Association study of IL10 and IL23R-IL12RB2 in Iranian patients with Behçet's disease. Arthritis Rheum. 2012;64(8):2761–72.
52. Jiang Z, Yang P, Hou S, Du L, Xie L, Zhou H, et al. IL-23R gene confers susceptibility to Behcet's disease in a Chinese Han population. Ann Rheum Dis. 2010;69(7):1325–8.
53. Kim ES, Kim SW, Moon CM, Park JJ, Kim TI, Kim WH, et al. Interactions between IL17A, IL23R, and STAT4 polymorphisms confer susceptibility to intestinal Behcet's disease in Korean population. Life Sci. 2012;90(19–20):740–6.
54. Yalçin B, Atakan N, Dogan S. Association of interleukin-23 receptor gene polymorphism with Behçet disease. Clin Exp Dermatol. 2014;39(8):881–7.
55. Sousa I, Shahram F, Francisco D, Davatchi F, Abdollahi BS, Ghaderibarmi F, et al. Brief report: association of CCR1, KLRC4, IL12A-AS1, STAT4, and ERAP1 with Behçet's disease in Iranians. Arthritis Rheumatol. 2015;67(10):2742–8.
56. Kirino Y, Zhou Q, Ishigatsubo Y, Mizuki N, Tugal-Tutkun I, Seyahi E, et al. Targeted resequencing implicates the familial Mediterranean fever gene MEFV and the toll-like receptor 4 gene TLR4 in Behçet disease. Proc Natl Acad Sci U S A. 2013;110(20):8134–9.

57. Cargill M, Schrodi SJ, Chang M, Garcia VE, Brandon R, Callis KP, et al. A large-scale genetic association study confirms IL12B and leads to the identification of IL23R as psoriasis-risk genes. Am J Hum Genet. 2007;80(2):273–90.
58. Duerr RH, Taylor KD, Brant SR, Rioux JD, Silverberg MS, Daly MJ, et al. A genome-wide association study identifies IL23R as an inflammatory bowel disease gene. Science. 2006;314(5804):1461–3.
59. Rueda B, Orozco G, Raya E, Fernandez-Sueiro JL, Mulero J, Blanco FJ, et al. The IL23R Arg381Gln non-synonymous polymorphism confers susceptibility to ankylosing spondylitis. Ann Rheum Dis. 2008;67(10):1451–4.
60. Iwakura Y, Ishigame H. The IL-23/IL-17 axis in inflammation. J Clin Invest. 2006;116(5):1218–22.
61. Wu Z, Zheng W, Xu J, Sun F, Chen H, Li P, et al. IL10 polymorphisms associated with Behçet's disease in Chinese Han. Hum Immunol. 2014;75(3):271–6.
62. Kang EH, Choi JY, Lee YJ, Lee EY, Lee EB, Song YW. Single nucleotide polymorphisms in IL-10-mediated signalling pathways in Korean patients with Behçet's disease. Clin Exp Rheumatol. 2014;32(4 Suppl 84):S27–32.
63. Wallace GR, Kondeatis E, Vaughan RW, Verity DH, Chen Y, Fortune F, et al. IL-10 genotype analysis in patients with Behçet's disease. Hum Immunol. 2007;68(2):122–7.
64. Temple SE, Lim E, Cheong KY, Almeida CA, Price P, Ardlie KG, et al. Alleles carried at positions -819 and -592 of the IL10 promoter affect transcription following stimulation of peripheral blood cells with Streptococcus pneumoniae. Immunogenetics. 2003;55(9):629–32.
65. Turner DM, Williams DM, Sankaran D, Lazarus M, Sinnott PJ, Hutchinson IV. An investigation of polymorphism in the interleukin-10 gene promoter. Eur J Immunogenet. 1997;24(1):1–8.
66. Moore KW, de Waal Malefyt R, Coffman RL, O'Garra A. Interleukin-10 and the interleukin-10 receptor. Annu Rev Immunol. 2001;19:683–765.
67. Chang JT, Shevach EM, Segal BM. Regulation of interleukin (IL)-12 receptor beta2 subunit expression by endogenous IL-12: a critical step in the differentiation of pathogenic autoreactive T cells. J Exp Med. 1999;189(6):969–78.
68. Kappen JH, Medina-Gomez C, van Hagen PM, Stolk L, Estrada K, Rivadeneira F, et al. Genome-wide association study in an admixed case series reveals IL12A as a new candidate in Behçet disease. PLoS One. 2015;10(3):e0119085.
69. Kirino Y, Bertsias G, Ishigatsubo Y, Mizuki N, Tugal-Tutkun I, Seyahi E, et al. Genome-wide association analysis identifies new susceptibility loci for Behçet's disease and epistasis between HLA-B*51 and ERAP1. Nat Genet. 2013;45(2):202–7.
70. Remmers EF, Plenge RM, Lee AT, Graham RR, Hom G, Behrens TW, et al. STAT4 and the risk of rheumatoid arthritis and systemic lupus erythematosus. N Engl J Med. 2007;357(10):977–86.
71. Korman BD, Alba MI, Le JM, Alevizos I, Smith JA, Nikolov NP, et al. Variant form of STAT4 is associated with primary Sjögren's syndrome. Genes Immun. 2008;9(3):267–70.
72. Hou S, Yang Z, Du L, Jiang Z, Shu Q, Chen Y, et al. Identification of a susceptibility locus in STAT4 for Behçet's disease in Han Chinese in a genome-wide association study. Arthritis Rheum. 2012;64(12):4104–13.
73. Morinobu A, Gadina M, Strober W, Visconti R, Fornace A, Montagna C, et al. STAT4 serine phosphorylation is critical for IL-12 induced IFN-gamma production but not for cell proliferation. Proc Natl Acad Sci U S A. 2002;99(19):12281–6.
74. Abelson AK, Delgado-Vega AM, Kozyrev SV, Sánchez E, Velázquez-Cruz R, Eriksson N, et al. STAT4 associates with systemic lupus erythematosus through two independent effects that correlate with gene expression and act additively with IRF5 to increase risk. Ann Rheum Dis. 2009;68(11):1746–53.
75. Conde-Jaldón M, Montes-Cano MA, García-Lozano JR, Ortiz-Fernández L, Ortego-Centeno N, González-León R, et al. Epistatic interaction of ERAP1 and HLA-B in Behçet disease: a replication study in the Spanish population. PLoS One. 2014;9(7):e102100.

76. Takeuchi M, Ombrello MJ, Kirino Y, Erer B, Tugal-Tutkun I, Seyahi E, et al. A single endoplasmic reticulum aminopeptidase-1 protein allotype is a strong risk factor for Behçet's disease in HLA-B*51 carriers. Ann Rheum Dis. 2016;75(12):2208–11.
77. Burton PR, Clayton DG, Cardon LR, Craddock N, Deloukas P, Duncanson A, et al. Association scan of 14,500 nonsynonymous SNPs in four diseases identifies autoimmunity variants. Nat Genet. 2007;39(11):1329–37.
78. Strange A, Capon F, Spencer CC, Knight J, Weale ME, Allen MH, et al. A genome-wide association study identifies new psoriasis susceptibility loci and an interaction between HLA-C and ERAP1. Nat Genet. 2010;42(11):985–90.
79. Sun LD, Cheng H, Wang ZX, Zhang AP, Wang PG, Xu JH, et al. Association analyses identify six new psoriasis susceptibility loci in the Chinese population. Nat Genet. 2010;42(11):1005–9.
80. Saric T, Chang SC, Hattori A, York IA, Markant S, Rock KL, et al. An IFN-gamma-induced aminopeptidase in the ER, ERAP1, trims precursors to MHC class I-presented peptides. Nat Immunol. 2002;3(12):1169–76.
81. Xavier JM, Shahram F, Sousa I, Davatchi F, Matos M, Abdollahi BS, et al. FUT2: filling the gap between genes and environment in Behçet's disease? Ann Rheum Dis. 2015;74(3):618–24.
82. Ferrer-Admetlla A, Sikora M, Laayouni H, Esteve A, Roubinet F, Blancher A, et al. A natural history of FUT2 polymorphism in humans. Mol Biol Evol. 2009;26(9):1993–2003.
83. Franke A, McGovern DP, Barrett JC, Wang K, Radford-Smith GL, Ahmad T, et al. Genome-wide meta-analysis increases to 71 the number of confirmed Crohn's disease susceptibility loci. Nat Genet. 2010;42(12):1118–25.
84. Hu DY, Shao XX, Xu CL, Xia SL, Yu LQ, Jiang LJ, et al. Associations of FUT2 and FUT3 gene polymorphisms with Crohn's disease in Chinese patients. J Gastroenterol Hepatol. 2014;29(10):1778–85.
85. Smyth DJ, Cooper JD, Howson JM, Clarke P, Downes K, Mistry T, et al. FUT2 nonsecretor status links type 1 diabetes susceptibility and resistance to infection. Diabetes. 2011;60(11):3081–4.
86. Lindesmith L, Moe C, Marionneau S, Ruvoen N, Jiang X, Lindblad L, et al. Human susceptibility and resistance to Norwalk virus infection. Nat Med. 2003;9(5):548–53.
87. Ruiz-Palacios GM, Cervantes LE, Ramos P, Chavez-Munguia B, Newburg DS. Campylobacter jejuni binds intestinal H(O) antigen (Fuc alpha 1, 2Gal beta 1, 4GlcNAc), and fucosyloligosaccharides of human milk inhibit its binding and infection. J Biol Chem. 2003;278(16):14112–20.
88. Wacklin P, Mäkivuokko H, Alakulppi N, Nikkilä J, Tenkanen H, Räbinä J, et al. Secretor genotype (FUT2 gene) is strongly associated with the composition of bifidobacteria in the human intestine. PLoS One. 2011;6(5):e20113.
89. Rausch P, Rehman A, Künzel S, Häsler R, Ott SJ, Schreiber S, et al. Colonic mucosa-associated microbiota is influenced by an interaction of Crohn disease and FUT2 (Secretor) genotype. Proc Natl Acad Sci U S A. 2011;108(47):19030–5.
90. Hayashi T, Imai K, Morishita Y, Hayashi I, Kusunoki Y, Nakachi K. Identification of the NKG2D haplotypes associated with natural cytotoxic activity of peripheral blood lymphocytes and cancer immunosurveillance. Cancer Res. 2006;66(1):563–70.
91. Hou S, Xiao X, Li F, Jiang Z, Kijlstra A, Yang P. Two-stage association study in Chinese Han identifies two independent associations in CCR1/CCR3 locus as candidate for Behçet's disease susceptibility. Hum Genet. 2012;131(12):1841–50.
92. Marzio PD, Sherry B, Thomas EK, Franchin G, Schmidtmayerova H, Bukrinsky M. beta-Chemokine production in CD40L-stimulated monocyte-derived macrophages requires activation of MAPK signaling pathways. Cytokine. 2003;23(3):53–63.
93. Fei Y, Webb R, Cobb BL, Direskeneli H, Saruhan-Direskeneli G, Sawalha AH. Identification of novel genetic susceptibility loci for Behçet's disease using a genome-wide association study. Arthritis Res Ther. 2009;11(3):R66.

94. Lee YJ, Horie Y, Wallace GR, Choi YS, Park JA, Choi JY, et al. Genome-wide association study identifies GIMAP as a novel susceptibility locus for Behcet's disease. Ann Rheum Dis. 2013;72(9):1510–6.
95. Ortiz-Fernández L, Conde-Jaldón M, García-Lozano JR, Montes-Cano MA, Ortego-Centeno N, Castillo-Palma MJ, et al. GIMAP and Behçet disease: no association in the European population. Ann Rheum Dis. 2014;73(7):1433–4.
96. Burillo-Sanz S, Montes-Cano MA, García-Lozano JR, Ortiz-Fernández L, Ortego-Centeno N, García-Hernández FJ, et al. Mutational profile of rare variants in inflammasome-related genes in Behçet disease: a next generation sequencing approach. Sci Rep. 2017;7(1):8453.
97. Kastelein RA, Hunter CA, Cua DJ. Discovery and biology of IL-23 and IL-27: related but functionally distinct regulators of inflammation. Annu Rev Immunol. 2007;25:221–42.
98. Carmona FD, González-Gay MA, Martín J. Genetic component of giant cell arteritis. Rheumatology (Oxford). 2014;53(1):6–18.
99. Eyre S, Orozco G, Worthington J. The genetics revolution in rheumatology: large scale genomic arrays and genetic mapping. Nat Rev Rheumatol. 2017;13(7):421–32.
100. Ortiz-Fernández L, Carmona FD, López-Mejías R, González-Escribano MF, Lyons PA, Morgan AW, et al. Cross-phenotype analysis of Immunochip data identifies. Ann Rheum Dis. 2018;77(4):589–95.
101. Ellinghaus D, Jostins L, Spain SL, Cortes A, Bethune J, Han B, et al. Analysis of five chronic inflammatory diseases identifies 27 new associations and highlights disease-specific patterns at shared loci. Nat Genet. 2016;48(5):510–8.
102. Carmona FD, Coit P, Saruhan-Direskeneli G, Hernández-Rodríguez J, Cid MC, Solans R, et al. Analysis of the common genetic component of large-vessel vasculitides through a meta-Immunochip strategy. Sci Rep. 2017;7:43953.
103. Coit P, Direskeneli H, Sawalha AH. An update on the role of epigenetics in systemic vasculitis. Curr Opin Rheumatol. 2018;30(1):4–15.
104. Serwold T, Gonzalez F, Kim J, Jacob R, Shastri N. ERAAP customizes peptides for MHC class I molecules in the endoplasmic reticulum. Nature. 2002;419(6906):480–3.

Sjögren's Syndrome

4

Laëtitia Le Pottier, Kahina Amrouche, Amandine Charras, Anne Bordron, and Jacques-Olivier Pers

Contents

L. Le Pottier · K. Amrouche · A. Charras · A. Bordron · J.-O. Pers (✉)
Univ Brest, UMR1227, Lymphocytes B et Autoimmunité, Brest, France
e-mail: laetitia.lepottier@univ-brest.fr; anne.bordron@univ-brest.fr; pers@univ-brest.fr

J. Martín, F. D. Carmona (eds.), *Genetics of Rare Autoimmune Diseases*,
Rare Diseases of the Immune System, https://doi.org/10.1007/978-3-030-03934-9_4

4.1 Introduction

Primary Sjögren's syndrome (pSS) is a systemic autoimmune disease characterized by sicca symptoms and a broad variety of systemic clinical manifestations. The prevalence in the general population is 0.02–0.1%, and middle-aged women are predominantly affected [1]. Indeed, even though keratoconjunctivitis sicca (KCS), resulting from the involvement of lacrimal glands, and xerostomia, resulting from the involvement of salivary glands (SGs), are usually prominent, pSS presents as a multifaceted and systemic condition with a broad variety of clinical manifestations. The spectrum of pSS extends from an organ-specific autoimmune disorder (referred to as an autoimmune exocrinopathy) to a systemic process that may involve the musculoskeletal system, nervous system, lungs, kidneys, and blood vessels. Biological abnormalities associated with B lymphocytes are also a hallmark of the disease, and these abnormalities are characterized by the presence of rheumatoid factor (RF), hypergammaglobulinemia, anti-sicca syndrome A/Ro (SSA) and anti-sicca syndrome B/La (SSB) antibodies, and an abnormal distribution of mature B lymphocytes in the peripheral blood [2], in addition to an increased risk of non-Hodgkin's lymphoma (NHL) in 5% of patients [3].

More than 50 years ago, genetic involvement was suggested in the etiology of pSS [4]. The idea that genetic and epigenetic factors contribute to the etiology of systemic autoimmune diseases such as pSS is supported by familial autoimmunity and poly-autoimmunity [5]. Indeed, some studies have reported familial forms of pSS [6] with some cases in twins. However, although the number of cases remains too low to evaluate the familial risk of pSS, several studies have been conducted based on the co-aggregation of autoimmune diseases in affected families [5, 7]. The clustering of autoimmune diseases such as systemic lupus erythematosus (SLE), rheumatoid arthritis (RA), autoimmune thyroid disease (AITD), psoriasis, multiple sclerosis, and pSS within families has frequently been reported.

Most of the genes associated with susceptibility to pSS have been identified because the proteins involved have been previously associated with the pathogenesis of pSS or because the genes had already been associated with another autoimmune disease such as SLE or RA. Consequently, in this chapter, we will first focus on the immunopathology of pSS in order to better understand the genetic and epigenetic alterations described in the disease. The last section will be dedicated to genetic alterations in pSS related to lymphoma.

4.2 Immunopathology of pSS

4.2.1 An Autoimmune Epithelitis

Lymphocytic infiltration is a histological hallmark of pSS. T and B lymphocytes indeed constitute the vast majority of the mononuclear cells infiltrating the salivary glands. Although the majority of infiltrating mononuclear cells are T cells in mild lesions, B-cell levels reach up to 50% in advanced lesions [8]. Epithelial cell

(EC) apoptosis induced by the lymphocytic infiltrates is considered a key factor in the decreased production of exocrine secretions. Fas-FasL mechanisms may explain the increased EC apoptosis mediated by T cells, but B cells also directly mediate EC death via a mechanism that is independent of Fas-FasL interactions but requires protein kinase C delta (PKC δ) translocation into the EC nucleus [9]. Immunohistochemical studies of inflammatory salivary gland tissue from patients with pSS have shown that the ECs contain high levels of several immunoactive molecules known to mediate lymphoid cell homing, antigen presentation, and the amplification of epithelial cell-immune cell interactions. ECs can secrete proinflammatory cytokines via a mechanism initially mediated by Toll-like receptor (TLR) activation. Several TLRs are expressed by ECs in salivary gland tissue (TLR2, TLR3, TLR4, and TLR7) [10]. Consequently, the most likely hypothesis is that EC activation in pSS may be related to the viral infection of the exocrine glands. Toll-like receptor signaling in the salivary gland ECs, which is achieved through epigenetic mechanisms [11], upregulates the expression of MHC-I, CD54/ICAM-I, CD40, CD95/Fas proteins, CD80, and CD86, thereby linking the innate and adaptive immune responses. Global DNA methylation is reduced in salivary gland ECs and could explain the aberrant transcription of many genes by these cells. Global DNA demethylation of ECs was accounted for by a decrease in the methylating enzyme DNMT1, which is associated with an increase in its demethylating partner Gadd45-alpha [12]. Thus, environmental factors may convert ECs to nonprofessional antigen-presenting cells (APCs) that also induce the polarization of naive T cells. Furthermore, interferon (IFN)-γ increases HLAII expression by ECs, thereby encouraging them to shift toward APCs. The functional expression of these immunoreactive molecules indicates that salivary gland ECs can probably mediate the presentation of antigen peptides and the transmission of activation signals to T cells. Furthermore, cytokines play a role in EC activation, as shown by the finding that IFN-γ and interleukin (IL)-1β induce CD40 expression by cultured ECs. Finally, nuclear autoantigens such as the Ro/SSA and La/SSB ribonucleoproteins may translocate from the nucleus to the membrane of ECs. These ribonucleoproteins are present in apoptotic bodies, whose numbers are increased in ECs taken from patients with pSS. Thus, ECs can present antigens to T and B cells. Cathepsin S, the activity of which is upregulated in the lacrimal glands of patients with pSS [13], is involved in class II MHC-mediated immune responses that promote the displacement of class II MHC molecules to the cell surface for presentation, thereby increasing antigen presentation by B cells and amplifying the autoimmune process. ECs also produce chemokines such as CXCL13, CCL19, and CCL21, which promote lymphocyte migration into the salivary glands. A relationship has been demonstrated linking CXCL13, salivary gland inflammation, and the loss of salivary function. Moreover, CXCL13 and CCL21 are directly involved in the organization of ectopic germinal centers. Finally, a link between CXCL13 and CCL11 and disease activity and lymphoma has been established [14]. Thus, by aberrantly expressing various immunoactive factors, ECs seem able to actively participate in and modulate the immune response within inflammatory lesions.

4.2.2 An Interferon Signature

Transcriptome analyses of salivary gland tissue and mononuclear cells from patients with pSS have shown the overexpression of type I IFN-induced genes, a phenomenon known as the IFN signature. In some patients, the IFN signature is associated with disease activity [15]. In addition to the increased expression of IFN-regulated genes, IRF5 polymorphisms have been described in association with pSS. These findings support a role on the part of IFN induction in the immunological activation seen in both the peripheral blood and the exocrine glands of patients with pSS. One of the most relevant IFN-induced genes encodes B-cell activating factor (BAFF) of the TNF ligand family. Thus, the IFN signature is associated with BAFF, the overexpression of which is a hallmark of pSS.

4.2.3 The Role of BAFF

Serum BAFF levels are elevated in patients with pSS and associated with the increased production of autoantibodies such as anti-SSA, anti-SSB, and rheumatoid factor. Moreover, elevated BAFF levels have been found in the salivary glands of patients with pSS and are produced by B cells, T cells, and ECs [16]. Also, another observation that is in keeping with a role for BAFF in the pathogenesis of SS is that most lymphomas associated with pSS arise from B cells. Among patients with SS, those with lymphoma have higher serum BAFF levels as compared to those without lymphoma [17]. BAFF overexpression may allow autoreactive B cells to survive stronger autoantigen-triggered death signals and produce autoantibodies. This BAFF-mediated survival mechanism is evident in the peripheral blood B cells of patients with pSS because apoptosis was significantly decreased in B cells taken from patients with SS, indicating the antiapoptotic and survival-extending effects of BAFF.

4.2.4 A Form of B-Cell Hyperactivity

In this context, B-cell hyperactivity is among the main features of pSS and acts by producing autoantibodies, cytokines, and antigen-presenting cells [18]. The presence of germinal cell-like structures in salivary gland biopsies from 25% of patients with pSS indicates that it may be a strong predictor of non-Hodgkin's lymphoma development, although this observation deserves further investigation [19]. Interestingly, the terminal differentiation of B cells into plasma cells and memory B cells occurs within germinal centers under the supervision of T follicular helper (Tfh) cells [20]. Although the development and control of Tfh cells remain debated, IL-21 production by dendritic cells is known as a major contributor to the terminal differentiation of Tfh cells. Importantly, abnormal Tfh cell function has deleterious effects, including triggering autoimmunity. Ectopic germinal centers serve as a conduit to recruit and expand autoreactive B cells and may also contribute to the emergence of high-affinity autoantibodies in the salivary glands [18]. Interestingly, an increased circulating Tfh cell count and increased IL-21 production in these cells are found in patients with pSS and may predict a more severe clinical course [21]. Recently, IL-22 was reported to regulate lymphoid chemokine production and the assembly of ectopic germinal centers [22].

4.2.5 A Defect of the Suppressive Immune Response

The evolution of pSS could also be associated with defects in the control of the immune response. Foxp3+ regulatory T cells (Treg) may play an important role in controlling autoimmunity. Foxp3+ Treg counts in minor salivary gland lesions in patients with SS are comparable to those in controls with non-SS sialadenitis, suggesting that the number of Foxp3+ Treg cells may not be decreased in SS. However, the counts of Foxp3+ T cells circulating in the blood correlate inversely with those of such cells infiltrating the salivary glands [23]. The fact that Treg cell counts are lower in advanced as compared to mild salivary gland infiltrates supports the view that dendritic cell-derived TGF-β induces Foxp3 in naive T cells and switches T-cell differentiation from the defective Treg cell pathway to a Th17 differentiation pathway in the presence of IL-6 [24]. Although B-cell overactivity is evident in pSS, a new category of B cells known as regulatory B cells (Breg) can blunt the development of autoimmune disorders [25]. The CD40-CD40L interaction between B and T cells is critical to the acquisition of Breg function upon Th1 differentiation through the production of IL-10, IL-35, and transforming growth factor β (TGF-β) or indoleamine 2,3-dioxygenase [26]. Various chronic inflammatory environments that can occur in pSS have been reported to induce Breg cell populations, and Breg cells seem to be efficient in controlling T-cell proliferation and Th1 differentiation in patients with pSS. Consequently, their depletion could explain the altered efficacy of B-cell depletion in pSS [27].

4.2.6 Evolution Toward Lymphoma

Malignancy is the most fatal complication experienced by pSS patients, with an eightfold risk of mortality in this population as compared to the normal population. In consequence of that critical impact, a great deal of effort has been made to identify predictable biomarkers for lymphoma development in patients affected by pSS. This research has provided several prognostic factors associated with lymphoma development in pSS patients, namely, the presence of rheumatoid factor, C4 hypocomplementemia, monoclonal gammopathy, lymphopenia, higher levels of disease activity, the abnormal presence of germinal center-like structures within the mucosal sites of the exocrine glands [28], and, more recently, higher serum levels of FMS-like tyrosine kinase 3 (FLT3) cytokine [29]. In addition, the risk of lymphoma establishment increases with disease duration, with a cumulative risk of 3.4% at 5 years and 9.8% at 15 years from diagnosis [30]. In contrast, among pSS patients, neither previous treatment for pSS nor male was associated with any effect on lymphoma occurrence [31].

4.3 Genetics of Sjögren's Syndrome

Genome-wide association studies (GWAS) of complex diseases, such as autoimmune diseases, have been successful in identifying new loci and confirming previously described genetic variations. Moreover, the gene association mapping is complicated by the linkage disequilibrium (LD) and haplotype block presence in the human genome, blurring the identification of the causal variant in the loci. The LD is particularly important in the HLA region [32]. To better understand how genetic variations, such as single-nucleotide polymorphisms (SNPs) in loci, contribute to the disease, more recent studies combine GWAS and global gene expression (microarray or RNA-sequencing analyses) to map gene expression as a quantitative trait (expression quantitative trait loci [eQTL] mapping) [33].

4.3.1 HLA Associations

Historically, the HLA region, located in chromosome 6p21.3, was the first associated with pSS [34]. It is not easy to summarize HLA association with pSS because, since 1975, the HLA nomenclature has changed and variant identification techniques have evolved. Moreover, the mapping of MHC (major histocompatibility complex) susceptibility variants is complex because (1) there are differences between populations other than pathological status; (2) there is a high and extensive LD in this region, and thus, the identification of causal and independent loci is complicated; and (3) some epistatic effects have been established between the MHC and other loci [35].

The extended MHC was divided into five subregions from telomeric to centromeric on the short arm of chromosome 6 (q21.3 region): extended class I region, class I region, class III region, class II region, and extended class II region (Fig. 4.1).

The main genes in subregions I, II, and III are mapped in Fig. 4.1, and their associations with pSS are identified by arrows (GWAS analyses) or by stars (identified otherwise than by GWAS).

4.3.1.1 MHC Class I

This subregion, with a spacing of 1.9 Mb, contains classical gene loci (HLA-A, HLA-B, and HLA-C) and nonclassical gene loci (HLA-E, HLA-F, and HLA-G).

HLA-A

An increased prevalence of HLA-A24 has been associated with pSS ($P = 0.009$; OR = 3.5). The GWAS identification in Caucasians has shown that the HLA-A*0101 allele frequency was higher in cases of pSS ($P_{meta} = 6.74 \times 10^{-35}$;

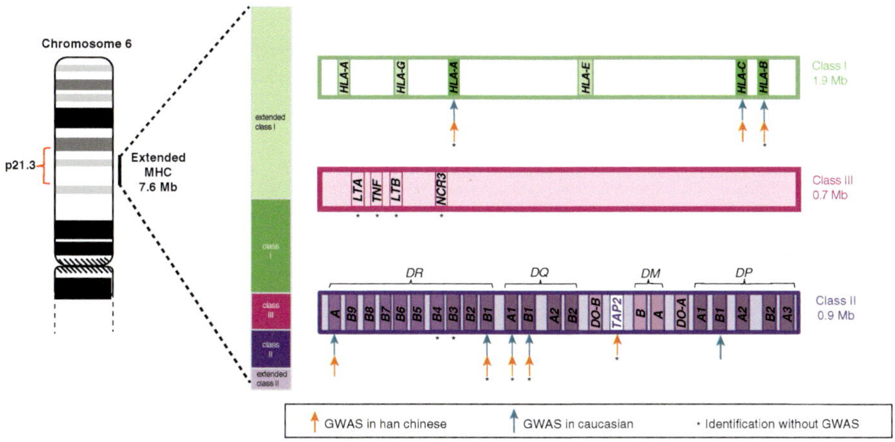

Fig. 4.1 Map of main genes in major histocompatibility complex (MHC) and association with Sjögren's syndrome (SS). The extended MHC is located on short arm of chromosome 6 (p21.3) and divided in five subregions spanning about 7.6 megabases (Mb). The arrows indicate locus susceptibility to SS identified by genome-wide association study (GWAS) in the Han Chinese population (orange) or in the Caucasian population (blue). Star (*) indicates locus susceptibility to SS identified without GWAS

OR_{meta} = 1.88) and that the cis-eQTL analysis was significant at rs113258639 (FDR = 5.02×10^{-11}) [36]. The HLA-A*0101 allele was associated with anti-La/SSB autoantibodies in Mexican patients with pSS ($P = 0.003$; OR = 4.75). Finally, the GWAS in the Han Chinese showed the most likely SNP at rs17186258 ($P = 1.73 \times 10^{-2}$; OR = 0.66) [37].

HLA-B

The prevalence of HLA-B8 was significantly increased in patients with pSS. The GWAS in the Han Chinese showed that the most likely SNP was at rs4992474 ($P = 8.21 \times 10^{-5}$; OR = 1.40) [37]. The GWAS in Caucasians identified the HLA-B*0801 allele with increased frequency ($P_{meta} = 1.09 \times 10^{-86}$; $OR_{meta} = 3.27$) and the HLA-B*1501 with decreased frequency in pSS cases ($P_{meta} = 4.09 \times 10^{-8}$; $OR_{meta} = 0.55$) [36]. No significant cis-eQTL was associated with the HLA-B gene [36]. In Mexican patients, HLA-B*3501 was significantly associated with pSS ($P = 0.004$; OR = 3.70).

HLA-C

The association of the HLA-C gene with pSS was only identified via GWAS. In the Han Chinese population, the most likely SNP was at rs3905495 ($P = 1.77 \times 10^{-4}$; OR = 0.75) [37]. In the Caucasian population, two alleles of HLA-C have been identified, HLA-C*0701 ($P_{meta} = 3.67 \times 10^{-81}$; $OR_{meta} = 2.72$) and HLA-C*0304 ($P_{meta} = 5.57 \times 10^{-10}$; OR = 0.59), the frequencies of which were higher and lower, respectively, in patients with pSS [36].

4.3.1.2 Class II

This subregion, with a spacing of 0.9 Mb, contains classical gene loci (HLA-DP, HLA-DQ, and HLA-DR) and nonclassical gene loci (HLA-DO and HLA-DM).

HLA-DR and HLA-DQ

These two genes are always associated because three of their loci are in very strong LD ($r^2 = 0.97$): HLA-DRB1, HLA-DQA1, and HLA-DQB1 [36]. In 1993, a study on HLA class II genes showed differing haplotype frequencies between Caucasian, Chinese, and Japanese populations. Thus, the HLA-DRB1*0301(-DRB3*0101)-DQA1*0501-DQB1*0201 haplotype was significantly more common in Caucasian patients, the HLA-DRB1*0405(-DRB4*0101)-DQA1*0301-DQB1*0401 haplotype was significantly more common in Japanese patients, and the HLA-DRB1*0803-DQA1*0103-DQB1*0601 haplotype was significantly more common in Chinese patients. The frequency increases of these alleles in the Caucasian population have been confirmed by several studies on a Finnish population, a Scandinavian population [38], a Colombian population, and a French population [39]. Moreover, the GWAS in Caucasians confirmed that HLA-DQB1*0201 ($P_{meta} = 1.38 \times 10^{-95}$; $OR_{meta} = 3.36$), HLA-DQA1*0501 ($P_{meta} = 8.50 \times 10^{-94}$; $OR_{meta} = 3.34$), and HLA-DRB1*0301 ($P_{meta} = 2.19 \times 10^{-74}$; ORmeta = 3.25) were the alleles most significantly associated with pSS [36]. Cis-eQTL analysis showed a significant association at rs112038669 in the HLA-DQA1 gene (FDR = 1.27×10^{-12}) and, surprisingly, at rs114846898 in the HLA-DRB6 gene (FDR = 2.57×10^{-31}). No significant eQTL has been identified in the HLA-DQB1 and HLA-DRB1 genes [36]. In the HLA-DQA1 gene, one SNP (rs9271588) has been identified in three GWAS analyses: one in a Caucasian population ($P_{meta} = 1.37 \times 10^{-85}$; $OR_{meta} = 0.41$) [36] and two in a Han Chinese population ($P = 9.50 \times 10^{-12}$; OR = 0.58 for the first and $P = 1.82 \times 10^{-5}$; OR = 1.57 for the second) [37, 40].

HLA-DP

Only the GWAS in Caucasians identified the HLA-DPB1*0101 allele, which was significantly higher in pSS cases as compared to controls ($P_{meta} = 8.42 \times 10^{-19}$; $OR_{meta} = 2.07$) [36]. Moreover, HLA-DPB1 at rs3128917 showed a significant cis-eQTL (FDR = 3.23×10^{-14}) [36]. In 1993, a study that compared HLA class II genes in Caucasian, Chinese, and Japanese patients with pSS showed no significant association with DPB1 alleles.

TAP2

TAP2 (transporter associated with antigen processing 2) is a crucial subunit for the molecular assembly of the MHC-I complex. A mutation in exon 9 of TAP2, which leads to a methionine-to-valine substitution at codon 577, has been observed in a Japanese population. This new TAP2 allele, named TAP2*Bky2, showed an increased frequency in patients with pSS ($P < 0.05$) and a strong association with anti-SSA production ($P = 0.001$) [41]. This association was not identified by GWAS, but two other SNPs have been found in a Han Chinese population, rs3763355

($P = 1.24 \times 10^{-4}$; OR = 0.50) [37] and rs211429 ($P = 9.88 \times 10^{-5}$; OR = 1.47) [40], both of which are located in the 5′ region upstream of the *TAP2* gene.

4.3.1.3 Class III

The genes located in the class III region are involved in inflammation, such as C2, C4, TNF, and lymphotoxins.

Lymphotoxin System and TNFα

TNFSF1 (lymphotoxin α) and *TNFSF3* (lymphotoxin β) are located in the same locus as *TNFSF2* (TNFα) on chromosome 6p21.33, in the HLA class III region. A study conducted on 1059 individuals comprised of a Norwegian (193 pSS and 213 healthy controls) and Swedish cohort (334 pSS and 319 healthy controls) identified 12 SNPs. Only four SNPs showed a significant association with pSS in the total cohort and in each independently after logistic regression: rs915654 (1379 bases upstream of *TNFSF1*) ($P_{total} = 1.13 \times 10^{-4}$), rs909253 (*TNFSF1* intron 1) ($P_{total} = 1.25 \times 10^{-7}$), rs2229094 (*TNFSF1* exon 2) ($P_{total} = 4.15 \times 10^{-4}$), and rs1800629 (319 bases upstream of *TNFSF2*) ($P_{total} = 2.48 \times 10^{-10}$). At the haplotype level, the researchers observed several significant associations, most of which involved the two SNPs with the lowest *P* values: rs909253 and rs1800629. Moreover, they identified a very significant association with the haplotype G/A (rs909253/rs1800629) ($P = 9.14 \times 10^{-17}$) with a nearly doubled frequency in pSS cases as compared to healthy controls [42].

An older study showed that the frequency of allele A at position −308 in the *TNFSF2* gene was higher in pSS cases than in controls [43].

NCR3

The *NCR3* gene encodes NKp30, an innate receptor expressed by natural killer cells and crucial for cross-talk with dendritic cells. A combined meta-analysis in a French and a Scandinavian cohort showed that two NCR3 SNPs, rs11575837 and rs2736191, were inversely associated with the risk of pSS (OR = 0.48, $P = 0.0039$ and OR = 0.56, $P = 0.0019$, respectively) [44].

4.3.2 Non-HLA Associations

Table 4.1 summarizes the non-HLA risk genes or susceptibility regions in Sjögren's syndrome.

4.3.2.1 Chemokines, Cytokines, and Receptors

CCL11/CCL7 Regions

Two SNPs, rs3091328 (G/A) (located between *CCL7* and *CCL11* genes) and rs1860184 (A/T) (located in the *CCL11* intron), have been associated with germinal center status in Swedish and Norwegian patients. They are in an intermediate LD ($r^2 = 0.66$), and the haplotypes of the major alleles (A and T, respectively) are the

Table 4.1 Summary of non-HLA association genes or regions in Sjögren's syndrome

	Gene or locus	CHR.	Variation	Population	Reference
Chemokines, cytokines, and receptors	**CCL11**	17q21.1–21.2	**rs1860184**	Swedish and Norwegian	[45]
	CCL7/CCL11 region	17q	**rs3091328**	Swedish and Norwegian	[45]
	CCR5	3q21.31	**delta32 rs333**	Caucasian Slovak origin	[46]
	CXCR5	11q23.3	**rs7119038 rs11217033**	*Meta-analysis Caucasian*	[36]
	IL-10	1q32.1	**GCC haplotype promoter**	Japanese	[49]
				Caucasian French	[43]
				Spanish	[48]
				Finnish	[47]
	IL-12A	3q25.33	**rs485497 rs4680536**	*Meta-analysis Caucasian*	[36]
	IL-2-IL-21 region	4q27	**rs6822844**	*Meta-analysis Caucasian*	[50]
Tumor necrosis factor and associated molecules	**TNFSF4**	1q25	**rs1234315 rs1234314 rs704840**	Swedish and Norwegian	[51]
			rs704840 rs2205960	Han Chinese	[52]
			rs2205960	Han Chinese	[53]
	TNFSF13B	13q33.3	**rs9514827 rs3759467 rs1041569 rs9514828**	Australian Caucasian	[54]
			rs9514827 rs9514828 rs1224141 rs12583006	Caucasian Greek ancestry	[28]
	TNFRSF13C	22q13.2	**His159Tyr**	Greek	[55]
	TNFRSF6	10q23.31	**−670(G/A)**	Australian	[57]
			−671	Swedish and Norwegian	[56]
	TNFAIP3	6q23.3	**rs2230926**	Caucasian	[58]
			rs2230926 rs5029939	Han Chinese	[37, 52]
	TNIP1	5q33.1	**rs6579837**	*Meta-analysis Caucasian*	[36]
			rs3792783 rs7708392	Meta-analysis Swedish, Norwegian, and UK	[59]

Table 4.1 (continued)

	Gene or locus	CHR.	Variation	Population	Reference
Transcription factors	**EBF1**	5q33.3	rs3843489 rs869593	Swedish and Norwegian	[59]
	GTF2I	7q11.23	**rs117026326**	Han Chinese	[37]
			rs117026326	Han Chinese	[40]
	IKZF1	7p12.2	**rs4917014** **rs4917129**	Han Chinese	[60]
	NFKBIA	14q13.2	**–826 C/T**	Taiwanese	[61]
	IRF5 (IRF5/ TNPO3 locus)	7q32.1	**CGGGG indel**	French Cohort *Assess*	[62]
			rs10488631 **CGGGG indel**	Swedish and Norwegian	[63]
			rs10488631 **rs13246321**	Swedish and Norwegian	[51]
			rs3757387	*Meta-analysis Caucasian*	[36]
	STAT4	2q32.3	**rs7574865**	Caucasian	[64]
			rs7582694	Swedish and Norwegian	[51, 63]
			rs10168266	Han Chinese	[37]
			rs10553577	*Meta-analysis Caucasian*	[36]
Immune system and others	**CHRM3**	1q43	**rs7548522** **rs4620530** **rs11578320** **rs6690809** **rs12072029**	Swedish and Norwegian	[65]
	CTLA4	2q33.2	**+49G allele** **CT60 allele**	Australian Caucasian	[66]
	FAM167A-BLK locus	8q23.1	**rs12549796** **rs12677843** **rs2736340** **rs13277113**	Swedish and Norwegian	[51]
			rs2736340 **rs13277113**	Han Chinese	[52]
			rs2736345 **rs2729935**	*Meta-analysis Caucasian*	[36]
			rs7812879 **rs2254546**	Han Chinese	[52]
	FCGR3B	1q23.3	**Copy number variation**	Paisa community (85% Caucasian and 15% Amerindian)	[68]
				Australian Caucasian	[69]
	MECP2	Xq28	**rs17435**	European	[70]
	OAS1	12q24.13	**rs10774671**	Meta-analysis	[71]
	PTPN22	1p13.2	**C1858T (R620W)**	Colombian	[72]
				Caucasian	[73]
	TRIM21	11p15.5	**C/T genotype**	Norwegian	[38]
			9571C/T	Japanese	[74]

CCL7/CCL11 risk haplotypes for ectopic germinal center formation in pSS ($p = 1.7 \times 10^{-4}$, OR 2.17) [45].

CCR5

CCR5 (CD195) is the receptor for CCL3 (MIP1α) and CCL4 (MIP1β), chemokines implicated in the pathogenesis of pSS. A truncated form of CCR5 called CCR5Δ32 due to the deletion of 32 bp in the coding sequence is famous for its protective effect against HIV infection (CCR5 is a co-receptor for HIV entry) in homozygotes. In 2002, *CCR5Δ32/CCR5* heterozygosis was associated with a reduced relative risk of pSS (OR = 0.35, $p = 0.043$) [46].

CXCR5

In 2013, a meta-analysis using GWAS and large-scale replication approaches identified a new risk locus in chromosome 11, near to the *CXCR5* gene. The authors observed an association with a variant ~16 kb 5′ of the coding region of *CXCR5* (receptor for CXCL13) at rs7119038 ($P_{meta} = 1.10 \times 10^{-8}$). However, no statistically significant cis-eQTL for *CXCR5* has been observed in this region [36].

Interleukin 10 (IL-10)

Three SNPs are described in the promoter region of the *IL-10* gene: G/A base-exchange polymorphism at −1082, −819 C/T polymorphism, and − 592 C/A polymorphism. The association between the GCC haplotype and pSS has been analyzed in four studies (Finnish, Spanish, French, and Japanese populations). In the Finnish population, the frequency of the *IL-10* GCC haplotype was increased ($P < 0.05$, OR = 1.90) in pSS as compared with healthy controls [47]. The same observation was reported by a French study and a Spanish study ($P = 0.003$, OR = 2.25, and $P = 0.006$, respectively), and no significant association was observed in patients with anti-SSA/SSB antibodies [43, 48]. The last study reported that the GCC haplotype, which is predominant among white subjects, was less common in the Japanese population. The most common *IL-10* haplotype in Japan is ATA. The frequency of the ATA haplotype was found to be increased in patients with pSS as compared with controls [49].

Interleukin 12A (p35)

Regarding CXCR5, a new risk locus in the *IL-12A* region was identified by GWAS. Seven variants were demonstrated, with the peak association occurring at 5.3 kb in the 3′ of *IL-12A* at rs485497 ($P_{meta} = 1.17 \times 10^{-10}$). This is the only locus that was associated with *IL-12A* transcript expression by cis-eQTL analysis. However, seven variants in the 3′ of *IL-12A* influenced expression more significantly, with the eQTL peaking at rs4680536 (FDR = 2.04×10^{-2}) [36].

IL-2/IL-21 Region

A meta-analysis performed in European and Colombian populations demonstrated that rs6822844 in the *IL-2-IL-21* region (chromosome 4q27) was strongly associated with multiple autoimmune diseases ($P_{meta} = 2.61 \times 10^{-25}$) and pSS in particular ($P = 0.033$) [50].

4.3.2.2 TNF, TNFR, and Associated Molecules

TNFSF4 (OX40L)

A combined analysis of Swedish and Norwegian cohorts identified SNPs in the *TNFSF4* gene locus that were associated with pSS. Two SNPs that were located in the 5′UTR region were in strong LD ($r^2 = 0.83$) and associated with pSS: rs1234315 ($P < 0.001$) and rs1234314 ($P < 0.01$). A third SNP, rs704840, which was located upstream of the *TNFSF4* gene in the 5′UTR region which had a lower LD (with SNP rs1234315, $r^2 = 0.37$) showed an association with pSS in a combined cohort ($P < 0.001$) [51]. This last SNP was also analyzed in a Han Chinese cohort, and no significative association with pSS was shown ($P = 0.068$) [52]. However, when genotype frequencies were analyzed, they identified a new SNP in the *TNFSF4* gene locus associated with pSS: rs2205960 (T/G) ($P = 0.026$ for T/T genotype). This new association was confirmed by another study in a Han Chinese cohort at the allelic and genotypic level (allele T and genotype T/T) [53].

BAFF (TNFSF13B) and BAFF-R (TNFRSF13C)

TNFSF13B, better known as BAFF, is a famous cytokine involved in autoimmune diseases. Thus, it is not surprising that some studies have attempted to analyze genetic variations in the *TNFSF13B* gene. In 2008, four SNPs located in the 5′ regulatory region of *TNFSF13B* were identified: rs9514827 (−2841 C/T), rs3759467 (−2704 C/T), rs1041569 (−2701 A/T), and rs9514828 (−871 C/T). These SNPs were studied in a haplotype block because they were in strong LD ($P < 0.000001$), with $r^2 = 0.94$ between rs9514827 and rs9514828, the two most distant SNPs. The CTAT haplotype was significantly increased in pSS patients ($P = 0.004$; OR = 2.12) as compared to the TTAC haplotype, which was most frequent in controls. Moreover, the CTAT haplotype association was apparently specific to SSA/SSB autoantibody-positive pSS patients ($P = 0.00004$, OR = 2.59), and its frequency was often decreased in SSA/SSB-negative pSS patients ($P = 0.16$, OR 0.47) [54]. During B-cell ontogenesis, BAFF signaling essentially acts through BAFF-R (TNFRSF13C). A mutation in the coding region of *TNFRSF13C* (missense substitution of tyrosine for histidine in codon 159 [His159Tyr]) seems to be more prevalent in pSS cases as compared to healthy controls (6.9% vs. 1.7%, respectively) and associated with MALT lymphoma development [55].

Fas (TNFRSF6)

Two studies reported genetic variations in the form of SNPs in the *TNFRSF6* gene located at −671 in the former study and at −670 in the latter study. In the first study, the authors observed a higher frequency of the G/G genotype at position −671 in pSS patients as compared to controls [56]. In the second study, they analyzed two common SNPs in the promoter region of the *TNFRSF6* gene: −1377 G/A and −670 A/G. No significant differences in allele or genotype frequencies were detected between patients and controls. However, the authors observed that A allele at −670 was more frequent in SSA/SSB-negative patients as compared to SSA/SSB-positive patients [57].

TNFAIP3

The TNFAIP3 (tumor necrosis factor, alpha-induced protein 3) gene is a key regulator of NF-kB signaling in activated T cells. Only 1 study in a Caucasian population identified an association between 1 SNP (rs2230926) and patients with pSS ($P = 0.038$; OR = 3.11), but the authors analyzed only 18 patients [58]. This SNP has been also identified in a Han Chinese population by GWAS ($P = 5.11 \times 10^{-2}$; OR = 1.38) [37]. The authors also identified another SNP at rs5029939 ($P = 3.69 \times 10^{-2}$; OR = 1.41) that was associated with pSS patients. However, another study in a Han Chinese population, which did not used GWAS, showed no significant difference between patients with pSS and controls for rs2230926 or rs5029939 [52]. The GWAS in the Caucasian population proposed TNFAIP3 as a region associated with pSS at rs6933404 ($P_{meta} = 6.53 \times 10^{-8}$; $OR_{meta} = 1.29$) and at rs35926684 ($P_{meta} = 7.21 \times 10^{-8}$; $OR_{meta} = 1.29$) [36].

TNIP1

TNIP1 (TNFAIP3 interacting protein 1) is implicated in the regulation of NF-kB signaling, and some SNPs of this gene have been associated with several autoimmune diseases. Three SNPs in the *TNIP1* locus (chromosome 5q33.1) have been identified by two different meta-analyses. The first analyzed Scandinavian (Swedish and Norwegian) and UK cohorts and detected two SNPs, rs3792783 and rs7708392, that were significantly associated with pSS ($P = 2.2 \times 10^{-4}$, OR = 1.26, and $P = 1.4 \times 10^{-3}$, OR = 1.19, respectively). Moreover, these two SNPs were significantly associated with SSA/SSB-positive pSS patients [59]. The second meta-analysis identified a new SNP in the *TNIP1* region, rs6579837, the only SNP of genome-wide significance ($P < 5 \times 10^{-8}$), with $P_{meta} = 3.3 \times 10^{-8}$ [36]. Nevertheless, 29 other SNPs showed evidence of association, with $P_{meta} < 5 \times 10^{-5}$, one of which was rs3792783 ($P_{meta} = 1.74 \times 10^{-6}$). The rs7708392 SNP ($P_{meta} = 9.5 \times 10^{-5}$) did not surpass the suggestive association threshold ($P < 5 \times 10^{-5}$). In the cis-eQTL analysis, the authors observed the most statistically significant SNP at rs73272842, which was located in *TNIP1* (FDR = 2.80×10^{-3}; $P_{meta} = 1.58 \times 10^{-5}$), where multiple regulatory elements have been identified [36].

4.3.2.3 Transcription Factors

EBF1

EBF1 (early B-cell factor 1) and PAX5 have been described as crucial keys in the development of B cells. Only one study performed using Swedish and Norwegian cohorts showed a significant association between genetic variation in the *EBF1* gene and pSS [51]. The authors identified two SNPs (among the 66 analyzed), rs3843489 (*EBF1* intron 10) ($P = 9.9 \times 10^{-5}$) and rs869593 (*EBF1* intron 6) ($P = 2.0 \times 10^{-3}$), which had a low LD ($r^2 = 0.12$).

GTF2I

One SNP in GTF2I (general transcription factor 2I) at rs117026326 has recently been associated with pSS by two studies in a Han Chinese population using GWAS.

The former study included a three-stage GWAS, and the combined analysis identified GTF2I at 7q11.23 ($P_{combined} = 1.31 \times 10^{-53}$, $OR_{combined} = 2.20$) [37]. The second GWAS, also performed in Han Chinese but only on females, confirmed this strong association between rs117026326 and pSS ($P = 1.10 \times 10^{-15}$, OR = 1.982) [40].

IKZF1

The IKZF1 (IKAROS family zinc finger 1) gene is located at 7p12.2 and encodes a transcription factor crucial for lymphocyte activation. A recent GWAS in a Han Chinese cohort identified two SNPs near the IKZF1 locus that were associated with pSS using an additive logistic regression model: rs4917014 ($P = 5.5 \times 10^{-4}$, OR = 0.72) and rs4917129 ($P = 1.2 \times 10^{-3}$, OR = 0.76) [60].

NFKBIA

Polymorphism in the promoter of *NFKBIA* (nuclear factor of kappa light polypeptide gene enhancer in B-cell inhibitor alpha), also called IκBα, NF-κB regulator, is particularly important. Five SNPs (−881 A/G, −826 C/T, −550 A/T, −519 C/T, and −297 C/T) have been analyzed via RFLP in a Taiwanese population. The authors demonstrated that the genotype frequency of *NFKBIA* −826 T/T was significantly higher in patients with pSS as compared to controls, who more frequently exhibited the *NFKBIA* −826 C/C genotype ($P < 0.001$ for both) [61].

IRF5 (IRF5-TNPO3 Locus)

The transcription factor IRF5 (interferon regulatory factor 5) has been involved in type I IFN production. Given the data on type I IFN involvement in autoimmune diseases, it was not surprising that several genetic variations of *IRF5* gene have been associated with pSS. The *IRF5* and *TNPO3* genes are in the same locus with a strong LD. The first variation described was a 5-bp insertion/deletion polymorphism (CGGGG indel) located in the promoter region of *IRF5*. Two alleles of *IRF5* CGGGG indel, consisting of three repeats (3R) or four repeats (4R) of the CGGGG sequence, were identified. The carriage of the *IRF5* 4R CGGGG allele was associated with a strongly increased risk of developing pSS ($P = 7 \times 10^{-5}$; OR = 2.67) [62]. The same year, this CGGGG indel polymorphism was also associated with pSS in a combined Swedish and Norwegian cohort ($P_{combined} = 2.41 \times 10^{-5}$, $OR_{combined} = 1.49$) [63]. Two years later, the same team identified two SNPs in this locus that are in perfect LD ($r^2 = 1$) and strongly associated with pSS in a combined Swedish and Norwegian cohort: rs10488631 (3′UTR of *IRF5*) and rs13246321 (located in the *TNPO3* gene) ($P_{combined} = 5.5 \times 10^{-6}$). In 2013, the first GWAS meta-analysis conducted on a Caucasian cohort showed that outside the HLA region, the *IRF5-TNO3* locus was the locus most statistically significantly associated with pSS. The authors identified 67 SNPs that exceeded the $P_{meta} < 5 \times 10^{-8}$ threshold, with a peak effect observed in the *IRF5* promoter region (rs3757387, $P_{meta} = 2.73 \times 10^{-19}$) [36]. Among these 67 SNPs significantly associated with pSS, they identified the two SNPs observed in the Swedish and Norwegian cohort: rs10488631 ($P_{meta} = 5.36 \times 10^{-16}$) and rs13246321 ($P_{meta} = 1.27 \times 10^{-13}$).

STAT4

The transcription factor STAT4 (signal transducer and activator of transcription 4) is an important regulator of adaptive immunity [64]. The first SNP in the *STAT4* gene to be associated with pSS has been described in a combined Swedish and Norwegian cohort: rs7582694 ($P_{combined} = 1.45 \times 10^{-3}$, OR = 1.41) [51, 63]. This association was confirmed in 2013, using GWAS meta-analysis in a Caucasian cohort ($P_{meta} = 1.27 \times 10^{-13}$) in which 12 variants showed a statistically significant association (exceeding the GWAS threshold), with a peak association located at rs10553577 ($P_{meta} = 6.80 \times 10^{-15}$) and characterized by an insertion/deletion polymorphism [36]. However, neither effect resulted in a statistically significant cis-eQTL. In a GWAS study preformed in a Han Chinese population, the authors identified a new SNP in the *STAT4* gene (not identified in the GWAS in a Caucasian cohort) associated with pSS: rs10168266 ($P_{combined} = 1.77 \times 10^{-17}$, $OR_{combined} = 1.44$) [37].

4.3.2.4 Immune System and Other Molecules

CHRM3

Ten years ago, antimuscarinic antibodies were described in pSS, which modulated salivary secretion by human submandibular acinar cells. Genetic variations in the *CHRM3* gene (encoding muscarinic receptor 3) have been investigated in the Swedish and Norwegian cohort. No copy number variation in the CHRM3 gene has been observed between pSS and controls, but five SNPs, located in introns 3 and 4, exhibited associations with pSS. The strongest association has been observed with rs7548522 (minor allele frequency (A) = 0.06, $P = 0.0033$; OR = 1.93) (rs11578320, $P = 0.0053$; rs6690809, $P = 0.0087$; rs6429157, $P = 0.015$; and rs4620530, $P = 0.0062$). However, none of these showed an association with common clinical parameters (focus score, presence of anti-SSA/SSB autoantibodies, presence of ANAs, and abnormal Schirmer's test) [65].

CTLA4

Cytotoxic T lymphocyte-associated antigen 4 (CTLA4) is a crucial negative regulator of T-cell activation and cytokine production, and some SNPs have been associated with susceptibility to autoimmune diseases. Two of these SNPs have been investigated in relation to pSS: +49A/G polymorphism in exon 1, resulting in threonine-to-alanine conversion at codon 17, and the noncoding CT60A/G polymorphism, located in the 3′ region of the *CTLA4* gene [66]. Significant differences were observed in the frequency of the *CTLA4* haplotype between patients and controls ($P = 0.032$). Relative to the +49G; CT60G haplotype, the frequencies of both the +49A; CT60A haplotype (OR = 1.53) and the +49A; CT60G haplotype (OR = 1.78) were increased in patients with pSS as compared to controls [66].

FAM167A (C8orf13)-BLK Locus

Several genetic variations of the *FAM167A-BLK* region (family with sequence similarity 167, member of the A-B lymphoid tyrosine kinase) have been identified and associated with pSS. In the combined Swedish and Norwegian cohort, four SNPs have been described ($P < 0.001$) as associated with pSS: rs12549796 (in the second intron of *FAM167A*, $P_{combined} = 4.7 \times 10^{-4}$, $OR_{combined} = 1.37$), rs12677843 (in first intron of *BLK*, $P_{combined} = 7.0 \times 10^{-4}$, $OR_{combined} = 1.37$), and two SNPs, located between these two genes, rs2736340 ($P_{combined} = 1.4 \times 10^{-3}$, $OR_{combined} = 1.36$) and rs13277113 ($P_{combined} = 2.2 \times 10^{-3}$, $OR_{combined} = 1.35$). The SNPs rs2736340 and rs13277113 are in a very strong LD ($r^2 = 0.98$) [51], and the frequencies of haplotype T and A were higher in pSS cases as compared to controls in a Han Chinese population ($P = 0.034$ and $P = 0.026$, respectively) [67]. These two SNPs have been also identified by a GWAS meta-analysis performed in 2013 in a Caucasian cohort (exceeded the $P_{meta} < 5 \times 10^{-8}$ threshold) and associated with pSS ($P_{meta} = 3.27 \times 10^{-9}$ for rs2736340 and $P_{meta} = 1.31 \times 10^{-9}$ for rs13277113) [36]. No significant association with pSS was shown in the *FAM167A-BLK* region via GWAS in two studies in Han Chinese populations [37, 40]. However, another study in a Han Chinese population identified two new SNPs (not identified by the previously mentioned studies), rs7812879 and rs2254546, the genotype frequencies of which showed associations with pSS ($P = 0.005$ and $P = 0.010$, respectively) [52].

FCGR3B

The *FCGR3B* (Fc fragment of IgG, low-affinity IIIb, receptor) gene, located in 1q23.3, encodes the CD16b protein, and copy number variations (CNVs) have been associated with susceptibility to systemic autoimmune diseases. Two studies investigated *FCGR3B* CNVs in pSS. The older study, conducted in the Paisa community, concluded that low (<2 copies) and high (>2 copies) CNVs of *FCGR3B* ($P = 0.074$, OR = 2.01, and $P = 0.048$, OR = 2.26, respectively) were associated with an increased risk of developing pSS [68]. The second study, conducted in an Australian population, showed that only low copy numbers of FCGR3 (<2 copies) were a risk factor for pSS ($p = 0.016$) [69].

MECP2

A genetic association between the *MECP2* gene (methyl-CpG binding protein 2) and in lupus has been reported. The following year, a SNP in *MECP2* located at rs17435 was shown to exhibit high allele (T) and genotype (TT) frequencies in pSS cases as compared with controls ($P = 0.0016$, OR = 1.33 for allele risk and $P = 0.0024$, OR = 2.17 for genotype risk) [70].

OAS1

A recent study combining GWAS (765 pSS and 3825 controls) and gene expression data (microarray on whole blood, 115 anti-Ro$^+$pSS cases vs. 56 healthy controls) has identified, through cis-eQTL analyses, an association between the rs10774671 SNP, located in OAS1 (2′5′-oligoadenylate synthetase 1) gene locus, and pSS. Microarray analyses (FDR < 0.05, −2 < FC>2) have identified 73 differentially expressed genes, among which 57 genes are regulated by type I IFN such as the *OAS1* gene [71]. This SNP is an A/G substitution within the consensus sequence of a splice acceptor site in the fifth intron of the *OAS1* gene, which is known to alter normal splicing and induce isoforms. The impact of the genotype at rs10774671 (GG, GA, or AA) on the transcript levels of four isoforms of *OAS1* (p46, p42, p44, and p48) has been determined by performing a RNA-seq analysis on whole blood (57 pSS cases and 27 healthy controls) [71]. The pSS risk allele A (genotype GA or AA) for this SNP was correlated with the increased expression of the p42 isoform ($P = 1.30 \times 10^{-7}$) and also that of the p44 and p48 isoforms ($P = 1.78 \times 10^{-3}$ and $P = 1.19 \times 10^{-5}$, respectively). In contrast, the expression of the p46 isoform was shown to be decreased in samples with the AA genotype ($P = 3.48 \times 10^{-10}$). Moreover, the in vitro type I IFN stimulation of EBV-immortalized B cells from pSS patients indicated the upregulated expression of p46 protein in GG and GA subjects [71].

PTPN22

The association between pSS and the polymorphism of *PTPN22* (protein tyrosine phosphatase non-receptor 22) is controversial. Two studies have assessed the *PTPN22* polymorphism C1858T in pSS as compared to controls. The first identified a significant association between the T allele and pSS (OR = 2.42) in a Colombian population [72], while the second, performed on Caucasians, showed no significant difference in the allele between pSS cases and controls [73].

TRIM21

A major characteristic of pSS is the production of autoantibodies against ribonucleoprotein complexes composed of the Ro/La protein (Ro 52 kDa, Ro 60 kDa, and La 48 kDa). A C/T polymorphism located in intron 3 of the Ro 52 gene was present at a significantly higher frequency in anti-Ro + pSS patients than in controls ($P = 0.00003$, 52.6% vs. 12.5%, respectively) [38]. This polymorphism was not associated with the presence of anti-Ro antibodies in Japanese patients [74].

4.4 Epigenetic Mechanisms in Sjögren's Syndrome

Epigenetic mechanisms are crucial in immune cell differentiation, function, and adaptation to external solicitations. Thus, these mechanisms play a pivotal role in the immune system and confer the cell plasticity needed to integrate and define a new transcriptional program. Epigenetics is defined by its capacity to modulate gene expression without affecting the DNA sequence, and this phenomenon is reversible and heritable. These mechanisms, which are specific to a given cell type, include DNA methylation, posttranslational histone modifications, and noncoding RNA, which affect chromatin structure and may either repress or enhance gene transcription. Important modifications of these processes have been observed in pathologies, particularly in cancer and autoimmune diseases [75].

4.4.1 Environmental Factors

The use of hydralazine and procainamide drugs interfering with DNA methylation leads to the appearance of pSS associated with lupus in humans and mice. Further observations support a role for other environmental factors in pSS via the alteration of the epigenetic machinery. In this context, ultraviolet light, smoking, chemicals, and psychological stress have been described as likely examples of this phenomenon. Other arguments could be made regarding, for example, the fact that monozygotic twins have a genetic pSS rate of only 15–25%, highlighting the role of epigenetics rather than that of genetics [76], as well as a pSS geoepidemiology distribution that reveal highest rates of this disease in Northern countries. Moreover, viruses have been incriminated in pSS development, such as the Epstein-Barr virus (EBV) and human herpes virus 6 (HHV6). This supposition was correlated with an increased prevalence of a specific IgG against EBV or HHV6 [77]. A cross-reaction with the SSB/La protein was also described for these two viruses because of the common epitopes shared with the viruses. Nevertheless, no direct proof was reported regarding the role of these viruses, which are frequently found in human populations. In any event, various studies have demonstrated their nonimplication in the pathophysiology of this disease.

As a whole, these observations strongly suggest a major role on the part of epigenetic mechanisms in the development of pSS [78].

4.4.2 Global Analysis of DNA Methylation

4.4.2.1 In pSS, DNA Demethylation Is Preponderant

As an epigenetic process, DNA methylation is a stable, heritable, and reversible change transmitted to the next cellular generations based on the covalent transfer, via DNA methyltransferases (DNMTs), of a methyl group to the fifth carbon of the cytosine pyrimidine ring in a CpG dinucleotide [79]. DNA methylation acts on gene transcription directly, by preventing the fixation of transcription factors on DNA, or indirectly, by encouraging the compaction of DNA through the recruitment of histone deacetylases (HDAC) and histone methyltransferases (HMT). Conversely, the demethylation of DNA can be a passive phenomenon occurring during cellular division or an active phenomenon initiated by the oxidative enzyme TET (ten eleven translocation). In mammals, chromatin is normally methylated, and areas that are demethylated are regulating and transcriptionally active. The global rate of methylation found is around 70–80% and depends on the cellular type. For example, low methylation rates have been found in immune system cells.

A global analysis of DNA methylation was realized on histological sections taken from minor salivary glands (MSG), epithelial cells isolated and cultured from MSG patients, and B and T cells from the peripheral blood [12]. These analyses demonstrated in cases of pSS: (1) a major reduction of global DNA methylation in salivary glands occurs, and this reduction was prominent in epithelial cells; (2) this default was conserved in culture and was associated with the repression of DNMT1 methylation enzyme expression; and (3) conversely, a difference in global DNA methylation was observed in T and B peripheral blood lymphocytes taken from patients and those taken from controls, indicating that these epigenetic modifications preferentially affect epithelial cells.

4.4.2.2 Implication of Lymphocytes in DNA Methylation from Minor Salivary Gland Epithelial Cells

The presence of a major lymphocyte infiltration in MSG was associated with a decrease in methylation. In fact, the methylation rate found was inversely proportional with the Tarpley score, which is used to grade the severity of inflammatory infiltrate [80]. During this process, a role for B lymphocytes was strongly suspected because DNA methylation anomalies could also be found when an immortalized human epithelial cell line (HSG, human salivary gland) was co-cultured with B lymphocytes, and conversely this anomaly could be inhibited with anti-B lymphocyte therapies [12]. This observation allows for important therapeutic perspectives.

4.4.3 Complete Analysis of Methylome

4.4.3.1 DNA Methylation Analysis of CpG Motifs from Peripheral Blood Cells

Three groups used HM450K technology to study DNA methylation across the entire genome in peripheral blood mononuclear cells (PBMC), T lymphocytes (naive and totals), and B lymphocytes from patients with pSS, as seen in Table 4.2 [81–83]. Despite the use of different analysis methods, several points can be underscored. Firstly, hypermethylated regions of DNA were found on type *I* and *II* antigen-presenting HLA genes and also on several genes regulated by interferon type I (*IFI44L, IFITMI*). Secondly, some specific signaling pathways regulated by DNA methylation were found in T lymphocytes (protein carrier of solutes and the transcription factor RUN2X) and in B lymphocytes (B-cell receptor, genes of development). Thirdly, this effect is prominent in patients with anti-SSA/SSB antibodies and B lymphocytes because the modifications of methylation are 50 times more important in these latter cells than in T lymphocytes [82].

4.4.3.2 Analysis of Methylation from DNA CpG Motifs of Minor Salivary Glands

Using HM450K beadchips, two groups analyzed DNA methylation in the MSGs of pSS patients. However, the limit of this approach is connected to the heterogeneity of the samples because the glands studied contained acinar and tubular epithelial cells and also immune cells. Despite this limitation, in GWAS, the IFN signaling pathway was found correlated with the expression of demethylated *OAS2*, a gene that is inducible by IFN. The other regions that were differentially methylated concern microRNAs and a wide variety of genes implicated in cellular activation, antigen presentation, and the production of autoantigens [84], as seen in Table 4.2. Moreover, these alterations of DNA methylation seem to be associated with the severity of the disease [84].

As indicated previously, these analyses, which were realized using a mixture of cells, do not fully reflect the impact of DNA changes in epithelial cells from MSGs.

Table 4.2 Global analysis of DNA methylation with 450 k HumanBeadChip from Illumina

Cell type or tissue	Minor salivary gland biopsies	Labial salivary gland biopsies	Salivary gland epithelial cells	Peripheral blood mononuclear cells	CD19+ B cells	CD19+ B cells	CD4+ naive T cells
Patients (control)	15 (13)	13 (13)	8 (4)	100 (400)	24 (47)	26 (22)	11 (11)
Reference	[83]	[84]	[85]	[83]	[83]	[82]	[81]
GO analysis of differentially methylated genes	–	Immune response (GO:0006955) Intrinsic to plasma membrane (GO:0031226) Immune system process (GO:0002376) Cell surface receptor linked signal transduction (GO:0007166) Signal transduction (GO:0007165)	Regulation of small GTPase-mediated signal transduction (GO:0051056) Positive regulation of GTPase activity (GO:0043547) Regulation of rho protein signal transduction (GO:0035023) Actin cytoskeleton organization (GO:0030036) Positive regulation of JNK cascade (GO:0046330) Filopodium assembly (GO:0046847) Wnt pathway Ca^{2+} pathway	TCR pathway T1 diabetes pathway Allograft rejection	–	BCR pathway T1 diabetes pathway Tight junction	Lymphocyte activation (GO:0046649) Leukocyte differentiation (GO:0002521) Immune response (GO:0006955) Chromatin organization (GO:0006325) T-cell differentiation (GO:0030217) Homophilic cell adhesion (GO:0007156) L-amino acid transport (GO:0015807) Antigen processing and Presentation (GO:0019882) T1 diabetes pathway

This limitation was indicated by the use of epithelial cells from MSGs that were cultured for 3 weeks to obtain a pure cellular population of salivary gland epithelial cells (SGECs) [85] (Table 4.2). Important differences were identified between SGECs taken from patients and those taken from controls using the HM450K bead-chips. The differences are primarily seen in a large number of the genes regulated by IFN (61%). Moreover, the calcium (implicated in the control of salivary flux) and Wnt (implicated in the survival and differentiation of epithelial cells) signaling pathways have also been highlighted.

4.4.4 Epigenetic Reprogramming and Its Consequences

4.4.4.1 miRNAs

MicroRNAs (miRNAs) are small RNA molecules that contain 18–25 nucleotides and regulate gene expression at the posttranscriptional level. Alterations in their expression levels play crucial roles in a wide range of physiological and pathological processes. miRNAs affect gene expression via (1) their binding to complementary sites on the 3′ tails of messenger RNA transcripts and their targeting of these transcripts for degradation by the RNA-induced silencing complex (RISC) [86], (2) the binding and destabilization of mRNAs without cleavage, (3) their ability to reduce the efficiency of ribosomal translation [86], and (4) their involvement in pSS pathology, which was investigated in MSGs, T lymphocytes, B lymphocytes, monocytes, and SGECs (Table 4.3).

4.4.4.2 Retrotransposons

Retrotransposons are groups of mobile DNA elements that copy and paste themselves using RNA molecules. More than 50% of our genome is composed of these elements, which correspond to DNA sequences, are invasive, and, after transcription, are randomly inserted into genome and thus increase their copy numbers [87]. In humans, long interspersed nuclear elements (LINEs, L1) represent 21% (500,000 copies) of the genome. They are the most active retroelement. However, 80–100 copies of these elements have maintained their mobility [87]. Alu elements are also heavily present in the genome (10%) and belong to the short interspersed nuclear element (SINE) family. These SINEs are nonautonomous elements that do not encode protein and, as a consequence, require LINEs to propagate [87]. Finally, human endogenous retrovirus represents 8% of the human genome.

In order to maintain genome integrity, control mechanisms are necessary, and DNA methylation is a help in this regard. For example, HRES-1 (human T-cell leukemia-related endogenous retrovirus) is inserted in the long arm of chromosome 1 at position 1q42 and controlled by DNA methylation. During the loss of this control, Gag p38 autoantigen is expressed, inducing the production of anti-Gag p38 autoantibodies. This phenomenon is observed in 10% of patients with pSS as compared to 1.5% of healthy controls. Moreover, Alu transcripts are found to be increased in pSS [88]. Induced by type I IFN, Alu allows its own production

Table 4.3 Deregulation expression of miRNAs in Sjögren's syndrome patients

miRNAs	Upregulated	Downregulated	Tissue/cell type	Target genes	Putative(s) function(s)	References
hsa-miR-146a-5p	yes	–	Peripheral blood mononuclear cells	IRAK1, TRAF6, IRF5, STAT1	– Preceding clinical symptoms	[112–114]
	yes	–	T lymphocytes CD4+		– Sustaining inflammation	
	–	yes	B lymphocytes CD19+		– Loss promote interferon expression in B cells	
hsa-miR-155-5p	–	yes	Peripheral blood mononuclear cells	SOCS-1, TAB-2, c-Maf	– Lead to production of many cytokines and downregulation of the expression of several anti-inflammatory cytokines	[113]
	yes	–	T lymphocytes CD4+		– Enhances differentiation and activation of Th1 and Th17 cells	[114, 115]
hsa-miR-200b-3p	yes	–	Long-term cultured salivary gland epithelial cells	TRIM21, TROVE2	– Negatively correlated with TRIM21 and TROVE2	[116, 117]
hsa-Let-7b	yes	–	Long-term cultured salivary gland epithelial cells	TRIM21, TROVE2, SSB, DICER	– Associated with SSB – Autoantigens	[116, 117]
ebv-miR-BART13-3p	yes	–	Minor salivary gland tissues	STIM, AQP5	– Impaired calcium signaling and salivary secretion	[118]
hsa-miR-150-5p	–	yes	Peripheral blood mononuclear cells	Unknown	– Inhibition of B-cell activation and differentiation – Might contribute to host defense against invading pathogenesis	[112]
hsa-miR-16	yes	–	Peripheral blood mononuclear cells	SMRT, TRIM21	–Regulator of TLR-mediated immune responses – Can promote NF-kB-regulated transactivation of IL-8 gene	[112, 116, 117]
	yes	–	Minor salivary gland tissues		– Autoantigen production	

(continued)

Table 4.3 (continued)

miRNAs	Upregulated	Downregulated	Tissue/cell type	Target genes	Putative(s) function(s)	References
hsa-miR-21-3p	yes	–	Peripheral blood mononuclear cells	Unknown	– DNA methylation-associated miRNAs – B- and T-cell activation	[112]
hsa-miR-32-5p	–	yes	B lymphocytes CD19+	PTEN	– Negative regulator of PTEN in PI3K signaling	[114]
hsa-miR-30b-5p	–	yes	B lymphocytes CD19+	BAFF	– Promotes B-cell maturation, proliferation, and survival	
hsa-let-7d-3p	–	yes	T lymphocytes CD4+	Unknown	Unknown	
hsa-miR-222-3p	–	yes	T lymphocytes CD4+	Unknown	Unknown	
		yes	B lymphocytes CD19+			
hsa-miR-30c-5p	–	yes	T lymphocytes CD4+	Unknown	Unknown	
hsa-miR-378a-3p	–	yes	T lymphocytes CD4+	Unknown	Unknown	
		yes	B lymphocytes CD19+			
hsa-miR-28-5p	–	yes	T lymphocytes CD4+	Unknown	Unknown	
hsa-miR-26a-5p	–	yes	B lymphocytes CD19+	Unknown	Unknown	
hsa-miR-19b-3p	–	yes	B lymphocytes CD19+	Unknown	Unknown	
hsa-miR-181a-2	yes	–	Peripheral blood mononuclear cells	Smad7	– Anti-inflammatory effects – Compromise maturation of B cells – Regulate differentiation of T-helper cells – Promote T-cell regulatory generation	[117, 119, 120]
	yes	–	Minor salivary gland tissues		– Associated with decreased salivary function	
hsa-miR-223	yes	–	Peripheral blood mononuclear cells	TROVE2	– Autoantigen production	[117]

hsa-miR-4524b-3p	yes	–	Minor salivary gland tissues	Unknown	Unknown	[121]
	yes	–	Human salivary gland cell line			
hsa-miR-4524b-5p	yes	–	Minor salivary gland tissues	Unknown	Unknown	
	yes	–	Human salivary gland cell line			
hsa-miR-5571-3p	yes	–	Minor salivary gland tissues	Unknown	Unknown	
	yes	–	Human salivary gland cell line			
hsa-miR-5571-5p	yes	–	Minor salivary gland tissues	Unknown	Unknown	
	yes	–	Human salivary gland cell line			
hsa-miR-5100	yes	–	Minor salivary gland tissues	Unknown	– Link with salivary flow decrease	
	yes	–	Human salivary gland cell line			
hsa-miR-5572	yes	–	Minor salivary gland tissues	Unknown	Unknown	
	yes	–	Human salivary gland cell line			
hsa-miR-4701-5p	yes	–	Peripheral blood CD14+ monocyte	Unknown	Unknown	[122]
hsa-miR-3162-3p	yes	–	Peripheral blood CD14+ monocyte	Unknown	Unknown	
hsa-miR-300	yes	–	Peripheral blood CD14+ monocyte	Unknown	Unknown	
hsa-miR-34b-3p	yes	–	Peripheral blood CD14+ monocyte	GRB2, P38/MAPK13, MEKK1/MAP3K1	– p38 MAPK pathway	
hsa-miR-609	yes	–	Peripheral blood CD14+ monocyte	TGFBR3, SMAD2	– TGFβ signaling – MAPK pathway	
hsa-miR-4701-5p	yes	–	Peripheral blood CD14+ monocyte	TGFBR3, SMAD2, SOS1, NRAS, ERK1/MAPK1, RAC1, HGK/MAP4K4, STAT6	– TGFβ signaling – MAPK pathway – Jak/STAT pathway	

(continued)

Table 4.3 (continued)

miRNAs	Upregulated	Downregulated	Tissue/cell type	Target genes	Putative(s) function(s)	References
hsa-miR-1207-5	–	yes	Minor salivary gland tissues	TRIM21	– Autoantigen production	[123]
hsa-miR-4695-3p	–	yes	Minor salivary gland tissues	TRIM21	– Autoantigen production	
hsa-miR-203a	yes	–	Saliva	Unknown	Unknown	[124]
hsa-miR-763-3p	yes	–	Saliva	Unknown	Unknown	[124, 125]
	yes	–	Minor salivary gland tissues		Unknown	
hsa-miR-574-3p	–	yes	Saliva	Unknown	Unknown	
	–	yes	Minor salivary gland tissues		Unknown	

and that of other proinflammatory cytokines. It also fixes the autoantigen Ro60 and the Alu-Ro60 complex, as well as anti-Ro60 autoantibodies, which are frequently found in lupus and pSS [89]. In MSGs, in addition to the expression of HRES-1, other retroviruses have also been found to be surexpressed, such as HERV-K113, HERV-5, and elements of HERV-E. Recently, Mavragani et al. confirmed decreased L1 promoter methylation and increased L1 expression in MSG tissues. They suspected a potential contributory role on the part of the altered methylation mechanisms and related lymphoproliferative processes observed in the disease [90].

4.4.4.3 Autoantigens

The demethylation of the *ssb/la* promoter is observed in patients with pSS, which induces the surexpression of this autoantigen transcription, as well as the translation, processing, and production of anti-SSB/La autoantibodies. This effect is found regarding the treatment of HSGs with 5-Aza, demonstrating the impact of DNA demethylation on this autoantigen in pSS cases [80]. Similar observations have been made regarding ICA1. In parallel, several studies on miRNAs underscored the potential involvement of hsa-miR-200b-3p, hsa-Let-7b, and hsa-miR-16 (Table 4.3) in TRIM21 transcription regulation.

4.4.4.4 Other Genes

The treatment of 5-Aza induces an increase in cytokeratin 19 expression in the HSG cell line [91] and also in the aquaporin 5 (*aq5*) gene. An analysis performed after the bisulfite sequencing of the *aq5* promoter shows the hypermethylation of the CpG islands at the level of binding sites for the transcriptional factor Sp1. 5-Aza, while demethylating these sites, allows Sp1 to be linked to DNA and initiate the transcription of *aq5*. Other gene promoters were analyzed, particularly that of the gene for dystonine (*dst*). The hypermethylation of this promoter is observed during the surexpression of an epithelial alternative splicing variant, antigen 1 from bullous pemphigoid, which is described as able to act as an autoantigen in other autoimmune diseases, such as multiple sclerosis.

4.4.5 Link Between Genetic and Epigenetic Risk Factors

More than 40 risk factors not associated with HLA were found in pSS, thanks to the development of sample genome analysis in Chinese and Caucasian populations. The genetic loci associated with pSS are also associated with the key pathological pathways, including antigen presentation (HLAI/II), genes inducible by type I IFN (*IRF5*, *STAT4*), the NF-kB pathway (*TNIP1*, *TNFAIP3*), and B lymphocyte activation (*CXCR5*, *BLK*) [92]. It seems interesting to analyze the expression of certain risk factors. In fact, these factors are suspected to control gene expression via various actions if they are present in promoter, enhancer, or insulator regions. These actions affect the transcriptional machinery; the spliceosome formation, which controls intron excision; the activation of nonsense RNA messengers; and the control of RNA messengers via microRNA. Moreover, they could be associated with a specific tissue and influence the autoreactivity of certain cell targets, notably B lymphocytes. It must be said that half of these factors are found in lupus and other autoimmune diseases and can be considered major immune elements in the development of these diseases (IL-10, IL-21, receptors (TNFSF4/CD252), transcription factors (IRF5), and specific proteins of B lymphocytes (BLK, BANK1)).

4.5 Genetic Alterations in Sjögren's Syndrome-Related Lymphoma

4.5.1 Lymphomagenesis Scenario in Primary Sjögren's Syndrome

In the current lymphomagenesis scenario of pSS, the evolution of a malignant proliferation of B lymphocytes from an inflammatory infiltration is certainly a complex and multistep process. On the one hand, pSS disease promotes chronic exposure to a range of unknown autoantigens in the salivary and lacrimal gland tissues, which leads to persistent proliferation and the clonal expansion of B cells. On the other hand, genetic predispositions, typically translocations involving immunoglobulin gene loci and proto-oncogenes or other genes involved in cell cycle regulation, promote the uncontrolled expansion of neoplastic B cells. Indeed, several genetic alterations have been suggested as possible mechanisms underlying neoplastic diversion in the setting of pSS such as the translocations involving the MALT1 gene t(11;18)(q21;q21) and t(14;18)(q32;q21) [93]. Moreover, the B cell itself undergoes several potentially dangerous genetic events during its development, including IGHV-IGHD-IGHJ recombination, class-switch recombination, and somatic hypermutation, all of which involve double-stranded breaks and hence an increased chance of generating genetic aberrations. In an interesting way, chromosomal translocations into Ig heavy-chain t(14;18) have been described in salivary gland biopsies of pSS cases who develop lymphoma but not in the biopsies of pSS cases without lymphoma. This translocation juxtaposes the bcl-2 gene with the Ig heavy-chain locus, leading to the deregulation of apoptosis and increased B-cell survival [93].

Furthermore, one of the hypotheses that has been put forward is that some genetic mutations controlling nuclear factor-kB (NF-kB) activation could contribute, along with many other factors, to propagating inflammation, favoring autoimmunity, and activating autoimmune B cells, with consequences in only those B cells that are continuously stimulated by immune complexes, promoting their escape as lymphoma B cells [94]. Thereby, genetic mutations involved in cellular proliferation and the nuclear factor NF-kB pathway were reported in pSS with MALT lymphoma. One example is at specific mutation of B-cell activating factor receptor (BAFF-R) (His159Tyr), which leads to the activation of the NF-kB_2 pathway or even genetic variations impacting the function of TNFAIP3 (A20) protein, which can be described as negative feedback for NF-kB activation [94].

Some studies also underscore that chronic active B-cell receptor signaling is strongly associated with lymphoma cell survival [95]. Considering the close connection between higher levels of disease activity and lymphoma development and the essential role of B cells in the pathogenesis of pSS, the same scenario probably occurs in the lymphomas that occur within this disease.

Finally, while MALT lymphoma is considered to be the main histological type of lymphoma in pSS, non-MALT lymphomas such as diffuse large B-cell lymphoma may also occur. Interestingly, MTHFR polymorphisms (an enzyme necessary for DNA synthesis and methylation) leading to genomic instability have been associated with only the non-MALT lymphoma subtype in pSS patients [96]. Another specific feature of pSS with non-MALT lymphoma is the translocation t(14;18)(q32;q21), which was absent in MALT lymphoma but was detected in five of seven pSS patients with the non-MALT lymphoma subtype. The development of lymphoma in pSS patients is not yet completely understood. In a broader context, the underlying pathogenic events leading from benign autoimmunity to malignant transformation remain elusive. It is clear that the buildup of genetic mutations, translocations, and polymorphism may lead to this malignant transformation. In the section below, we will further describe the few studies that have explored this issue in pSS patients with lymphoma.

4.5.2 Chromosomal Translocation of MALT1

Histologically, MALT lymphomas are characterized by the proliferation of neoplastic marginal zone-related cells that infiltrate epithelial structures to generate lymphoepithelial lesions and colonize reactive lymphoid follicles.

This lymphoid tissue becomes genetically unstable due to the acquisition of abnormalities. Two chromosomal aberrations, t(11;18) and t(14;18), which are mutually exclusive and involved the MALT1 gene, located on chromosome 18, have been reported as genetic events specific to MALT lymphoma.

The translocation t(11;18)(q21;q21) is the result of the fusion of the apoptosis inhibitor-2 (API2) gene and the MALT1 gene at the 11q21 and 18q21 breakpoints, respectively [97]. On the one hand, API2 inhibits the biological activity of caspases 3, 7, and 9 and is described as an apoptosis inhibitor, while, on the other hand, MALT1 is involved in antigen-receptor-mediated nuclear factor-kB activation [97]. Consequently, the upregulation of these molecules promotes cellular proliferation and resistance to apoptotic signals. It has been reported that patients with gastric MALT lymphoma who carry this t(11;18)(q21;q21) translocation display more aggressive clinical courses.

The (14;18)(q32;q21) translocation is the result of the fusion of the Ig heavy-chain gene and the MALT1 gene at the 14q32 and 18q21 breakpoints, respectively. This translocation causes an overexpression of MALT1 that is controlled by the Ig heavy-chain gene. Consequently, this chromosomal translocation leads to the overexpression of MALT1, likely promoting the dysregulation of the NF-kB activation pathway [98].

Moreover, it has been reported that a high incidence of t(11;18)(q21;q21) translocation is detected in gastric MALT lymphomas, whereas this translocation is rarely found in MALT lymphomas outside of the gastrointestinal tract. In contrast, the translocation t(14;18)(q32;q21) has been observed more frequently in non-gastrointestinal MALT lymphomas, mainly those of the liver, lung, and ocular adnexa [99]. Interestingly, this dichotomy is also found in pSS patients with MALT lymphomas. Indeed, Streubel et al. evaluated the frequency of these translocations in 26 pSS patients with MALT lymphoma and found the translocation t(11;18)(q21;q21) in 6 of 9 (67%) patients with gastric MALT lymphoma and pSS, as opposed to only 1 of 17 patients (6%) with extra-gastrointestinal lymphoma. In contrast, regarding the patients who were positive for t(14;18)(q32; q21), three had extra-gastrointestinal lymphomas, and only one had gastric lymphoma [93].

To summarize, the frequency of translocations involving *MALT1* appears to be low in patients with extra-gastrointestinal MALT lymphoma associated with pSS. In contrast, *MALT1* rearrangement is frequently present in patients with gastric MALT lymphoma and pSS (78%).

These translocations, which involve immunoglobulin gene loci, a gene involved in cell cycle regulation, and the NF-kB activation pathway, likely contribute to the uncontrolled expansion of B cells and malignant expansion.

4.5.3 BAFF Genetic Variants and BAFF Receptor Mutation

BAFF, a member of the TNF family, is a key regulator of B-cell development from the T1 to the T2 stage and survival, conferring resistance to apoptosis [100].

BAFF plays a key role in malignant B-cell survival. BAFF production has been correlated with histological grade and patient survival in a study on NHL patients. BAFF is also implicated in the pathogenesis of pSS and is believed to be a major player in pSS lymphomagenesis based on its potent inducer effect on B lymphocyte activation and proliferation. Quartuccio et al. reported an increase in serum BAFF levels in pSS patients with either lymphoma or pre-lymphomatous manifestations, as compared to those with a low risk of lymphoma. Furthermore, BAFF levels have been found to be associated with B-cell clonal expansion in the salivary glands and also with disease activity scores [17]. BAFF is highly overexpressed in several autoimmune diseases, with increased mean serum levels in pSS patients, even higher than those in SLE or RA patients. The underlying abnormalities involved in the deregulation of BAFF may be explained, in part, by genetic variations. For instance, the rs9514828 polymorphism in the promoter of the BAFF gene (−871C/T) has previously been linked to heightened BAFF transcription levels [101]. Nezos et al. reported that the pSS population that was at a high-risk of lymphoma development had a higher prevalence of the rs9524828 T allele in the BAFF promoter as compared to HC [28]. Even more interestingly, the authors also demonstrated, for the first time, the contribution of BAFF gene polymorphisms to the pathogenesis of pSS-related lymphomagenesis. They identified a lower frequency of the AA genotype of the rs12583006 polymorphism in the high-risk pSS group as compared to low-risk pSS patients. These authors hypothesized that this allele has a potential protective effect against lymphoma development in a pSS setting. They also suggest that another polymorphism or mutations of the BAFF gene or other related immune genes may cooperate with this risk allele, mentioning in their conclusions the example of the deregulated expression of BAFF receptors [28].

In this respect, a strong link was recently demonstrated between a His159Tyr BAFF-R mutation and both pSS and pSS-related lymphoma [55]. Papageorgiou et al. identified an increased prevalence of the BAFF-R His159Tyr mutation in patients with pSS, particularly in those with pSS complicated by MALT lymphoma whose disease onset occurred at a younger age. Therefore, this mutation of BAFF-R has been associated with a high risk of lymphoproliferation in patients with NHL through the activation of the NF-kB pathway [102]. Interestingly, the presence of the His159Tyr mutation in the pSS-lymphoma patients group was also associated with faster lymphoma development, whereas in non-lymphoma pSS patients, the mutation was associated with hypergammaglobulinemia and rheumatoid factor positivity [55]. This mutation is more frequent among the pSS patient population as compared to patients with other autoimmune diseases, such as SLE and RA. The authors propose that this could account for the higher prevalence of pSS-related lymphoproliferative diseases seen among all autoimmune disease populations [103].

Finally, because the presence of the BAFF-R mutation has been strongly associated with a shorter interval between pSS diagnosis and lymphoma development, as well as B-cell hyperactivity and rheumatoid factor positivity, the authors suggest that genetically determined enhanced B-cell signaling could accelerate disease onset, providing a plausible explanation for the increased prevalence of the His159Tyr BAFF-R mutation in the younger disease subset [55].

4.5.4 TNFAIP3 (A20) Inactivation

Protein A20, which is coded by the gene TNFAIP3, functions as a negative feedback regulator for NF-kB in many immune cells, and it is described as a potent endogenous anti-inflammatory molecule. Reduced A20 activity has been observed in several lymphoma subtypes that are associated with somatic mutations and chromosomal deletions in the TNFAIP3 region, as well as with epigenetic methylation in the promoter region. *TNFAIP3*-knockout mice develop an autoimmune phenotype and have high rates of lymphoma. The TNFAIP3 gene locus also appears to play other roles in autoimmune diseases [58], and the dysregulation of the protein A20 has been observed in various human autoimmune diseases [104]. Interestingly, the ablation of A20 in the B-cell lineage in mice increased the number of germinal center B cells and led to spontaneous autoimmune disease, but lymphomas did not develop spontaneously [105].

Genome-wide association studies have demonstrated associations between TNFAIP3 polymorphisms and the risk of other autoimmune diseases [58]. Many of these studies have demonstrated an association with the exonic SNP rs2230926, which is located in exon 3, leading to the replacement of phenylalanine by cysteine at amino acid position 127 (rs2230926 T.G; F127C). In 2013, Nocturne et al. demonstrated that the rs2230926 SNP was significantly associated with lymphoma development in pSS patients but no association was found between the rs2230926G variant and the risk of pSS among patients without lymphoma [106]. In a cohort of pSS patients with lymphoma, 12 (60%) of the 20 patients had functional abnormalities of A20: 6 of germinal origin (germline DNA), 5 of somatic origin (in lymphoma DNA), and 1 of both. Among patients with MALT lymphoma complicated with pSS, this frequency reached 77%. This prevalence in pSS patients with MALT lymphoma is higher than that generally described in MALT lymphoma alone, which ranged between 22 and 28% [107]. Consequently, this supports the idea of the specific involvement of A20 inactivation in lymphoma-complicated autoimmune disease. In another work, the authors studied the association between a germline coding variant (rs2230926) of TNFAIP3 and the development of lymphoma in patients with pSS in two large cohorts of European subjects and confirmed that this germline missense variant was not associated with pSS in general but with a specific lymphoma complication of the disease. The rs2230926 minor (G) allele was more common in French controls as compared to UK controls. The same trend was seen among French patients with pSS as compared with UK pSS patients, including the subset of patients with lymphoma. However, this exonic variant was associated with pSS-associated lymphoma in both cohorts.

In addition, functional analyses have shown that cells with mutated A20 variants were less effective in reducing NF-kB activation after TNFa stimulation. The high prevalence of functional A20 defects in pSS-related MALT lymphomas indicates that reduced A20 function may be a relevant element over the course of lymphomagenesis in pSS [108].

In summary, TNFAIP3 is a transcriptional target of NF-kB that serves as a global feedback regulator to attenuate NF-kB activity. In this respect, polymorphisms and mutations of TNFAIP3 have an impact on A20 deficiency, which can lead to exaggerated NF-kB signaling and/or increased cell death. Because enhanced NF-kB signaling has been linked to several types of human B-cell lymphoma, the A20mediated restriction of this crucial signaling cascade may explain the tumor-suppressive function of A20 in B cells.

4.5.5 MTHFR Polymorphism in Non-MALT Lymphoma

The methylenetetrahydrofolate reductase (MTHFR) gene encodes for an enzyme that is essential in DNA synthesis and methylation. On the one hand, MTHFR catalyzes the irreversible reduction of 5,10-methylenetetrahydrofolate (5,10-MTHF) to 5-methyltetrahydrofolate (5-MTHF), which then gives rise to S-adenosylmethionine (SAM) formation, the global methyl group donor that is essential for the majority of biological methylation reactions. On the other hand, this process reduces the bioavailability of 5,10-MTHF, which ultimately allows uracil levels to decrease.

This is a critical point during DNA replication given that elevated uracil levels significantly enhance uracil misincorporation into DNA, resulting in increased DNA double-stranded breaks during the normal repair process. In contrast, dysfunction in the MTHFR enzyme can lead to aberrant gene expression by disturbing the process of DNA methylation via the reduction of SAM formation and, at the same time, to reduced DNA damage through decreased uracil levels, leading to incorrect DNA synthesis and repair. Two of the most well-studied common SNPs in the MTHFR gene occur at nucleotide position 677, where there is a cytosine-to-thymine base change (rs1801133; 677C N T), and at nucleotide position 1298, where there is an adenine-to-cytosine base change (rs1801131; 1298A N C). Both polymorphisms result in a missense mutation, conferring a different protein conformation with lowered enzyme activity. The MTHFR c. 677C > T TT genotype has been associated with reduced DNA methylation levels, while the MTHFR c. 1298A > C AC genotype has been associated with reduced DNA double-stranded break levels [109]. Genetic polymorphisms leading to dysfunction in the MTHFR enzyme have been associated with both the onset of cancer susceptibility and an increased risk of both autoimmune disorders and NHL development [110].

Recently, Fragkioudaki et al. explored, for the first time, the potential role of these MTHFR polymorphisms in both pSS and pSS-related lymphomagenesis. Three hundred and fifty-six pSS patients, of whom 75 had extranodal marginal zone lymphoma and 19 had non-MALT NHL, and 600 HC patients were genotyped for the detection of MTHFR polymorphisms. Similar rates of both MTHFR c. 677C > T and c. 1298A > C polymorphisms were found among the pSS, pSS-lymphoma, and HC groups. Interestingly, regarding lymphoma subtype, the frequency of the MTHFR c. 677C > T TT homozygous genotype was higher in the pSS non-MALT group than in the pSS and HC groups. In contrast, the occurrence of the MTHFR c. 1298A > C AC and CC genotypes was lower in the pSS non-MALT group in comparison to the pSS and HC groups. Furthermore, an allele analysis of the studied MTHFR variants has shown that the pSS non-MALT group exhibited increased MTHFR c. 677C > T T allele prevalence as compared to the HC group, with allele frequencies of 52.6% and 36.6%, respectively. On the other hand, a reduced rate of the minor MTHFR c. 1298A > C C allele was found in the pSS non-MALT group as compared to both the HC and pSS groups.

Finally, since double-stranded DNA breaks promote chromosomal instability, translocations, and aberrations that may contribute to increased cancer risk [111], Jackson and Bartek explored the functional implications of these variants linked to increase DNA damage levels, providing a plausible biological scenario for their observed association with non-MALT lymphomagenesis in a pSS setting. Double-stranded DNA break levels were quantified in PBMCs derived from 13 pSS patients, and double-stranded DNA break levels were found significantly decreased in individuals carrying the MTHFR c. 1298A > C AC genotype, suggesting that the MTHFR variant may play a protective role against non-MALT development by restricting double-stranded DNA break formation [96].

Taken together, MTHFR polymorphisms may promote genomic instability by disturbing the methylation of DNA and allowing improper DNA synthesis and repair. All of these genetic variations may lead to either the overexpression of oncogenes or the defective expression of tumor suppressor genes, likely constituting an important pathogenic mechanism underlying the lymphoproliferative disorders that manifested in pSS.

4.6 Conclusions

The emerging data linking pSS with lymphoma development have given rise to new pathogenesis scenario. We suggest that pathogenesis is based on the association of two pathological processes that share a common target in common tissues. This target is the B lymphocyte, and the preferred tissues are the salivary glands and mucosal tissues.

On the one hand, we have a process of malignant transformation, mainly on a genetic basis (chromosomal aberrations and polymorphisms), and on the other, we have a multifactorial autoimmune process, which is prototypical of B-cell-mediated autoimmune disease. These two processes are reciprocal inductors; therefore, one of the processes (autoimmunity) can trigger or reveal a dormant malignant process. The latter may exacerbate and prolong the deleterious impact of the former on their common target, which is the B lymphocyte. The final result of these pathologic processes is the development of B-cell lymphoma in patients with a severe form of pSS. Nevertheless, despite efforts to identify risk factors for lymphoma development in pSS patients, neither the onset of its development nor which patients will develop lymphoma and have poor prognoses can be predicted effectively. Considering the fact that strategies to eliminate cancer cells by reducing tolerance can result in autoimmunity and that suppressing immune function to inhibit autoimmune response can allow malignancy development, there is a clear need for new and more specific therapeutic approaches. Undoubtedly, the genetic alterations that occur in this complex process may be a highly valuable source of information and should not be neglected in the future.

References

1. Cornec D, Chiche L. Is primary Sjogren's syndrome an orphan disease? A critical appraisal of prevalence studies in Europe. Ann Rheum Dis. 2015;74(3):e25. https://doi.org/10.1136/annrheumdis-2014-206860.
2. Binard A, Le Pottier L, Devauchelle-Pensec V, Saraux A, Youinou P, Pers JO. Is the blood B-cell subset profile diagnostic for Sjogren syndrome? Ann Rheum Dis. 2009;68(9):1447–52. https://doi.org/10.1136/ard.2008.096172.
3. Voulgarelis M, Dafni UG, Isenberg DA, Moutsopoulos HM. Malignant lymphoma in primary Sjogren's syndrome: a multicenter, retrospective, clinical study by the European Concerted Action on Sjogren's syndrome. Arthritis Rheum. 1999;42(8):1765–72. https://doi.org/10.1002/1529-0131(199908)42:8<1765::AID-ANR28>3.0.CO;2-V.
4. Gayral L, Gayral J. A familial strain of 11 cases of the Marinesco-Sjogren syndrome. J Genet Hum. 1966;15(1):63–9.

5. Cardenas-Roldan J, Rojas-Villarraga A, Anaya JM. How do autoimmune diseases cluster in families? A systematic review and meta-analysis. BMC Med. 2013;11:73. https://doi.org/10.1186/1741-7015-11-73.
6. Longhi BS, Appenzeller S, Centeville M, Gusmao RJ, Marini R. Primary Sjogren's syndrome in children: is a family approach indicated? Clinics (Sao Paulo). 2011;66(11):1991–3.
7. Kuo CF, Grainge MJ, Valdes AM, See LC, Luo SF, Yu KH, et al. Familial risk of Sjogren's syndrome and co-aggregation of autoimmune diseases in affected families: a Nationwide population study. Arthritis Rheumatol. 2015;67(7):1904–12. https://doi.org/10.1002/art.39127.
8. Christodoulou MI, Kapsogeorgou EK, Moutsopoulos HM. Characteristics of the minor salivary gland infiltrates in Sjogren's syndrome. J Autoimmun. 2010;34(4):400–7. https://doi.org/10.1016/j.jaut.2009.10.004.
9. Varin MM, Guerrier T, Devauchelle-Pensec V, Jamin C, Youinou P, Pers JO. In Sjogren's syndrome, B lymphocytes induce epithelial cells of salivary glands into apoptosis through protein kinase C delta activation. Autoimmun Rev. 2012;11(4):252–8. https://doi.org/10.1016/j.autrev.2011.10.005.
10. Zheng L, Zhang Z, Yu C, Yang C. Expression of Toll-like receptors 7, 8, and 9 in primary Sjogren's syndrome. Oral Surg Oral Med Oral Pathol Oral Radiol Endod. 2010;109(6):844–50. https://doi.org/10.1016/j.tripleo.2010.01.006.
11. Konsta OD, Thabet Y, Le Dantec C, Brooks WH, Tzioufas AG, Pers JO, et al. The contribution of epigenetics in Sjogren's syndrome. Front Genet. 2014;5:71. https://doi.org/10.3389/fgene.2014.00071.
12. Thabet Y, Le Dantec C, Ghedira I, Devauchelle V, Cornec D, Pers JO, et al. Epigenetic dysregulation in salivary glands from patients with primary Sjogren's syndrome may be ascribed to infiltrating B cells. J Autoimmun. 2013;41:175–81. https://doi.org/10.1016/j.jaut.2013.02.002.
13. Hamm-Alvarez SF, Janga SR, Edman MC, Madrigal S, Shah M, Frousiakis SE, et al. Tear cathepsin S as a candidate biomarker for Sjogren's syndrome. Arthritis Rheumatol. 2014;66(7):1872–81. https://doi.org/10.1002/art.38633.
14. Nocturne G, Seror R, Fogel O, Belkhir R, Boudaoud S, Saraux A, et al. CXCL13 and CCL11 serum levels and lymphoma and disease activity in primary Sjogren syndrome. Arthritis Rheumatol. 2015;67(12):3226–33. https://doi.org/10.1002/art.39315.
15. Brkic Z, Versnel MA. Type I IFN signature in primary Sjogren's syndrome patients. Expert Rev Clin Immunol. 2014;10(4):457–67. https://doi.org/10.1586/1744666X.2014.876364.
16. Ittah M, Miceli-Richard C, Gottenberg JE, Sellam J, Eid P, Lebon P, et al. Viruses induce high expression of BAFF by salivary gland epithelial cells through TLR- and type-I IFN-dependent and -independent pathways. Eur J Immunol. 2008;38(4):1058–64. https://doi.org/10.1002/eji.200738013.
17. Quartuccio L, Salvin S, Fabris M, Maset M, Pontarini E, Isola M, et al. BLyS upregulation in Sjogren's syndrome associated with lymphoproliferative disorders, higher ESSDAI score and B-cell clonal expansion in the salivary glands. Rheumatology (Oxford). 2013;52(2):276–81. https://doi.org/10.1093/rheumatology/kes180.
18. Le Pottier L, Devauchelle V, Fautrel A, Daridon C, Saraux A, Youinou P, et al. Ectopic germinal centers are rare in Sjogren's syndrome salivary glands and do not exclude autoreactive B cells. J Immunol. 2009;182(6):3540–7. https://doi.org/10.4049/jimmunol.0803588.
19. Haacke EA, van der Vegt B, Vissink A, Spijkervet FKL, Bootsma H, Kroese FGM. Germinal centres in diagnostic labial gland biopsies of patients with primary Sjogren's syndrome are not predictive for parotid MALT lymphoma development. Ann Rheum Dis. 2017;76(10):1781–4. https://doi.org/10.1136/annrheumdis-2017-211290.
20. Goodnow CC, Vinuesa CG, Randall KL, Mackay F, Brink R. Control systems and decision making for antibody production. Nat Immunol. 2010;11(8):681–8. https://doi.org/10.1038/ni.1900.
21. Szabo K, Papp G, Barath S, Gyimesi E, Szanto A, Zeher M. Follicular helper T cells may play an important role in the severity of primary Sjogren's syndrome. Clin Immunol. 2013;147(2):95–104. https://doi.org/10.1016/j.clim.2013.02.024.

22. Barone F, Nayar S, Campos J, Cloake T, Withers DR, Toellner KM, et al. IL-22 regulates lymphoid chemokine production and assembly of tertiary lymphoid organs. Proc Natl Acad Sci U S A. 2015;112(35):11024–9. https://doi.org/10.1073/pnas.1503315112.
23. Christodoulou MI, Kapsogeorgou EK, Moutsopoulos NM, Moutsopoulos HM. Foxp3+ T-regulatory cells in Sjogren's syndrome: correlation with the grade of the autoimmune lesion and certain adverse prognostic factors. Am J Pathol. 2008;173(5):1389–96. https://doi.org/10.2353/ajpath.2008.080246.
24. Nguyen CQ, Hu MH, Li Y, Stewart C, Peck AB. Salivary gland tissue expression of interleukin-23 and interleukin-17 in Sjogren's syndrome: findings in humans and mice. Arthritis Rheum. 2008;58(3):734–43. https://doi.org/10.1002/art.23214.
25. Lemoine S, Morva A, Youinou P, Jamin C. Regulatory B cells in autoimmune diseases: how do they work? Ann N Y Acad Sci. 2009;1173:260–7. https://doi.org/10.1111/j.1749-6632.2009.04651.x.
26. Nouel A, Pochard P, Simon Q, Segalen I, Le Meur Y, Pers JO, et al. B-cells induce regulatory T cells through TGF-beta/IDO production in A CTLA-4 dependent manner. J Autoimmun. 2015;59:53–60. https://doi.org/10.1016/j.jaut.2015.02.004.
27. Devauchelle-Pensec V, Mariette X, Jousse-Joulin S, Berthelot JM, Perdriger A, Puechal X, et al. Treatment of primary Sjogren syndrome with rituximab: a randomized trial. Ann Intern Med. 2014;160(4):233–42. https://doi.org/10.7326/M13-1085.
28. Nezos A, Papageorgiou A, Fragoulis G, Ioakeimidis D, Koutsilieris M, Tzioufas AG, et al. B-cell activating factor genetic variants in lymphomagenesis associated with primary Sjogren's syndrome. J Autoimmun. 2014;51:89–98. https://doi.org/10.1016/j.jaut.2013.04.005.
29. Tobon GJ, Renaudineau Y, Hillion S, Cornec D, Devauchelle-Pensec V, Youinou P, et al. The Fms-like tyrosine kinase 3 ligand, a mediator of B cell survival, is also a marker of lymphoma in primary Sjogren's syndrome. Arthritis Rheum. 2010;62(11):3447–56. https://doi.org/10.1002/art.27611.
30. Solans-Laque R, Lopez-Hernandez A, Bosch-Gil JA, Palacios A, Campillo M, Vilardell-Tarres M. Risk, predictors, and clinical characteristics of lymphoma development in primary Sjogren's syndrome. Semin Arthritis Rheum. 2011;41(3):415–23. https://doi.org/10.1016/j.semarthrit.2011.04.006.
31. Nishishinya MB, Pereda CA, Munoz-Fernandez S, Pego-Reigosa JM, Rua-Figueroa I, Andreu JL, et al. Identification of lymphoma predictors in patients with primary Sjogren's syndrome: a systematic literature review and meta-analysis. Rheumatol Int. 2015;35(1):17–26. https://doi.org/10.1007/s00296-014-3051-x.
32. Kauppi L, Stumpf MP, Jeffreys AJ. Localized breakdown in linkage disequilibrium does not always predict sperm crossover hot spots in the human MHC class II region. Genomics. 2005;86(1):13–24. https://doi.org/10.1016/j.ygeno.2005.03.011.
33. Westra HJ, Peters MJ, Esko T, Yaghootkar H, Schurmann C, Kettunen J, et al. Systematic identification of trans eQTLs as putative drivers of known disease associations. Nat Genet. 2013;45(10):1238–43. https://doi.org/10.1038/ng.2756.
34. Gershwin ME, Terasaki I, Graw R, Chused TM. Increased frequency of HL-A8 in Sjogren's syndrome. Tissue Antigens. 1975;6(5):342–6.
35. Matzaraki V, Kumar V, Wijmenga C, Zhernakova A. The MHC locus and genetic susceptibility to autoimmune and infectious diseases. Genome Biol. 2017;18(1):76. https://doi.org/10.1186/s13059-017-1207-1.
36. Lessard CJ, Li H, Adrianto I, Ice JA, Rasmussen A, Grundahl KM, et al. Variants at multiple loci implicated in both innate and adaptive immune responses are associated with Sjogren's syndrome. Nat Genet. 2013;45(11):1284–92. https://doi.org/10.1038/ng.2792.
37. Li Y, Zhang K, Chen H, Sun F, Xu J, Wu Z, et al. A genome-wide association study in Han Chinese identifies a susceptibility locus for primary Sjogren's syndrome at 7q11.23. Nat Genet. 2013;45(11):1361–5. https://doi.org/10.1038/ng.2779.

38. Nakken B, Jonsson R, Bolstad AI. Polymorphisms of the Ro52 gene associated with anti-Ro 52-kd autoantibodies in patients with primary Sjogren's syndrome. Arthritis Rheum. 2001;44(3):638–46. https://doi.org/10.1002/1529-0131(200103)44:3<638::AID-ANR112>3.0.CO;2-J.
39. Gottenberg JE, Busson M, Loiseau P, Cohen-Solal J, Lepage V, Charron D, et al. In primary Sjogren's syndrome, HLA class II is associated exclusively with autoantibody production and spreading of the autoimmune response. Arthritis Rheum. 2003;48(8):2240–5. https://doi.org/10.1002/art.11103.
40. Song IW, Chen HC, Lin YF, Yang JH, Chang CC, Chou CT, et al. Identification of susceptibility gene associated with female primary Sjogren's syndrome in Han Chinese by genome-wide association study. Hum Genet. 2016;135(11):1287–94. https://doi.org/10.1007/s00439-016-1716-0.
41. Kumagai S, Kanagawa S, Morinobu A, Takada M, Nakamura K, Sugai S, et al. Association of a new allele of the TAP2 gene, TAP2*Bky2 (Val577), with susceptibility to Sjogren's syndrome. Arthritis Rheum. 1997;40(9):1685–92. https://doi.org/10.1002/1529-0131(199709)40:9<1685::AID-ART19>3.0.CO;2-I.
42. Bolstad AI, Le Hellard S, Kristjansdottir G, Vasaitis L, Kvarnstrom M, Sjowall C, et al. Association between genetic variants in the tumour necrosis factor/lymphotoxin alpha/lymphotoxin beta locus and primary Sjogren's syndrome in Scandinavian samples. Ann Rheum Dis. 2012;71(6):981–8. https://doi.org/10.1136/annrheumdis-2011-200446.
43. Gottenberg JE, Busson M, Loiseau P, Dourche M, Cohen-Solal J, Lepage V, et al. Association of transforming growth factor beta1 and tumor necrosis factor alpha polymorphisms with anti-SSB/La antibody secretion in patients with primary Sjogren's syndrome. Arthritis Rheum. 2004;50(2):570–80. https://doi.org/10.1002/art.20060.
44. Rusakiewicz S, Nocturne G, Lazure T, Semeraro M, Flament C, Caillat-Zucman S, et al. NCR3/NKp30 contributes to pathogenesis in primary Sjogren's syndrome. Sci Transl Med. 2013;5(195):195ra96. https://doi.org/10.1126/scitranslmed.3005727.
45. Reksten TR, Johnsen SJ, Jonsson MV, Omdal R, Brun JG, Theander E, et al. Genetic associations to germinal centre formation in primary Sjogren's syndrome. Ann Rheum Dis. 2014;73(6):1253–8. https://doi.org/10.1136/annrheumdis-2012-202500.
46. Petrek M, Cermakova Z, Hutyrova B, Micekova D, Drabek J, Rovensky J, et al. CC chemokine receptor 5 and interleukin-1 receptor antagonist gene polymorphisms in patients with primary Sjogren's syndrome. Clin Exp Rheumatol. 2002;20(5):701–3.
47. Hulkkonen J, Pertovaara M, Antonen J, Lahdenpohja N, Pasternack A, Hurme M. Genetic association between interleukin-10 promoter region polymorphisms and primary Sjogren's syndrome. Arthritis Rheum. 2001;44(1):176–9. https://doi.org/10.1002/1529-0131(200101)44:1<176::AID-ANR23>3.0.CO;2-K.
48. Font J, Garcia-Carrasco M, Ramos-Casals M, Aldea AI, Cervera R, Ingelmo M, et al. The role of interleukin-10 promoter polymorphisms in the clinical expression of primary Sjogren's syndrome. Rheumatology (Oxford). 2002;41(9):1025–30.
49. Origuchi T, Kawasaki E, Ide A, Kamachi M, Tanaka F, Ida H, et al. Correlation between interleukin 10 gene promoter region polymorphisms and clinical manifestations in Japanese patients with Sjogren's syndrome. Ann Rheum Dis. 2003;62(11):1117–8.
50. Maiti AK, Kim-Howard X, Viswanathan P, Guillen L, Rojas-Villarraga A, Deshmukh H, et al. Confirmation of an association between rs6822844 at the Il2-Il21 region and multiple autoimmune diseases: evidence of a general susceptibility locus. Arthritis Rheum. 2010;62(2):323–9. https://doi.org/10.1002/art.27222.
51. Nordmark G, Kristjansdottir G, Theander E, Appel S, Eriksson P, Vasaitis L, et al. Association of EBF1, FAM167A(C8orf13)-BLK and TNFSF4 gene variants with primary Sjogren's syndrome. Genes Immun. 2011;12(2):100–9. https://doi.org/10.1038/gene.2010.44.
52. Sun F, Li P, Chen H, Wu Z, Xu J, Shen M, et al. Association studies of TNFSF4, TNFAIP3 and FAM167A-BLK polymorphisms with primary Sjogren's syndrome in Han Chinese. J Hum Genet. 2013;58(7):475–9. https://doi.org/10.1038/jhg.2013.26.

53. Kong F, Li JX, Li P, Li YZ, Zhang FC, Zhang J. Association of TNFSF4 polymorphisms with susceptibility to primary Sjogren's syndrome and primary biliary cirrhosis in a Chinese Han population. Clin Exp Rheumatol. 2013;31(4):546–51.
54. Nossent JC, Lester S, Zahra D, Mackay CR, Rischmueller M. Polymorphism in the 5′ regulatory region of the B-lymphocyte activating factor gene is associated with the Ro/La autoantibody response and serum BAFF levels in primary Sjogren's syndrome. Rheumatology (Oxford). 2008;47(9):1311–6. https://doi.org/10.1093/rheumatology/ken246.
55. Papageorgiou A, Mavragani CP, Nezos A, Zintzaras E, Quartuccio L, De Vita S, et al. A BAFF receptor His159Tyr mutation in Sjogren's syndrome-related lymphoproliferation. Arthritis Rheumatol. 2015;67(10):2732–41. https://doi.org/10.1002/art.39231.
56. Bolstad AI, Wargelius A, Nakken B, Haga HJ, Jonsson R. Fas and Fas ligand gene polymorphisms in primary Sjogren's syndrome. J Rheumatol. 2000;27(10):2397–405.
57. Mullighan CG, Heatley S, Lester S, Rischmueller M, Gordon TP, Bardy PG. Fas gene promoter polymorphisms in primary Sjogren's syndrome. Ann Rheum Dis. 2004;63(1):98–101.
58. Musone SL, Taylor KE, Nititham J, Chu C, Poon A, Liao W, et al. Sequencing of TNFAIP3 and association of variants with multiple autoimmune diseases. Genes Immun. 2011;12(3):176–82. https://doi.org/10.1038/gene.2010.64.
59. Nordmark G, Wang C, Vasaitis L, Eriksson P, Theander E, Kvarnstrom M, et al. Association of genes in the NF-kappaB pathway with antibody-positive primary Sjogren's syndrome. Scand J Immunol. 2013;78(5):447–54. https://doi.org/10.1111/sji.12101.
60. Qu S, Du Y, Chang S, Guo L, Fang K, Li Y, et al. Common variants near IKZF1 are associated with primary Sjogren's syndrome in Han Chinese. PLoS One. 2017;12(5):e0177320. https://doi.org/10.1371/journal.pone.0177320.
61. Ou TT, Lin CH, Lin YC, Li RN, Tsai WC, Liu HW, et al. IkappaBalpha promoter polymorphisms in patients with primary Sjogren's syndrome. J Clin Immunol. 2008;28(5):440–4. https://doi.org/10.1007/s10875-008-9212-5.
62. Miceli-Richard C, Gestermann N, Ittah M, Comets E, Loiseau P, Puechal X, et al. The CGGGG insertion/deletion polymorphism of the IRF5 promoter is a strong risk factor for primary Sjogren's syndrome. Arthritis Rheumatol. 2009;60(7):1991–7. https://doi.org/10.1002/art.24662.
63. Nordmark G, Kristjansdottir G, Theander E, Eriksson P, Brun JG, Wang C, et al. Additive effects of the major risk alleles of IRF5 and STAT4 in primary Sjogren's syndrome. Genes Immun. 2009;10(1):68–76. https://doi.org/10.1038/gene.2008.94.
64. Korman BD, Kastner DL, Gregersen PK, Remmers EF. STAT4: genetics, mechanisms, and implications for autoimmunity. Curr Allergy Asthma Rep. 2008;8(5):398–403.
65. Appel S, Le Hellard S, Bruland O, Brun JG, Omdal R, Kristjansdottir G, et al. Potential association of muscarinic receptor 3 gene variants with primary Sjogren's syndrome. Ann Rheum Dis. 2011;70(7):1327–9. https://doi.org/10.1136/ard.2010.138966.
66. Downie-Doyle S, Bayat N, Rischmueller M, Lester S. Influence of CTLA4 haplotypes on susceptibility and some extraglandular manifestations in primary Sjogren's syndrome. Arthritis Rheum. 2006;54(8):2434–40. https://doi.org/10.1002/art.22004.
67. Sun F, Xu J, Wu Z, Li P, Chen H, Su J, et al. Polymorphisms in the FAM167A-BLK, but not BANK1, are associated with primary Sjogren's syndrome in a Han Chinese population. Clin Exp Rheumatol. 2013;31(5):704–10.
68. Mamtani M, Anaya JM, He W, Ahuja SK. Association of copy number variation in the FCGR3B gene with risk of autoimmune diseases. Genes Immun. 2010;11(2):155–60. https://doi.org/10.1038/gene.2009.71.
69. Nossent JC, Rischmueller M, Lester S. Low copy number of the Fc-gamma receptor 3B gene FCGR3B is a risk factor for primary Sjogren's syndrome. J Rheumatol. 2012;39(11):2142–7. https://doi.org/10.3899/jrheum.120294.
70. Cobb BL, Fei Y, Jonsson R, Bolstad AI, Brun JG, Rischmueller M, et al. Genetic association between methyl-CpG binding protein 2 (MECP2) and primary Sjogren's syndrome. Ann Rheum Dis. 2010;69(9):1731–2. https://doi.org/10.1136/ard.2009.122903.

71. Li H, Reksten TR, Ice JA, Kelly JA, Adrianto I, Rasmussen A, et al. Identification of a Sjogren's syndrome susceptibility locus at OAS1 that influences isoform switching, protein expression, and responsiveness to type I interferons. PLoS Genet. 2017;13(6):e1006820. https://doi.org/10.1371/journal.pgen.1006820.
72. Gomez LM, Anaya JM, Gonzalez CI, Pineda-Tamayo R, Otero W, Arango A, et al. PTPN22 C1858T polymorphism in Colombian patients with autoimmune diseases. Genes Immun. 2005;6(7):628–31. https://doi.org/10.1038/sj.gene.6364261.
73. Ittah M, Gottenberg JE, Proust A, Hachulla E, Puechal X, Loiseau P, et al. No evidence for association between 1858 C/T single-nucleotide polymorphism of PTPN22 gene and primary Sjogren's syndrome. Genes Immun. 2005;6(5):457–8. https://doi.org/10.1038/sj.gene.6364229.
74. Imanishi T, Morinobu A, Hayashi N, Kanagawa S, Koshiba M, Kondo S, et al. A novel polymorphism of the SSA1 gene is associated with anti-SS-A/Ro52 autoantibody in Japanese patients with primary Sjogren's syndrome. Clin Exp Rheumatol. 2005;23(4):521–4.
75. Brooks WH, Le Dantec C, Pers JO, Youinou P, Renaudineau Y. Epigenetics and autoimmunity. J Autoimmun. 2010;34(3):J207–19. https://doi.org/10.1016/j.jaut.2009.12.006.
76. Le Dantec C, Varin MM, Brooks WH, Pers JO, Youinou P, Renaudineau Y. Epigenetics and Sjogren's syndrome. Curr Pharm Biotechnol. 2012;13(10):2046–53.
77. Kivity S, Arango MT, Ehrenfeld M, Tehori O, Shoenfeld Y, Anaya JM, et al. Infection and autoimmunity in Sjogren's syndrome: a clinical study and comprehensive review. J Autoimmun. 2014;51:17–22. https://doi.org/10.1016/j.jaut.2014.02.008.
78. Thabet Y, Canas F, Ghedira I, Youinou P, Mageed RA, Renaudineau Y. Altered patterns of epigenetic changes in systemic lupus erythematosus and auto-antibody production: is there a link? J Autoimmun. 2012;39(3):154–60. https://doi.org/10.1016/j.jaut.2012.05.015.
79. Brooks WH, Renaudineau Y. Epigenetics and autoimmune diseases: the X chromosome-nucleolus nexus. Front Genet. 2015;6:22. https://doi.org/10.3389/fgene.2015.00022.
80. Konsta OD, Le Dantec C, Charras A, Cornec D, Kapsogeorgou EK, Tzioufas AG, et al. Defective DNA methylation in salivary gland epithelial acini from patients with Sjogren's syndrome is associated with SSB gene expression, anti-SSB/LA detection, and lymphocyte infiltration. J Autoimmun. 2016;68:30–8. https://doi.org/10.1016/j.jaut.2015.12.002.
81. Altorok N, Coit P, Hughes T, Koelsch KA, Stone DU, Rasmussen A, et al. Genome-wide DNA methylation patterns in naive CD4+ T cells from patients with primary Sjogren's syndrome. Arthritis Rheumatol. 2014;66(3):731–9. https://doi.org/10.1002/art.38264.
82. Miceli-Richard C, Wang-Renault SF, Boudaoud S, Busato F, Lallemand C, Bethune K, et al. Overlap between differentially methylated DNA regions in blood B lymphocytes and genetic at-risk loci in primary Sjogren's syndrome. Ann Rheum Dis. 2016;75(5):933–40. https://doi.org/10.1136/annrheumdis-2014-206998.
83. Imgenberg-Kreuz J, Sandling JK, Almlof JC, Nordlund J, Signer L, Norheim KB, et al. Genome-wide DNA methylation analysis in multiple tissues in primary Sjogren's syndrome reveals regulatory effects at interferon-induced genes. Ann Rheum Dis. 2016;75(11):2029–36. https://doi.org/10.1136/annrheumdis-2015-208659.
84. Cole MB, Quach H, Quach D, Baker A, Taylor KE, Barcellos LF, et al. Epigenetic signatures of salivary gland inflammation in Sjogren's syndrome. Arthritis Rheumatol. 2016;68(12):2936–44. https://doi.org/10.1002/art.39792.
85. Charras A, Konsta OD, Le Dantec C, Bagacean C, Kapsogeorgou EK, Tzioufas AG, et al. Cell-specific epigenome-wide DNA methylation profile in long-term cultured minor salivary gland epithelial cells from patients with Sjogren's syndrome. Ann Rheum Dis. 2017;76(3):625–8. https://doi.org/10.1136/annrheumdis-2016-210167.
86. Pratt AJ, MacRae IJ. The RNA-induced silencing complex: a versatile gene-silencing machine. J Biol Chem. 2009;284(27):17897–901. https://doi.org/10.1074/jbc.R900012200.
87. Goodier JL, Kazazian HH Jr. Retrotransposons revisited: the restraint and rehabilitation of parasites. Cell. 2008;135(1):23–35. https://doi.org/10.1016/j.cell.2008.09.022.
88. Mavragani CP, Sagalovskiy I, Guo Q, Nezos A, Kapsogeorgou EK, Lu P, et al. Expression of long interspersed nuclear element 1 retroelements and induction of type I interferon in

patients with systemic autoimmune disease. Arthritis Rheumatol. 2016;68(11):2686–96. https://doi.org/10.1002/art.39795.
89. Hung T, Pratt GA, Sundararaman B, Townsend MJ, Chaivorapol C, Bhangale T, et al. The Ro60 autoantigen binds endogenous retroelements and regulates inflammatory gene expression. Science. 2015;350(6259):455–9. https://doi.org/10.1126/science.aac7442.
90. Mavragani CP, Nezos A, Sagalovskiy I, Seshan S, Kirou KA, Crow MK. Defective regulation of L1 endogenous retroelements in primary Sjogren's syndrome and systemic lupus erythematosus: role of methylating enzymes. J Autoimmun. 2018;88:75–82. https://doi.org/10.1016/j.jaut.2017.10.004.
91. Konsta OD, Charras A, Le Dantec C, Kapsogeorgeou E, Bordron A, Brooks WH, et al. Epigenetic modifications in salivary glands from patients with Sjogren's syndrome affect cytokeratin 19 expression. Bull Group Int Rech Sci Stomatol Odontol. 2016;53(1):e01.
92. Burbelo PD, Ambatipudi K, Alevizos I. Genome-wide association studies in Sjogren's syndrome: what do the genes tell us about disease pathogenesis? Autoimmun Rev. 2014;13(7):756–61. https://doi.org/10.1016/j.autrev.2014.02.002.
93. Streubel B, Huber D, Wohrer S, Chott A, Raderer M. Frequency of chromosomal aberrations involving MALT1 in mucosa-associated lymphoid tissue lymphoma in patients with Sjogren's syndrome. Clin Cancer Res. 2004;10(2):476–80.
94. Nocturne G, Mariette X. Sjogren syndrome-associated lymphomas: an update on pathogenesis and management. Br J Haematol. 2015;168(3):317–27. https://doi.org/10.1111/bjh.13192.
95. Sutton LA, Agathangelidis A, Belessi C, Darzentas N, Davi F, Ghia P, et al. Antigen selection in B-cell lymphomas—tracing the evidence. Semin Cancer Biol. 2013;23(6):399–409. https://doi.org/10.1016/j.semcancer.2013.07.006.
96. Fragkioudaki S, Nezos A, Souliotis VL, Chatziandreou I, Saetta AA, Drakoulis N, et al. MTHFR gene variants and non-MALT lymphoma development in primary Sjogren's syndrome. Sci Rep. 2017;7(1):7354. https://doi.org/10.1038/s41598-017-07347-w.
97. Dierlamm J, Baens M, Wlodarska I, Stefanova-Ouzounova M, Hernandez JM, Hossfeld DK, et al. The apoptosis inhibitor gene API2 and a novel 18q gene, MLT, are recurrently rearranged in the t(11;18)(q21;q21) associated with mucosa-associated lymphoid tissue lymphomas. Blood. 1999;93(11):3601–9.
98. Du MQ. MALT lymphoma: a paradigm of NF-kappaB dysregulation. Semin Cancer Biol. 2016;39:49–60. https://doi.org/10.1016/j.semcancer.2016.07.003.
99. Murga Penas EM, Hinz K, Roser K, Copie-Bergman C, Wlodarska I, Marynen P, et al. Translocations t(11;18)(q21;q21) and t(14;18)(q32;q21) are the main chromosomal abnormalities involving MLT/MALT1 in MALT lymphomas. Leukemia. 2003;17(11):2225–9. https://doi.org/10.1038/sj.leu.2403122.
100. Lahiri A, Pochard P, Le Pottier L, Tobon GJ, Bendaoud B, Youinou P, et al. The complexity of the BAFF TNF-family members: implications for autoimmunity. J Autoimmun. 2012;39(3):189–98. https://doi.org/10.1016/j.jaut.2012.05.009.
101. Novak AJ, Grote DM, Ziesmer SC, Kline MP, Manske MK, Slager S, et al. Elevated serum B-lymphocyte stimulator levels in patients with familial lymphoproliferative disorders. J Clin Oncol. 2006;24(6):983–7. https://doi.org/10.1200/JCO.2005.02.7938.
102. Hildebrand JM, Luo Z, Manske MK, Price-Troska T, Ziesmer SC, Lin W, et al. A BAFF-R mutation associated with non-Hodgkin lymphoma alters TRAF recruitment and reveals new insights into BAFF-R signaling. J Exp Med. 2010;207(12):2569–79. https://doi.org/10.1084/jem.20100857.
103. Zintzaras E, Voulgarelis M, Moutsopoulos HM. The risk of lymphoma development in autoimmune diseases: a meta-analysis. Arch Intern Med. 2005;165(20):2337–44. https://doi.org/10.1001/archinte.165.20.2337.
104. Zhang M, Peng LL, Wang Y, Wang JS, Liu J, Liu MM, et al. Roles of A20 in autoimmune diseases. Immunol Res. 2016;64(2):337–44. https://doi.org/10.1007/s12026-015-8677-6.

105. Tavares RM, Turer EE, Liu CL, Advincula R, Scapini P, Rhee L, et al. The ubiquitin modifying enzyme A20 restricts B cell survival and prevents autoimmunity. Immunity. 2010;33(2):181–91. https://doi.org/10.1016/j.immuni.2010.07.017.
106. Nocturne G, Boudaoud S, Miceli-Richard C, Viengchareun S, Lazure T, Nititham J, et al. Germline and somatic genetic variations of TNFAIP3 in lymphoma complicating primary Sjogren's syndrome. Blood. 2013;122(25):4068–76. https://doi.org/10.1182/blood-2013-05-503383.
107. Bi Y, Zeng N, Chanudet E, Huang Y, Hamoudi RA, Liu H, et al. A20 inactivation in ocular adnexal MALT lymphoma. Haematologica. 2012;97(6):926–30. https://doi.org/10.3324/haematol.2010.036798.
108. Nocturne G, Tarn J, Boudaoud S, Locke J, Miceli-Richard C, Hachulla E, et al. Germline variation of TNFAIP3 in primary Sjogren's syndrome-associated lymphoma. Ann Rheum Dis. 2016;75(4):780–3. https://doi.org/10.1136/annrheumdis-2015-207731.
109. van Krieken JH. New developments in the pathology of malignant lymphoma: a review of the literature published from May to August 2017. J Hematopathol. 2017;10(2):65–73. https://doi.org/10.1007/s12308-017-0303-1.
110. Lee KM, Lan Q, Kricker A, Purdue MP, Grulich AE, Vajdic CM, et al. One-carbon metabolism gene polymorphisms and risk of non-Hodgkin lymphoma in Australia. Hum Genet. 2007;122(5):525–33. https://doi.org/10.1007/s00439-007-0431-2.
111. Jackson SP, Bartek J. The DNA-damage response in human biology and disease. Nature. 2009;461(7267):1071–8. https://doi.org/10.1038/nature08467.
112. Chen JQ, Papp G, Poliska S, Szabo K, Tarr T, Balint BL, et al. MicroRNA expression profiles identify disease-specific alterations in systemic lupus erythematosus and primary Sjogren's syndrome. PLoS One. 2017;12(3):e0174585. https://doi.org/10.1371/journal.pone.0174585.
113. Shi H, Zheng LY, Zhang P, Yu CQ. miR-146a and miR-155 expression in PBMCs from patients with Sjogren's syndrome. J Oral Pathol Med. 2014;43(10):792–7. https://doi.org/10.1111/jop.12187.
114. Wang-Renault SF, Boudaoud S, Nocturne G, Roche E, Sigrist N, Daviaud C, et al. Deregulation of microRNA expression in purified T and B lymphocytes from patients with primary Sjogren's syndrome. Ann Rheum Dis. 2018;77(1):133–40. https://doi.org/10.1136/annrheumdis-2017-211417.
115. Lopez-Ramirez MA, Wu D, Pryce G, Simpson JE, Reijerkerk A, King-Robson J, et al. MicroRNA-155 negatively affects blood-brain barrier function during neuroinflammation. FASEB J. 2014;28(6):2551–65. https://doi.org/10.1096/fj.13-248880.
116. Gourzi VC, Kapsogeorgou EK, Kyriakidis NC, Tzioufas AG. Study of microRNAs (miRNAs) that are predicted to target the autoantigens Ro/SSA and La/SSB in primary Sjogren's syndrome. Clin Exp Immunol. 2015;182(1):14–22. https://doi.org/10.1111/cei.12664.
117. Kapsogeorgou EK, Gourzi VC, Manoussakis MN, Moutsopoulos HM, Tzioufas AG. Cellular microRNAs (miRNAs) and Sjogren's syndrome: candidate regulators of autoimmune response and autoantigen expression. J Autoimmun. 2011;37(2):129–35. https://doi.org/10.1016/j.jaut.2011.05.003.
118. Gallo A, Jang SI, Ong HL, Perez P, Tandon M, Ambudkar I, et al. Targeting the Ca2+ sensor STIM1 by exosomal transfer of Ebv-miR-BART13-3p is associated with Sjogren's syndrome. EBioMedicine. 2016;10:216–26. https://doi.org/10.1016/j.ebiom.2016.06.041.
119. Ghorbani S, Talebi F, Chan WF, Masoumi F, Vojgani M, Power C, et al. MicroRNA-181 variants regulate T cell phenotype in the context of autoimmune neuroinflammation. Front Immunol. 2017;8:758. https://doi.org/10.3389/fimmu.2017.00758.
120. Peng L, Ma W, Yi F, Yang YJ, Lin W, Chen H, et al. MicroRNA profiling in Chinese patients with primary Sjogren syndrome reveals elevated miRNA-181a in peripheral blood mononuclear cells. J Rheumatol. 2014;41(11):2208–13. https://doi.org/10.3899/jrheum.131154.
121. Tandon M, Gallo A, Jang SI, Illei GG, Alevizos I. Deep sequencing of short RNAs reveals novel microRNAs in minor salivary glands of patients with Sjogren's syndrome. Oral Dis. 2012;18(2):127–31. https://doi.org/10.1111/j.1601-0825.2011.01849.x.

122. Williams AE, Choi K, Chan AL, Lee YJ, Reeves WH, Bubb MR, et al. Sjogren's syndrome-associated microRNAs in CD14(+) monocytes unveils targeted TGFbeta signaling. Arthritis Res Ther. 2016;18(1):95. https://doi.org/10.1186/s13075-016-0987-0.
123. Yang Y, Peng L, Ma W, Yi F, Zhang Z, Chen H, et al. Autoantigen-targeting microRNAs in Sjogren's syndrome. Clin Rheumatol. 2016;35(4):911–7. https://doi.org/10.1007/s10067-016-3203-3.
124. Michael A, Bajracharya SD, Yuen PS, Zhou H, Star RA, Illei GG, et al. Exosomes from human saliva as a source of microRNA biomarkers. Oral Dis. 2010;16(1):34–8. https://doi.org/10.1111/j.1601-0825.2009.01604.x.
125. Alevizos I, Alexander S, Turner RJ, Illei GG. MicroRNA expression profiles as biomarkers of minor salivary gland inflammation and dysfunction in Sjogren's syndrome. Arthritis Rheum. 2011;63(2):535–44. https://doi.org/10.1002/art.30131.

Polymyositis/Dermatomyositis

5

Ana Márquez, Ernesto Trallero-Araguás,
and Albert Selva-O'Callaghan

Contents

5.1 Introduction

The idiopathic inflammatory myopathies (IIM) represent a group of autoimmune disorders, all of them characterized by weakness of proximal muscles but showing heterogeneous system manifestations, including skin rashes, interstitial lung disease, and malignancy [1]. According to the presence of extramuscular and histopathological features, IIM can be subdivided into different subsets, including dermatomyositis (DM),

A. Márquez (✉)
Systemic Autoimmune Disease Unit, Instituto de Investigación Biosanitaria de Granada (ibs.GRANADA), Granada, Spain
e-mail: anamaort@ipb.csic.es

E. Trallero-Araguás
Department of Rheumatology, Vall d'Hebron General Hospital, Barcelona, Spain
e-mail: etrallero@vhebron.net

A. Selva-O'Callaghan
Internal Medicine Department, Autonomous University of Barcelona, Barcelona, Spain
e-mail: aselva@vhebron.net

J. Martín, F. D. Carmona (eds.), *Genetics of Rare Autoimmune Diseases*,
Rare Diseases of the Immune System, https://doi.org/10.1007/978-3-030-03934-9_5

polymyositis (PM), inclusion body myositis (IBM), immune-mediated necrotizing myopathies (IMNM), and DM/PM overlapping with other connective tissue diseases, which are correlated with the presence of disease-specific autoantibodies [1].

Although IIM are rare diseases, they represent the most common cause of acquired muscle disease in adults. The incidence of myositis has been estimated in 50–100 cases per million [1]. The precise cause of IIM is still unclear, but as other autoimmune diseases, these disorders present a complex etiology in which exposure to environmental risk factors results in chronic immune activation in individuals with a predisposing genetic background along with other epigenetic mechanisms. This genetic basis is supported by the identification of increased risk of autoimmune diseases in first-degree relatives of patients with IIM and rare case reports of familial aggregation [2, 3].

In this chapter, we summarize the current knowledge about the genetic architecture of IIM, with a particular focus on DM and PM, as well as the recent progress in the elucidation of the epigenetic factors influencing their development.

5.2 Immunopathogenesis of DM/PM

The pathogenesis of DM/PM is not fully understood. Both immune and nonimmune processes have been implicated in the development of muscle damage. In addition, muscle weakness seems to be mediated by different mechanisms in the different subgroups of IIM.

On one hand, the complement cascade has been shown to play a crucial role in the DM pathogenesis. Specifically, it has been proposed that the disease begin when putative antibodies directed against endothelial cells activate the C5b-9 complement membrane attack complex (MAC). Once activated, MAC is deposited on the surface of endothelial cells leading to necrosis of these cells, capillary ischemia, and muscle-fiber destruction, which results in the characteristic perifascicular atrophy found in muscle biopsy of DM patients [4]. In addition, the complement activation induces the production of pro-inflammatory cytokines, chemokines, and adhesion molecules, which are responsible for the recruitment of activated lymphocytes, including CD4+ T cells, B cells, and plasmacytoid dendritic cells (pDCs), to the site of inflammation. Moreover, increasing evidences suggest a relevant role of pDCs in DM through the production of type 1 interferons (IFNs) [5]. On the other hand, CD8+ T cells are considered as the primary effector cells mediating muscle damage in PM. These lymphocytes can invade healthy non-necrotic muscle fibers that aberrantly express major histocompatibility complex (MHC) class I molecules and release perforin granules toward the surface of the muscle fibers causing necrosis [4].

Nonimmune mechanisms have also been implicated in the IIM pathogenesis. The overexpression of MHC class I occurring in muscle fibers of myositis patients seems to act as a potential inducer of endoplasmic reticulum (EM) stress, which results in nuclear transcription factor κ-beta (NF-κB) activation and the subsequent production of pro-inflammatory cytokines [6]. Additionally, two potent inducers of autophagy, Toll-like receptor (TLR) 3 and TLR4, were found significantly overexpressed in IIM [7]. Moreover, these receptors co-localized with LC3, an autophagy-related protein, in IIM patients, thus suggesting a role of the autophagy pathway in myositis [7].

5.3 Genetics of DM/PM

In the last years, two main approaches have been used to elucidate the genetic basis of these disorders, both of which involve genotyping of genetic variations, mainly single-nucleotide polymorphisms (SNPs), in cases and controls. Initially, the genetic component of IIM was explored by candidate-gene association studies, which examine a set of SNPs within *loci* selected on the basis of their biological functions (functional candidates) or their location within genomic regions previously implicated by association or linkage studies (positional candidates). In contrast to this strategy, the more recently developed genome-wide association studies (GWASs) investigate the entire genome in a hypothesis-free manner, thus revolutionizing the possibilities of identifying the genetic component of complex diseases [8]. Subsequently, the success of GWAS spurred the design of targeted genotyping platforms, such as the Immunochip. Immunochip is specifically designed for fine-mapping of established autoimmune-associated *loci*, with a particular focus on the human leukocyte antigen (HLA) region [9]. In the last years, the application of the GWAS and Immunochip strategies to the study of the genetic basis of IIM together with international collaborative efforts to gather larger cohorts of IIM patients has led to significant advances in the knowledge of the molecular mechanisms underlying these disorders.

5.3.1 HLA Associations

The HLA region, encompassing 7.6 Mb on chromosome 6p21, is the most gene dense region within the human genome, including genes involved in the immune response. Similarly to that observed for other autoimmune diseases, allelic variants within the HLA region represent the strongest and most consistent genetic associations for IIM.

During the last years, several studies have investigated the role of the HLA in the IIM susceptibility. As result of these studies, the 8.1 ancestral haplotype (8.1 AH) was identified as the highest risk factor within this region [10–12] (Table 5.1). 8.1 AH, formed by the combination of the alleles HLA-A*01:01, -C*07:01, -B*08:01, -DRB1*03:01, -DQA1*05:01, and -DQB1*02:01, represents an evolutionary highly conserved haplotype that contains hundreds of immunologically relevant genes. Nevertheless, the independent impact of alleles forming the 8.1 AH could not be fully elucidated, probably due to the strong linkage disequilibrium (LD) within this region.

In 2006, a large immunogenetic study of HLA allelic associations with particular myositis-specific autoantibody (MSA) and myositis-associated autoantibody (MAA) groups of IIM patients identified the 8.1 AH-associated alleles B*08:01 and

Table 5.1 Main risk HLA alleles for overall idiopathic inflammatory myopathies (IIM), dermatomyositis (DM), and polymyositis (PM) in different populations

Population	IIM	DM	PM	Study
European	8.1 AH (**DRB1*03:01** and **B*08:01**)	8.1 AH (**B*08:01,** AA_DQB1_57, DQB1*04:02)	8.1 AH (**DRB1*03:01** and **B*08:01**)	[10–12]
Chinese	–	DQA1*01:04 DRB1*07	–	[15]
Japanese	DRB1*08:03	–	DRB1*08:03	[16]
African American	A*68:02 **DQA1*05:01** **DRB1*03**	**DRB1*03:01** DQA1*06:01	**DQA1*05:01**	[17]

IIM idiopathic inflammatory myopathies, *DM* dermatomyositis, *PM* polymyositis, *AH* ancestral haplotype
HLA alleles included in the 8.1 AH are marked in bold. Independent signals within the HLA region are shown in brackets

DRB1*03:01 as the main HLA risk markers [11]. In addition, several HLA susceptibility factors appeared to be specifically associated with particular MSA and MAA serogroups [11].

More recently, two large-scale genetic analyses have thoroughly explored the role of the HLA in different subgroups of Caucasian IIM patients by imputation of classical HLA alleles and amino acids from SNP genotype data [10, 12]. In 2015, a GWAS performed on 1710 patients with DM, PM, and juvenile DM (JDM), and DM, JDM, or PM cases with anti-histidyl-tRNA synthetase (anti-Jo-1) autoantibodies confirmed the previously described association between the 8.1 AH and myositis [10]. However, the stratified analysis according to the different clinical phenotypes showed that the DRB1*03:01 allele was the strongest signal in DM and JDM patients, whereas the B*08:01 allele represented the main risk factor for PM and myositis with anti-Jo autoantibodies.

Interestingly, an Immunochip study published a year later, which included the larger cohort of IIM patients analyzed so far, specifically 2566 patients with DM, JDM, PM, and IBM, yielded contradictory results [12]. In this study, DRB1*03:01 and B*08:01 were identified as independent association signals in PM, whereas three independent signals, B*08:01, amino acid position 57 of DQβ1, and DQB1*04:02, were detected in the DM subgroup. Regarding the JDM subset, DRB1*03:01 was identified as the strongest association and the C*02:02 allele (which is not included in the 8.1 AH) showed an independent effect after conditioning on DRB1*03:01. On the other hand, in this Immunochip study, the association with DRB1*03:01 was presumably attributed to amino acid residues that are only present at this classical allele, asparagine at position 77 and arginine at position 74 [12]. Interestingly, position 74 is structurally involved in the peptide-binding groove of the HLA-DRβ molecule, and the presence of arginine has been reported to modify the three-dimensional structure of pocket 4 of the binding cleft in a way that probably enables presentation of autoantigens [13, 14].

Although 8.1 AH is a risk factor for IIM among individuals of European origin, such association has not been clearly established in other ethnic groups (Table 5.1).

A study performed in Chinese population reported a susceptibility effect of DQA1*01:04 and DRB1*07 and a protective effect of DRB1*03 in DM patients [15]. In Japanese IIM patients, the strongest signal within the HLA region corresponded to the DRB1*08:03 classical allele [16]. Finally, a study performed in African Americans evidenced both shared and distinct immunogenetic susceptibility factors between this ethnic group and European American patients [17]. However, these studies included small sample sizes and lacked replication cohorts. Therefore, studies on well-powered case-control sets are required to definitively confirm or discard these associations.

On the other hand, the class III region of the HLA complex includes genes encoding several components of the complement system (C4, C2, and factor B), which is involved in the muscle damage occurring in DM. Most human chromosomes carry two *C4* genes, *C4A* and *C4B*; however, the number of expressed *C4* genes can range from none to four. Remarkably, the 8.1 AH is associated with a single *C4B* and the absence of a *C4A* gene, which leads to a genetic defect of complement function. A candidate-gene study published in 2016 analyzed gene copy-numbers (GCNs) for total *C4*, *C4A*, *C4B*, and HLA-DRB1 genotypes in 105 JDM patients and 500 healthy controls, all of them from European origin [18]. They found an association of presence of HLA-DRB1*03:01 and deficiency of *C4A* with JDM. However, the co-existence of both DRB1*03:01 and *C4A* deficiency conferred higher risk than either individual risk factor. In addition, they also observed that JDM patients with *C4A* deficiency had higher levels of multiple serum muscle enzymes compared with controls [18]. These findings suggest that deficiency of *C4A* represents a risk factor for JDM.

5.3.2 Non-HLA Associations

5.3.2.1 Genome-Wide Association Studies in DM/PM Research

Four GWAS on IIM, two in European population and two in Asian population, have been published so far [10, 19–21]. The application of this approach to the study of the genetic background of IIM has led to the discovery of several novel risk *loci* for both DM and PM (Table 5.2). However, the impact of GWAS on deciphering the genetic component of IIM has not been as relevant as for other autoimmune diseases. This may be due to a relatively weaker genetic influence on IIM predisposition or, more likely, to a higher disease heterogeneity compared to other immune-mediated disorders.

In 2013, the International Myositis Genetics Consortium (MYOGEN) published the first GWAS on DM, including 1178 cases and 4724 controls of European origin [20]. This study confirmed the HLA region as the main genetic risk factor for DM but failed to identify genome-wide associations outside this region. However, the analysis of 141 genetic variants previously associated with autoimmune disorders, specifically rheumatoid arthritis (RA), systemic lupus erythematosus (SLE), type 1 diabetes, Crohn's disease, thyroid disease, gluten-sensitive enteropathy, and multiple sclerosis, led to the identification of three new risk loci for DM, phospholipase

Table 5.2 Main non-HLA susceptibility factors for overall idiopathic inflammatory myopathies (IIM), dermatomyositis (DM), and polymyositis (PM)

Susceptibility locus	Chromosomic region	Phenotype	Population	Approach	Overlap with ADs	Study
YDJC/ UBE2L3	22q11.21	IIM	European	Immunochip	CeD, CD, JIA, MS, Ps, RA, SLE, UC	[12]
DGKQ	4p16.3	IIM	European	Immunochip	PBC, SJO	[12]
STAT4	2q32.2	IIM	European, Japanese	Immunochip, candidate-gene	CeD, CD, JIA, MS, PBC, RA, SLE, T1D, UC, SSc, SJO	[12, 40]
MGAT4A	2q11.2	IIM	European	Immunochip	–	[12]
PRR5L/ TRAF6	11p12	IIM	European	Immunochip	RA	[12]
CCL17	16q21	IIM	European	Immunochip	–	[12]
EOMES	3p24.1	IIM	European	Immunochip	MS, RA	[12]
CD28	2q33.2	IIM	European	Immunochip	CeD, RA, T1D	[12]
RPL31P10	12p13.31	IIM	European	Immunochip	–	[12]
BLK	8p23.1	DM/PM	European, Chinese, Japanese	GWAS, Immunochip, candidate-gene	RA, SLE, SSC, SJO	[12, 20, 23, 24]
CCL21	9p13.3	DM/PM	European, Chinese	GWAS, Candidate-gene	RA	[20, 25].
TNFAIP3	6q23.3	DM/PM	Chinese	Candidate-gene	CeD, CD, MS, PBC, Ps, RA, SLE, T1D, UC, SSc, SJO	[42]
IRF5	7q32.1	DM/PM	Chinese	Candidate-gene	CD, PBC, RA, SLE, UC, SSc, SJO	[42]
PLCL1	2q33.1	DM	European, Chinese	GWAS, Candidate-gene	CD, UC	[20, 22]
TYK2	19p13.2	DM	European	GWAS follow-up study	AS, CeD, CD, JIA, MS, PBC, Ps, RA, SLE, T1D, UC	[31]
CPN1	10q24.2	DM	Chinese	GWAS	–	[21]
PIP	7q34	DM	Chinese	GWAS	–	[21]

Table 5.2 (continued)

Susceptibility locus	Chromosomic region	Phenotype	Population	Approach	Overlap with ADs	Study
PTPN22	**1p13.2**	**PM**	**European**	**Candidate-gene, Immunochip**	**CD, JIA, RA, SLE, T1D, UC, SSc**	[38, 12]
LOC728073/ RPL38	17q25.1	PM	European	Immunochip	–	[12]
UBE3B/ MMAB	12q24.11	PM	European	Immunochip	–	[12]
NAB1	2q32.2	PM	European	Immunochip	PBC	[12]
IL18R1	2q12.1	PM	European	Immunochip	CeD, CD, PBC, UC	[12]
SLC26A1/ IDUA	4p16.3	PM	European	Immunochip	PBC	[12]
RGS1	1q31.2	PM	European	Immunochip	CeD, MS, T1D	[12]
ROPN1L/ ANKRD33B	5p15.2	DM+JDM	European	Immunochip	–	[12]
PTTG1/ ATP10B	5q33.3	DM+JDM	European	Immunochip	SLE, SJO	[12]
GSDMB	17q21.1	DM+JDM	European	Immunochip	CD, MS, PBC, RA, SLE, T1D, UC	[12]
WDFY4	10q11.23	CADM	Japanese	GWAS	RA, SLE	[19]

IIM idiopathic inflammatory myopathies, *DM* dermatomyositis, *PM* polymyositis, *JDM* juvenile dermatomyositis, *CADM* clinically amyopathic dermatomyositis, *GWAS* genome-wide association study, *ADs* autoimmune diseases, *AS* ankylosing spondylitis, *CeD* celiac disease, *CD* Crohn disease, *JIA* juvenile idiopathic arthritis, *MS* multiple sclerosis, *PBC* primary biliary cirrhosis, *Ps* psoriasis, *RA* rheumatoid arthritis, *SLE* systemic lupus erythematosus, *T1D* type 1 diabetes, *UC* ulcerative colitis, *SSc* systemic sclerosis, *SJO* Sjögren syndrome
Loci associated at the genome-wide significance level are indicated in bold

C like 1 (*PLCL1*), B lymphoid tyrosine kinase (*BLK*), and chemokine (C-C motif) ligand 21 (*CCL21*). Subsequently, candidate-gene studies performed in Asian population confirmed the association between *PLCL1* and DM [22] and described associations between *BLK* and *CCL21* and other myositis subgroups, specifically *BLK* was associated with DM and PM in Japanese and Chinese patients [23, 24], and *CCL21* was associated with PM in a Chinese cohort [25].

PLCL1 encodes a protein involved in an inositol phospholipid-based intracellular signaling cascade. Although its exact role in the pathogenesis of DM is not clear, this protein acts as a component in the phospho-dependent endocytosis process of GABA A receptor and regulates the turnover of receptors, thus contributing to the maintenance of the muscle tone [26]. *BLK* encodes a tyrosine kinase of the src family of proto-oncogenes which is involved in B-cell receptor signaling and B-cell development. Several lines of evidence support a key role of B lymphocytes in IIM, such as the presence of this cell type in DM skin and muscle biopsies [27], the existence of disease-specific autoantibodies [1], and the efficacy of anti-B-cell therapies [28]. Interestingly, the most strongly associated polymorphism in the genome-wide scan was in high LD with a genetic variant reported to downregulate both *BLK* mRNA and protein expression in naïve B cells [29]. Regarding *CCL21*, this gene encodes a protein that inhibits hemopoiesis and stimulates chemotaxis for thymocytes and activated T cells. In addition, this cytokine plays a role in mediating homing of lymphocytes to secondary lymphoid organs and acts as a high-affinity ligand for chemokine receptor 7 that is expressed on T and B cells [30].

Since this first GWAS revealed the existence of genetic overlap between DM and other autoimmune diseases, a follow-up study to test association between IIM (adult and juvenile DM and PM) and immune-related variants not captured through the DM GWAS was subsequently performed [31]. Using this candidate-gene association approach, tyrosine kinase 2 (*TYK2*) was identified as a new genetic risk *locus* for DM. *TYK2* encodes a member of the Janus kinases (JAKs) protein family with a crucial role in interleukin and IFN signaling [32].

In 2015, the MYOGEN Consortium published another GWAS including 1710 IIM cases and 4724 controls of European origin, which represented the first genome-wide scan in PM and myositis patients with anti-Jo-1 autoantibodies [10]. As mentioned above, this study confirmed the association between the 8.1 AH and IIM and identified specific HLA associations with the different IIM subgroups. Nevertheless, although the number of patients was increased with respect to the first GWAS, no genetic signals at the genome-wide level of significance were observed outside the HLA region.

Two large-scale genotyping studies in IIM patients of non-European origin have also been recently published. In 2016, a GWAS performed in 127 patients with DM and 1566 healthy controls from Han Chinese population identified two non-HLA signals that almost reached genome-wide significance [21]. These signals mapped on the prolactin-induced protein (*PIP*) and cytochrome P450 family 11 subfamily B member 1 (*CPN1*) *loci*. PIP has been shown to bind to CD4, a T-cell co-receptor molecule with a crucial role in activation of Th cells [33, 34], whereas the *CPN1* gene encodes a member of the cytochrome P450 superfamily of enzymes involved in de novo synthesis of glucocorticoids, essential regulators of T-cell development and function [35]. On the other hand, this GWAS failed to replicate previously reported IIM associations in Han Chinese population, including those described at the *PLCL1*, *BLK*, and *CCL21 loci*. However, these results should be taken with caution, considering the limited sample size of this study.

Finally, 576 IIM cases, including PM, DM, and clinically amyopathic DM (CADM), and 6270 controls from Japan were analyzed in a very recent GWAS by Kochi and colleagues [19]. No significant association signals for IIM, PM, or DM patients were found. However, when CADM patients were evaluated independently, an intronic variant within the WDFY family member 4 (*WDFY4*) gene appeared to be associated with this specific subgroup. *WDFY4* encodes a protein expressed in dendritic cells, neutrophils, B cells, and macrophages, and it has been previously identified as a susceptibility *locus* for RA [36] and SLE [37].

5.3.2.2 Findings from the Immunochip Approach

In 2016, the Immunochip platform was used to analyzed the largest cohort of IIM patients to date, including 2566 cases with DM, JDM, PM, and IBM and 15,651 controls of Caucasian descent [12]. Protein tyrosine phosphatase, non-receptor type 22 (*PTPN22*) was identified as a genetic risk factor for IIM, representing the only association at genome-wide level of significance in myositis thus far. Although an association between *PTPN22* and IIM was detected in the overall analysis, stratification by clinical subgroups revealed that this signal was mainly driven by the PM subset. A role of this gene in PM predisposition was previously reported in a candidate-gene association study including 381 British patients with adult or juvenile IIM [38], which overlapped with part of the samples included in the Immunochip study. *PTPN22* encodes a tyrosine phosphatase known as LYP that is involved in several signaling pathways associated with the immune response, including the T-cell receptor (TCR) pathway and the humoral activity of B cells. The PM-associated SNP (rs2476601) has been implicated in several autoimmune diseases, representing the clearest example of common genetic risk factor in autoimmunity. This SNP is a functional variant that results in a non-synonymous arginine (R) to tryptophan (W) amino acid change at position 620. Although its functional consequences have not been clearly elucidated yet, it has been reported that humans carrying the rs2476601 risk allele displayed enhanced B lymphocyte autoreactivity, deregulated TCR signaling, and reduced capacity for TLR-induced type 1 IFN production [39].

Furthermore, nine suggestive associations within the *YDJC/UBE2L3*, *DGKQ*, *STAT4*, *MGAT4A*, *PRR5L/TRAF6*, *CCL17*, *EOMES*, *CD28*, and *RPL31P10 loci* were also identified through the Immunochip approach [12]. Notably, the association between *STAT4* (signal transducer and activator of transcription 4) and IIM was described in a previous candidate-gene association study performed in Japanese population [40], supporting the implication of this gene in the myositis susceptibility. The protein encoded by *STAT4* is a member of the STAT family of transcription factors, which is crucial for mediating responses to interleukin-12, interleukin-23, and type 1 IFNs and regulating the differentiation of T helper cells into the Th1 and Th17 lineages [41].

Finally, specific non-HLA associations with the PM and DM/JDM subgroups were identified for seven (*LOC728073/RPL38*, *UBE3B/MMAB*, *NAB1*, *BLK*, *IL18R1*, *SLC26A1/IDUA*, *RGS1*) and three (*ROPN1L/ANKRD33B*, *PTTG1/ATP10B*, *GSDMB*) *loci*, respectively [12]. Although these signals did not reach genome-wide significance, this finding points to the existence of genetic differences between clinical subgroups.

During the last years, polymorphisms at common susceptibility *loci* in autoimmunity, such as *TNFAIP3*, *IRF5*, *IFNG*, *IL1*, or *TNF*, have been implicated in the IIM susceptibility by candidate-gene association studies [42–44]. However, no SNPs within these regions showed evidence of association with IIM in the Immunochip study, even though this platform is designed for dense genotyping of immune-related loci. This seems to indicate that they could be false-positive associations, mainly taking into account the low statistical power of these genetic studies. However, considering that some of these signals, such as those located within the *TNFAIP3* and *IRF5 loci* [42], were detected in non-European population, they may represent population-specific associations, and, therefore, a role in the IIM susceptibility cannot be discarded.

5.4 Biological Insights from GWAS and Immunochip Associations

Over the last few years, the translation of GWAS/Immunochip findings into biological implications has been challenging, mainly due to the difficulty of identifying causal variants as well as by the fact that most of the disease-associated SNPs are located in noncoding regions. Nevertheless, substantial effort has been recently directed toward the functional characterization of the large amount of genetic data generated by large-scale scans. In this line, different in silico approaches have been developed to understand biological meaning behind GWAS and Immunochip findings. These methods are usually based on the search for overrepresentation of disease-associated genes in protein-protein interaction networks or specific biological pathways, as well as for overlapping of associated variants with regulatory elements, such as DNase I hypersensitive sites, histone modifications associated with active promoters/enhancers, transcription factor-binding sites (TFBSs), or expression quantitative trait *loci* (eQTL), among others.

A number of approaches have been conducted to characterize the biological functions connected to myositis susceptibility. A first application of network-based methods in the context of IIM was reported in 2016. Following the Immunochip study, Parkes and colleagues conducted protein-protein interaction (PPI) and pathway enrichment analyses using both proteins encoded by genes associated with IIM (significant and suggestive signals) and autoantibody targets, in order to identify molecular mechanisms involved in myositis [45]. PPI analysis identified several genes, including *TRAF6*, *HSPA1A/B*, *UBE3B*, and *PSMD3*, as potentially relevant for IIM. TRAF6 (TNF receptor-associated factor 6) acted as a hub protein interacting with both autoantibody targets and IIM-associated proteins. This protein is a member of the TNF receptor-associated factor (TRAF) protein family that is involved in the development, homeostasis, and/or activation of B cells, T cells, macrophages, and dendritic cells, as well as in the organogenesis of thymic and secondary lymphoid tissues [46]. In addition, TRAF6 function is crucial for both a proper activation of the immune response and the maintenance of immune tolerance [46]. Remarkably, a pivotal role of TRAF6 in homeostasis of satellite cells, a stem cell population responsible for myofiber regeneration upon injury, has been recently described [47]. On the other hand, the remaining four genes identified in the PPI analysis encode proteins related to the ubiquitin proteasome pathway (UPP). Furthermore, pathway enrichment analysis evidenced ubiquitination as a relevant mechanism in IIM. It has been proposed that ER stress activates downstream UPPs in myositis, thus activating NF-kB, which leads to upregulation of MHC class I, production of pro-inflammatory cytokines, and suppression of myoblast differentiation [6]. Consequently, UPP inhibition has been proposed as a potential therapeutic target for myositis [48].

On the other hand, Kochi and colleagues performed in silico analyses using both publicly available datasets and in vitro studies to examine the causal mechanism of the CADM-associated variant in the Japanese GWAS [19]. First, an eQTL analysis using data from the Geuvadis project showed that the *WDFY4* SNP acted as a splicing QTL for a truncated *WDFY4* isoform in lymphoblastoid B cells [19]. In addition, using trans-eQTL and weighted parametric gene set analyses, the authors determined that the associated variant correlated with an increase expression of NF-κB associated genes, such as *TYK2* and *PTPN6*. They also demonstrated that the truncated isoform interacted with several pattern recognition receptors, especially MDA5, thus increasing NF-κB activation and apoptosis [19]. This finding is consistent with the presence of anti-MDA5 autoantibodies characteristic of patients with CADM [49] and suggests a role of both inflammatory signals and apoptosis in the pathogenesis of this condition.

5.5 Epigenetics Studies in DM/PM

Although the etiology of DM/PM is still unknown, it has become clear that both genetic and environmental factors may interact in the pathophysiology of these disorders. Epigenetic mechanisms, which include DNA methylation, histone modifications, nucleosome positioning, and noncoding RNA regulation, among others, represent the link between environmental triggers and genetic modulation. In this regard, several epigenetic studies have been conducted in PM and DM so far.

Genome-wide methylation profile of muscle biopsies from 20 JDM patients and four controls identified 27 genes differentially methylated, which allowed to distinguish cases from controls using supervised hierarchical clustering [50]. The set of differentially methylated genes was enriched in transcription factors and cell cycle regulators, including homeobox and *WT1* genes. These results were subsequently confirmed by pyrosequencing in patients with JPM and other IIM. Considering these findings, Wang and colleagues proposed that children with IIM may have an enhanced ability to self-renewal of damaged muscles and that this repair process would be facilitated through epigenetic modifications of homeobox and *WT1* genes [50].

Moreover, increased levels of a group of microRNAs (miRNAs) known as myomiRs, including miR-1, miR-133a/b, miR-206, miR-208, miR-208b, miR-486, and miR-499, were found in skeletal and cardiac muscle [51]. These muscle-specific miRNAs regulate diverse aspects of muscle function, and, therefore, they could be involved in muscle diseases. Indeed, a high number of miRNAs have been found to be deregulated in IIM.

Specifically, using array technology, Eisenberg and colleagues identified a high number of miRNAs deregulated in ten major muscular disorders, including DM and PM [52]. Specifically, they detected 37 miRNAs upregulated and 1 downregulated in PM patients and 35 miRNAs upregulated and 2 downregulated in DM. The set of miRNAs deregulated in patients with DM was enriched in pathways related to the immune response [52]. In addition, five miRNAs, miR-146b, miR-155, miR-214, miR-221, and miR-222, were consistently deregulated across all the muscle diseases analyzed, indicating a common regulatory mechanism for all of them [52]. Remarkably, miR-146b and miR-155 play key roles in the immune system [53]. Moreover, these two miRNAs, together with miR-146a (also involved in innate immunity [53]), miR-21, miR-432, and miR-378, were also overexpressed in muscle biopsies from myositis patients in two subsequent studies [54, 55], supporting their role in IIM.

On the other hand, a decreased expression of several miRNAs known to be absolutely critical for adult muscle differentiation and maintenance, specifically miR-1, miR-133a, miR-133b, and miR-206, has been detected in muscle biopsy samples from patients with myositis [54, 55].

Finally, long noncoding RNAs (lncRNAs) have also been implicated in IIM. A transcriptomic profiling of lncRNAs performed in muscle tissue identified 1198 lncRNAs deregulated (322 upregulated and 876 downregulated) in DM patients compared with controls [56]. Then, by constructing mRNA-lncRNA co-expression networks, they predicted the target genes of the differentially expressed lncRNAs. Interestingly, a lncRNA named linc-DGCR6-1 appeared to target USP18, a type 1 IFN-inducible protein considered as a key regulator of IFN signaling. In addition, an upregulated expression of USP18 protein was observed in perifascicular atrophy myofibers of DM patients using immunohistochemistry staining [56].

5.6 Conclusions

The past decade has seen a huge advance in the identification of genetic factors that predispose individuals to complex diseases, largely thanks to the development of high-throughput genotyping platforms such as GWAS and Immunochip. IIM have benefited from that genome-wide era, which has led to the discovery of several consistent genetic risk *loci*. However, despite the international collaborative efforts carried out, genetic studies conducted in IIM were still underpowered to detect variants with moderate effects, and only genome-wide associations at the *HLA* and *PTPN22 loci* have been identified thus far. In addition, the existence of genetic heterogeneity among the different myositis subgroups has probably also been an obstacle to the identification of robust susceptibility signals. Therefore, further genetic studies in larger and more homogeneous cohorts would definitively improve the consistency of the results, thus providing information on the missing heritability of IIM. In addition, the identification of the functional implications and mechanisms of the associated genetic *loci* will be critical to translate genetic findings into medical practice.

On the other hand, recent studies have shown that epigenetic regulation also plays a pivotal role in the IIM pathogenesis; this seems to indicate that certain environmental factors would trigger epigenetic modifications in genetically susceptible individuals, who would develop myositis. Integration of genetics and epigenetics has emerged as a useful approach to unravel the mechanisms behind complex diseases. Thus, a better understanding of the interplay between both factors will allow to obtain a clearer picture of the molecular network involved in the IIM pathogenesis.

References

1. Rider LG, Miller FW. Deciphering the clinical presentations, pathogenesis, and treatment of the idiopathic inflammatory myopathies. JAMA. 2011;305(2):183–90. https://doi.org/10.1001/jama.2010.1977.
2. Ginn LR, Lin JP, Plotz PH, Bale SJ, Wilder RL, Mbauya A, et al. Familial autoimmunity in pedigrees of idiopathic inflammatory myopathy patients suggests common genetic risk factors for many autoimmune diseases. Arthritis Rheum. 1998;41(3):400–5. https://doi.org/10.1002/1529-0131(199803)41:3<400::AID-ART4>3.0.CO;2-5.
3. Niewold TB, Wu SC, Smith M, Morgan GA, Pachman LM. Familial aggregation of autoimmune disease in juvenile dermatomyositis. Pediatrics. 2011;127(5):e1239–46. https://doi.org/10.1542/peds.2010-3022.
4. Dalakas MC. Inflammatory muscle diseases. N Engl J Med. 2015;373(4):393–4. https://doi.org/10.1056/NEJMc1506827.
5. de Padilla CM, Reed AM. Dendritic cells and the immunopathogenesis of idiopathic inflammatory myopathies. Curr Opin Rheumatol. 2008;20(6):669–74. https://doi.org/10.1097/BOR.0b013e3283157538.
6. Nagaraju K, Casciola-Rosen L, Lundberg I, Rawat R, Cutting S, Thapliyal R, et al. Activation of the endoplasmic reticulum stress response in autoimmune myositis: potential role in muscle fiber damage and dysfunction. Arthritis Rheum. 2005;52(6):1824–35. https://doi.org/10.1002/art.21103.
7. Cappelletti C, Galbardi B, Kapetis D, Vattemi G, Guglielmi V, Tonin P, et al. Autophagy, inflammation and innate immunity in inflammatory myopathies. PLoS One. 2014;9(11):e111490. https://doi.org/10.1371/journal.pone.0111490.
8. Visscher PM, Wray NR, Zhang Q, Sklar P, McCarthy MI, Brown MA, et al. 10 Years of GWAS discovery: biology, function, and translation. Am J Hum Genet. 2017;101(1):5–22. https://doi.org/10.1016/j.ajhg.2017.06.005.
9. Cortes A, Brown MA. Promise and pitfalls of the Immunochip. Arthritis Res Ther. 2011;13(1):101. https://doi.org/10.1186/ar3204.
10. Miller FW, Chen W, O'Hanlon TP, Cooper RG, Vencovsky J, Rider LG, et al. Genome-wide association study identifies HLA 8.1 ancestral haplotype alleles as major genetic risk factors for myositis phenotypes. Genes Immun. 2015;16(7):470–80. https://doi.org/10.1038/gene.2015.28.
11. O'Hanlon TP, Carrick DM, Targoff IN, Arnett FC, Reveille JD, Carrington M, et al. Immunogenetic risk and protective factors for the idiopathic inflammatory myopathies: distinct HLA-A, -B, -Cw, -DRB1, and -DQA1 allelic profiles distinguish European American patients with different myositis autoantibodies. Medicine. 2006;85(2):111–27. https://doi.org/10.1097/01.md.0000217525.82287.eb.
12. Rothwell S, Cooper RG, Lundberg IE, Miller FW, Gregersen PK, Bowes J, et al. Dense genotyping of immune-related loci in idiopathic inflammatory myopathies confirms HLA alleles as the strongest genetic risk factor and suggests different genetic background for major clinical subgroups. Ann Rheum Dis. 2016;75(8):1558–66. https://doi.org/10.1136/annrheumdis-2015-208119.
13. Ban Y, Davies TF, Greenberg DA, Concepcion ES, Osman R, Oashi T, et al. Arginine at position 74 of the HLA-DR beta1 chain is associated with Graves' disease. Genes Immun. 2004;5(3):203–8. https://doi.org/10.1038/sj.gene.6364059.
14. Menconi F, Monti MC, Greenberg DA, Oashi T, Osman R, Davies TF, et al. Molecular amino acid signatures in the MHC class II peptide-binding pocket predispose to autoimmune

thyroiditis in humans and in mice. Proc Natl Acad Sci U S A. 2008;105(37):14034–9. https://doi.org/10.1073/pnas.0806584105.
15. Gao X, Han L, Yuan L, Yang Y, Gou G, Sun H, et al. HLA class II alleles may influence susceptibility to adult dermatomyositis and polymyositis in a Han Chinese population. BMC Dermatol. 2014;14:9. https://doi.org/10.1186/1471-5945-14-9.
16. Furuya T, Hakoda M, Tsuchiya N, Kotake S, Ichikawa N, Nanke Y, et al. Immunogenetic features in 120 Japanese patients with idiopathic inflammatory myopathy. J Rheumatol. 2004;31(9):1768–74.
17. O'Hanlon TP, Rider LG, Mamyrova G, Targoff IN, Arnett FC, Reveille JD, et al. HLA polymorphisms in African Americans with idiopathic inflammatory myopathy: allelic profiles distinguish patients with different clinical phenotypes and myositis autoantibodies. Arthritis Rheum. 2006;54(11):3670–81. https://doi.org/10.1002/art.22205.
18. Lintner KE, Patwardhan A, Rider LG, Abdul-Aziz R, Wu YL, Lundstrom E, et al. Gene copy-number variations (CNVs) of complement C4 and C4A deficiency in genetic risk and pathogenesis of juvenile dermatomyositis. Ann Rheum Dis. 2016;75(9):1599–606. https://doi.org/10.1136/annrheumdis-2015-207762.
19. Kochi Y, Kamatani Y, Kondo Y, Suzuki A, Kawakami E, Hiwa R, et al. Splicing variant of WDFY4 augments MDA5 signalling and the risk of clinically amyopathic dermatomyositis. Ann Rheum Dis. 2018;77(4):602–11. https://doi.org/10.1136/annrheumdis-2017-212149.
20. Miller FW, Cooper RG, Vencovsky J, Rider LG, Danko K, Wedderburn LR, et al. Genome-wide association study of dermatomyositis reveals genetic overlap with other autoimmune disorders. Arthritis Rheum. 2013;65(12):3239–47. https://doi.org/10.1002/art.38137.
21. Zhang CE, Li Y, Wang ZX, Gao JP, Zhang XG, Zuo XB, et al. Variation at HLA-DPB1 is associated with dermatomyositis in Chinese population. J Dermatol. 2016;43(11):1307–13. https://doi.org/10.1111/1346-8138.13397.
22. Wang Q, Chen S, Li Y, Li P, Wu C, Wu Z, et al. Positive association of genetic variations in the phospholipase C-like 1 gene with dermatomyositis in Chinese Han. Immunol Res. 2016;64(1):204–12. https://doi.org/10.1007/s12026-015-8738-x.
23. Chen S, Wu W, Li J, Wang Q, Li Y, Wu Z, et al. Single nucleotide polymorphisms in the FAM167A-BLK gene are associated with polymyositis/dermatomyositis in the Han Chinese population. Immunol Res. 2015;62(2):153–62. https://doi.org/10.1007/s12026-015-8646-0.
24. Sugiura T, Kawaguchi Y, Goto K, Hayashi Y, Gono T, Furuya T, et al. Association between a C8orf13-BLK polymorphism and polymyositis/dermatomyositis in the Japanese population: an additive effect with STAT4 on disease susceptibility. PLoS One. 2014;9(3):e90019. https://doi.org/10.1371/journal.pone.0090019.
25. Chen S, Wang Q, Wu CY, Wu QJ, Li Y, Wu ZY, et al. A single-nucleotide polymorphism of CCL21 rs951005 T>C is associated with susceptibility of polymyositis and such patients with interstitial lung disease in a Chinese Han population. Clin Exp Rheumatol. 2015;33(5):639–46.
26. Watanabe M, Maemura K, Kanbara K, Tamayama T, Hayasaki H. GABA and GABA receptors in the central nervous system and other organs. Int Rev Cytol. 2002;213:1–47.
27. Nagaraju K, Lundberg IE. Polymyositis and dermatomyositis: pathophysiology. Rheum Dis Clin North Am. 2011;37(2):159–71., v. https://doi.org/10.1016/j.rdc.2011.01.002.
28. Fasano S, Gordon P, Hajji R, Loyo E, Isenberg DA. Rituximab in the treatment of inflammatory myopathies: a review. Rheumatology (Oxford). 2017;56(1):26–36. https://doi.org/10.1093/rheumatology/kew146.
29. Simpfendorfer KR, Olsson LM, Manjarrez Orduno N, Khalili H, Simeone AM, Katz MS, et al. The autoimmunity-associated BLK haplotype exhibits cis-regulatory effects on mRNA and protein expression that are prominently observed in B cells early in development. Hum Mol Genet. 2012;21(17):3918–25. https://doi.org/10.1093/hmg/dds220.
30. Hauser MA, Legler DF. Common and biased signaling pathways of the chemokine receptor CCR7 elicited by its ligands CCL19 and CCL21 in leukocytes. J Leukoc Biol. 2016;99(6):869–82. https://doi.org/10.1189/jlb.2MR0815-380R.

31. Jani M, Massey J, Wedderburn LR, Vencovsky J, Danko K, Lundberg IE, et al. Genotyping of immune-related genetic variants identifies TYK2 as a novel associated locus for idiopathic inflammatory myopathies. Ann Rheum Dis. 2014;73(9):1750–2. https://doi.org/10.1136/annrheumdis-2014-205440.
32. Ghoreschi K, Laurence A, O'Shea JJ. Janus kinases in immune cell signaling. Immunol Rev. 2009;228(1):273–87. https://doi.org/10.1111/j.1600-065X.2008.00754.x.
33. Autiero M, Cammarota G, Friedlein A, Zulauf M, Chiappetta G, Dragone V, et al. A 17-kDa CD4-binding glycoprotein present in human seminal plasma and in breast tumor cells. Eur J Immunol. 1995;25(5):1461–4. https://doi.org/10.1002/eji.1830250550.
34. Autiero M, Gaubin M, Mani JC, Castejon C, Martin M, el Marhomy S, et al. Surface plasmon resonance analysis of gp17, a natural CD4 ligand from human seminal plasma inhibiting human immunodeficiency virus type-1 gp120-mediated syncytium formation. Eur J Biochem. 1997;245(1):208–13.
35. Baschant U, Tuckermann J. The role of the glucocorticoid receptor in inflammation and immunity. J Steroid Biochem Mol Biol. 2010;120(2–3):69–75. https://doi.org/10.1016/j.jsbmb.2010.03.058.
36. Okada Y, Wu D, Trynka G, Raj T, Terao C, Ikari K, et al. Genetics of rheumatoid arthritis contributes to biology and drug discovery. Nature. 2014;506(7488):376–81. https://doi.org/10.1038/nature12873.
37. Yang W, Shen N, Ye DQ, Liu Q, Zhang Y, Qian XX, et al. Genome-wide association study in Asian populations identifies variants in ETS1 and WDFY4 associated with systemic lupus erythematosus. PLoS Genet. 2010;6(2):e1000841. https://doi.org/10.1371/journal.pgen.1000841.
38. Chinoy H, Platt H, Lamb JA, Betteridge Z, Gunawardena H, Fertig N, et al. The protein tyrosine phosphatase N22 gene is associated with juvenile and adult idiopathic inflammatory myopathy independent of the HLA 8.1 haplotype in British Caucasian patients. Arthritis Rheum. 2008;58(10):3247–54. https://doi.org/10.1002/art.23900.
39. Bottini N, Peterson EJ. Tyrosine phosphatase PTPN22: multifunctional regulator of immune signaling, development, and disease. Annu Rev Immunol. 2014;32:83–119. https://doi.org/10.1146/annurev-immunol-032713-120249.
40. Sugiura T, Kawaguchi Y, Goto K, Hayashi Y, Tsuburaya R, Furuya T, et al. Positive association between STAT4 polymorphisms and polymyositis/dermatomyositis in a Japanese population. Ann Rheum Dis. 2012;71(10):1646–50. https://doi.org/10.1136/annrheumdis-2011-200839.
41. Watford WT, Hissong BD, Bream JH, Kanno Y, Muul L, O'Shea JJ. Signaling by IL-12 and IL-23 and the immunoregulatory roles of STAT4. Immunol Rev. 2004;202:139–56. https://doi.org/10.1111/j.0105-2896.2004.00211.x.
42. Chen S, Wang Q, Wu Z, Li Y, Li P, Sun F, et al. Genetic association study of TNFAIP3, IFIH1, IRF5 polymorphisms with polymyositis/dermatomyositis in Chinese Han population. PLoS One. 2014;9(10):e110044. https://doi.org/10.1371/journal.pone.0110044.
43. Chinoy H, Salway F, John S, Fertig N, Tait BD, Oddis CV, et al. Interferon-gamma and interleukin-4 gene polymorphisms in Caucasian idiopathic inflammatory myopathy patients in UK. Ann Rheum Dis. 2007;66(7):970–3. https://doi.org/10.1136/ard.2006.068858.
44. Mamyrova G, O'Hanlon TP, Sillers L, Malley K, James-Newton L, Parks CG, et al. Cytokine gene polymorphisms as risk and severity factors for juvenile dermatomyositis. Arthritis Rheum. 2008;58(12):3941–50. https://doi.org/10.1002/art.24039.
45. Parkes JE, Rothwell S, Day PJ, McHugh NJ, Betteridge ZE, Cooper RG, et al. Systematic protein-protein interaction and pathway analyses in the idiopathic inflammatory myopathies. Arthritis Res Ther. 2016;18(1):156. https://doi.org/10.1186/s13075-016-1061-7.
46. Walsh MC, Lee J, Choi Y. Tumor necrosis factor receptor- associated factor 6 (TRAF6) regulation of development, function, and homeostasis of the immune system. Immunol Rev. 2015;266(1):72–92. https://doi.org/10.1111/imr.12302.
47. Hindi SM, Kumar A. TRAF6 regulates satellite stem cell self-renewal and function during regenerative myogenesis. J Clin Invest. 2016;126(1):151–68. https://doi.org/10.1172/JCI81655.

48. Rayavarapu S, Coley W, Van der Meulen JH, Cakir E, Tappeta K, Kinder TB, et al. Activation of the ubiquitin proteasome pathway in a mouse model of inflammatory myopathy: a potential therapeutic target. Arthritis Rheum. 2013;65(12):3248–58. https://doi.org/10.1002/art.38180.
49. Li L, Wang Q, Yang F, Wu C, Chen S, Wen X, et al. Anti-MDA5 antibody as a potential diagnostic and prognostic biomarker in patients with dermatomyositis. Oncotarget. 2017;8(16):26552–64. https://doi.org/10.18632/oncotarget.15716.
50. Wang M, Xie H, Shrestha S, Sredni S, Morgan GA, Pachman LM. Methylation alterations of WT1 and homeobox genes in inflamed muscle biopsy samples from patients with untreated juvenile dermatomyositis suggest self-renewal capacity. Arthritis Rheum. 2012;64(10):3478–85. https://doi.org/10.1002/art.34573.
51. van Rooij E, Liu N, Olson EN. MicroRNAs flex their muscles. Trends Genet. 2008;24(4):159–66. https://doi.org/10.1016/j.tig.2008.01.007.
52. Eisenberg I, Eran A, Nishino I, Moggio M, Lamperti C, Amato AA, et al. Distinctive patterns of microRNA expression in primary muscular disorders. Proc Natl Acad Sci U S A. 2007;104(43):17016–21. https://doi.org/10.1073/pnas.0708115104.
53. Saba R, Sorensen DL, Booth SA. MicroRNA-146a: A Dominant, Negative Regulator of the Innate Immune Response. Front Immunol. 2014;5:578. https://doi.org/10.3389/fimmu.2014.00578.
54. Georgantas RW, Streicher K, Greenberg SA, Greenlees LM, Zhu W, Brohawn PZ, et al. Inhibition of myogenic microRNAs 1, 133, and 206 by inflammatory cytokines links inflammation and muscle degeneration in adult inflammatory myopathies. Arthritis Rheumatol. 2014;66(4):1022–33. https://doi.org/10.1002/art.38292.
55. Zhu W, Streicher K, Shen N, Higgs BW, Morehouse C, Greenlees L, et al. Genomic signatures characterize leukocyte infiltration in myositis muscles. BMC Med Genomics. 2012;5:53. https://doi.org/10.1186/1755-8794-5-53.
56. Peng QL, Zhang YM, Yang HB, Shu XM, Lu X, Wang GC. Transcriptomic profiling of long non-coding RNAs in dermatomyositis by microarray analysis. Sci Rep. 2016;6:32818. https://doi.org/10.1038/srep32818.

ANCA-Associated Vasculitis

6

Francesco Bonatti, Alessia Adorni, Antonio Percesepe, Augusto Vaglio, and Davide Martorana

Contents

F. Bonatti
Department of Medicine and Surgery, University of Parma, Parma, Italy
e-mail: francesco.bonatti@unipr.it

A. Adorni
Hematology and Clinical Immunology, Department of Medicine, University of Perugia, Perugia, Italy
e-mail: alessia.adorni@unipg.it

A. Percesepe
Department of Medicine and Surgery, University of Parma, Parma, Italy

Unit of Medical Genetics, University Hospital of Parma, Parma, Italy
e-mail: antonio.percesepe@unipr.it

A. Vaglio (✉)
Nephrology Unit, Meyer Children's Hospital, Florence, Italy
e-mail: augusto.vaglio@meyer.it

D. Martorana
Unit of Medical Genetics, University Hospital of Parma, Parma, Italy
e-mail: dmartorana@ao.pr.it

J. Martín, F. D. Carmona (eds.), *Genetics of Rare Autoimmune Diseases*,
Rare Diseases of the Immune System, https://doi.org/10.1007/978-3-030-03934-9_6

6.1 Introduction

Vasculitis is a group of rare diseases that have in common inflammation of blood vessels. It is a multi-system inflammatory-autoimmune disease that affects both arteries and veins with consequent tissue damage, especially to the respiratory tract and the kidneys [1].

On the basis of the size of the affected vessel, small-, medium-, and large-vessel vasculitides are usually distinguished. Small-vessel vasculitides are characterized by necrotizing inflammation of the vessel wall, in particular small arteries, arterioles, capillaries, and venules; its association with circulating antineutrophil cytoplasmic antibody (ANCA) has led to these conditions being grouped together as ANCA-associated vasculitis (AAV) [2].

AAV has a worldwide reported annual incidence ranging from 1.2 to 2.0 cases per 100,000 individuals and a prevalence of 4.6–18.4 cases per 100,000 individuals [3].

AAV includes microscopic polyangiitis (MPA), granulomatosis with polyangiitis (GPA, formerly Wegener's granulomatosis), and eosinophilic granulomatosis with polyangiitis (EGPA, formerly Churg-Strauss syndrome) [2].

GPA and MPA partially overlap clinically and have been historically considered different forms of the same disease spectrum and therefore are frequently included together in clinical trials [4]. About 80–90% of individuals with GPA and MPA show ANCA positivity [5]; two types of ANCA are seen in AAV patients, perinuclear (P)-ANCA and cytoplasmic (C)-ANCA, usually tested using indirect immunofluorescence and then confirmed using ELISA [6].

GPA is usually associated with C-ANCA, directed against proteinase 3 (PR3), whereas MPA with P-ANCA, directed against myeloperoxidase (MPO), even if a significant overlap exists with regard to the ANCA status. Although ANCA results are often useful to confirm the diagnosis of AAV, PR3 or MPO-ANCA cannot be used to identify GPA versus MPA [7].

Although the etiopathogenesis of AAVs is not fully understood, they are considered complex diseases with a proposed role for environmental and infectious factors as well as dysregulation of the immune system [8].

The report of rare familial cases of AAV has drawn attention to the role of genetic factors in the pathogenesis of AAV, supporting the theory of a multifactorial nature of the disease [9–12].

In recent years, high-throughput technologies in the fields of genomics, transcriptomics, and proteomics for biomarker discovery have expanded enormously [13]. The identification of biomarkers linked to AAV would allow a better understanding of disease pathogenesis and risk factors; additionally, molecular biomarkers may be applied for diagnosis, prognosis, and selecting appropriate therapy [14]. Furthermore, the identification of genetic variants associated with AAV and their specific clinical features would allow a clearer classification with a potential impact on the management of the disease.

In this chapter, we summarize and discuss the results of genetic studies in AAV. We also present novel approaches aimed at identifying the causal variants in complex susceptibility loci. Finally, we discuss the limitations of current methods and the challenges that we still have to face in order to incorporate genomic data into clinical practice.

6.2 Molecular Genetics Approaches to Complex Traits

Genetic research in AAV has mainly focused on association studies between genetic variants, such as single-nucleotide polymorphisms (SNPs) and copy number variations (CNVs), and the risk of developing the disease [15]. SNPs and CNV are variants located both in coding and noncoding regions that may directly impact on gene function and gene expression; in fact, differences in allele or genotype frequencies between patients and controls may suggest an association with a specific disease.

The first studies investigated candidate-gene variants using a case-control approach. These studies explore the possible association between the disease and one or a small number of genes, usually highlighted by earlier studies or because they are considered of potential biological interest [16].

The development of new generation molecular analysis methods dramatically lowered the costs and analysis time, allowing the screening of many genes in the same experiment, identifying a large number of disease-associated variants [17]. The main tool used for this purpose is genome-wide association study (GWAS). GWAS routinely assays SNPs tagging 90% of the human genome [18]. This approach is highly informative; however, to avoid spurious associations, a very high level of statistical significance ($p < 5 \times 10^{-8}$) is required. The number of identified associations is in fact proportional to the cohort size, and therefore the larger the study, the higher the probability of obtaining useful information [19]. In order to reduce the risk of associations identified by chance, a correction is strongly suggested (i.e., Bonferroni's multiple test correction) [20]. Such studies need large numbers of cases and controls to avoid missing potential associations due to underpowered cohorts, and generally, in the field of rare diseases, this requires a multicenter approach. Furthermore, in both candidate-gene studies and GWAS, replication of the findings in an independent cohort of subjects is essential in order to avoid spurious findings [21].

Another case-control approach is based on the use of chips exploring a large set of SNPs identified a priori as of potential interest. The main example in the field of rare immunological diseases is the *Immunoarray*, which investigates about 200,000 genetic variants, including SNPs and small CNVs previously found as associated with autoimmune and inflammatory diseases, including a dense coverage of the HLA variants [22]. An advantage of this approach is a relatively lower cost compared to conventional GWAS chips; furthermore, Immunoarray is a feasible and economically sustainable tool able to provide useful information probably more meaningful than candidate-gene approach studies but yet lacking the wide exploratory nature of the ones provided by GWASs.

In the near future, other genomic approaches may be performed in the study of rare diseases, such as whole-exome/whole-genome sequencing; these tools are not yet routinely employed in complex diseases, but may have a big potential especially in the investigation of familial cases or clusters of extreme phenotypes [23].

6.3 Genetics of GPA and MPA

6.3.1 Candidate-Gene Approach: The Pre-GWAS Era

6.3.1.1 Associations with the HLA

The hypothesis of an autoimmune nature of AAV drove attention to the role of the HLA as a potential risk factor for AAV [24]. The HLA locus maps on chromosome 6 (6p21–31) and contains more than 200 genes divided in 3 classes, HLA class I (A, B, C), class II (DR, DQ, and DP), and class III [25]. The HLA locus is characterized by high polymorphism and CNV, and its study is quite complex due to the presence of strong linkage disequilibrium across the genes [26].

In 2004, a study investigating a cohort of 150 Northern German patients with GPA was performed, reporting an association with the *HLA-DP* locus [27]. In particular, the *DPB1**0401 allele is strongly associated with the risk of developing GPA with the extended *DPB1*0401/RXRB03* haplotype, found to be even more significantly associated ($p = 7.13 \times 10^{-17}$; OR: 6.41). This finding was then replicated in 282 German patients, and the association was more striking when the analysis was restricted to the ANCA-positive subgroup ($p = 1.26 \times 10^{-22}$).

In a Dutch cohort of 304 AAV patients, an association with *HLA-DR4* has been reported ($p < 0.0001$; OR: 1.7), and the association was more striking considering only GPA patients. Finally, two recent studies showed association of AAV with *HLA-DRB1* in African American [28] and Chinese [29] populations; interestingly, a different genetic background emerged for the PR3-ANCA-positive subgroup in both studies.

6.3.1.2 Non-HLA Associations

Outside of HLA locus, few genetic risk factors for AAV have been proposed, such as the protein tyrosine phosphatase N22 (PTPN22) and the cytotoxic T-lymphocyte antigen 4 (CTLA4); furthermore, more recent studies highlighted an association with toll-like receptor 9 (TLR9).

The *PTPN22* gene (1p13.2) encodes for lymphoid tyrosine phosphatase (Lyp) which may be aberrant in the form encoded by the genetic variant associated with autoimmunity; it can cause abnormal regulatory T-cell (T_{reg}) activity, increased humoral activity, and enhanced neutrophil function [30]. *PTPN22* SNPs were found to be associated with several autoimmune diseases, including type 1 diabetes, rheumatoid arthritis (RA), and systemic lupus erythematosus (SLE) [31–33]. The proposed mechanism of action is that an alteration of the interaction of Lyp with a protein kinase involved in T-cell receptor activation leads to abnormal CD4 Treg function and increased humoral activity [34]. In 2005, an association was demonstrated between the *PTPN22* 620W polymorphism (rs2476601) and GPA in a cohort of 199 German patients: the SNP was significantly increased in GPA ($p = 0.002$; OR:1.75), with a stronger association documented in the ANCA-positive subgroup ($p = 0.0002$; OR 2.01) [35]. This finding was then confirmed in an independent cohort of 641 British GPA and MPA patients and 344 Italian AAV cases [36, 37].

The *CTLA4* gene (2q33) encodes for a protein that functions as a T-cell inhibitor, competing with the co-stimulatory protein CD28 for the binding of CD80/CD86 [38]. Several studies highlighted associations between different *CTLA4* SNPs and AAV, suggesting a role for this molecule in AAV pathogenesis. In a study performed in 2002, an association was found between a SNP in the promoter region of the *CTLA4* gene (at position -318) and GPA [39]. Furthermore, CTLA4 has also been explored as potential therapeutic target in a pilot trial of patients with non-severe GPA treated with abatacept, a monoclonal antibody including the binding region of CTLA4, with good results in terms of safety and disease response [40].

TLR genes encode for the toll-like receptor (TLR) family, a group of proteins able to recognize microbiological structures and activating the innate immune response [41].

TLRs are usually overexpressed during infections and provide a potential link between infections and the pathogenesis and development of AAV. TLR9 stimulation in ex vivo neutrophils was associated with increased MPO release and PR3 surface expression; moreover, degranulation was induced after stimulation with PR3-ANCA in neutrophils primed by TLR9 ligand [42].

In order to investigate the genetic contribution of TLR9 on the susceptibility of AAV, four SNPs in *TLR9* have been genotyped in 863 German AAV cases and 1344 controls. In the replication analysis, significant results were investigated in a cohort of 426 Dutch and British AAV cases. Interestingly, in GPA patients, the association with genotypes and haplotypes was predisposing (OR > 1), while in MPA it was protective (OR < 1). When cases were stratified according to ANCA status rather than to clinical entity, the results showed a strong overall difference in TLR9 allele/haplotype frequencies between PR3-ANCA and MPO-ANCA cases [43]. Table 6.1 summarizes the genes reported as associated with GPA and/or MPA.

Table 6.1 Genes associated with the risk of developing AAV

Gene	Disease	Phenotype resulting from the variant associated with the disease
HLA-DPB1	GPA	Abnormal antigen presentation
HLA-DQ	MPA	Abnormal antigen presentation
PRTN3	GPA	Increased expression of PR3 on neutrophil cell surface
SERPINA1	GPA	Reduced activity of alpha1-antitrypsin, main inhibitor of PR3 activity
PTPN22	GPA	Abnormal T_{reg} function, increased B-cell and neutrophil function
CTLA4	GPA	Increased T-cell activity

GPA granulomatosis with polyangiitis, *MPA* microscopic polyangiitis, *PR3* proteinase 3

6.3.2 The GWAS Era

To date, three GWASs have been carried out in GPA and MPA. The first was performed by the European Vasculitis Genetics Consortium (EVGC) and involved 2687 Caucasian GPA and MPA subjects [44]; the second was performed on 1020 American GPA patients of European descent by the Vasculitis Clinical Research Consortium (VCRC) [45]. Recently, a third GWAS was conducted on a 1986 AAV cases and 4723 healthy controls [46].

In the EVGC GWAS, the analysis of the discovery and replication cohorts revealed that four SNPs were statistically associated with AAV, three of which mapped in the *HLA* locus. The most significant signal was reported in the *HLA-DPB1* gene. *HLA-DPB1* is a common predisposing factor for several autoimmune diseases, such as rheumatoid arthritis, systemic sclerosis, and ankylosing spondylitis [47–50]. The fourth associated SNP was in the *SERPINA1* (14q32) gene, which encodes for α1-antitrypsin, a neutral serine protease inhibitor whose enzymatic targets include proteinase 3 [51]. Subsequently, AAV patients were stratified according to the clinical syndromes and ANCA specificities. The comparison between the subgroup of PR3-ANCA-positive patients and the MPO-ANCA-positive subgroup showed significant differences at the *HLA*, *SERPINA1*, and *PRTN3* loci, demonstrating a genetic association with PR3-ANCA but not with MPO-ANCA. In particular, within the GPA subgroup, the associations with *HLA-DP* and the related SNPs in the *SERPINA1* and *PRTN3* loci were seen in subjects with PR3-ANCA, not in MPO-ANCA patients. In the MPA subgroup, although much smaller than the GPA subgroup, the findings were similar, resulting in an association between PR3-ANCA and the *HLA-DP* and *SERPINA1* SNPs. The most significant non-HLA association with both the PR3-ANCA and GPA subgroups was found at *SERPINA1* SNP (rs7151526). The SNP associated with the risk of developing GPA was identified as encoding a variant of the enzyme with null activity (called "Z" allele).

The importance of alpha-1 antitrypsin deficiency in the pathogenesis of AAV was already postulated by candidate-gene studies in the pre-GWAS era. In fact, in a group of 433 GPA patients and 421 controls, the carriers of two of the alleles with null or reduced enzymatic activity ("Z" and "S" allele) had an increased probability of developing the disease, with an odds ratio of 14.58 [52].

The second significant non-HLA association was found between *PRTN3* SNP (rs62132295) and GPA (OR: 0.78, $p = 2.6 \times 10^{-5}$). As observed for the abovementioned HLA association, the strength of the *PRTN3* SNP signal increased in the PR3-ANCA-positive subgroup, independently of the clinical diagnosis (OR: 0.73, $p = 2.6 \times 10^{-7}$). No association with *PRTN3* emerged in the MPO-ANCA-positive patients, indicating a role for *PRTN3* only in the pathogenesis of anti-PR3-positive AAV.

PRTN3 gene encodes for the serum protease PR3, and the finding that patients with GPA are more often PR3-ANCA positive already suggested that this enzyme plays a central role in GPA pathogenesis [53]. PR3 is expressed on the surface of neutrophils, and it has been described that only in this membrane-bound form it is able to interact with ANCA, facilitating neutrophil activation [54]. In addition, PR3 may mediate direct tissue damage once it is released by the neutrophils [55]. Interestingly, the SNP associated with GPA was found to be linked to the levels of PR3 expression with the carriers of the susceptibility genotype characterized by higher expression of the protein. This is in line with studies describing that neutrophils with high expression of the membrane-bound PR3 were found more frequently in GPA patients compared to controls [56].

The major result of the EVGC GWAS was the finding that the primary association of all these genetic variants appeared to be with ANCA specificity rather than with the clinically defined syndromes; the genetic differences between PR3-ANCA and MPO-ANCA may have immunopathogenic and therapeutic implications. On the basis of these findings, the distinct genetic background in patients with different with autoantibody specificity suggested that AAV could be better classified into PR3-ANCA and MPO-ANCA-related forms.

The role of the *HLA* in the pathogenesis of AAV was confirmed by the VCRC GWAS performed in GPA patients [57], which also identified an association with SNPs mapping in the *HLA-DPB1* (rs9277554) and *HLA-DPA1* (rs9277341) loci. In addition, this study also reported a non-HLA association at the *SEMA6A* locus (rs26595), which encodes for semaphorin 6A. Comparisons of the *HLA-DPB1*, *HLA-DPA1*, and *SEMA6A* signals between PR3-ANCA-positive subgroup (88% of GPA included in the study) and the ANCA-negative subgroup revealed that all three associations were restricted to the PR3-ANCA-positive group, suggesting genetic divergence between ANCA-positive and ANCA-negative GPA.

In 2017, Merkel and colleagues published a further GWAS including a total of 1986 cases of AAV and 4723 healthy controls [46]. Also in this case, genetic variants of *HLA* locus constitute the major risk in developing GPA; in particular, the most associated signal resulted from the HLA-*DPB1* locus, namely, the rs141530233 ($p = 3.80 \times 10^{-93}$; OR: 3.82) and rs1042169 (1.09×10^{-90}; OR: 2.99) variants. Furthermore, significant associations were also observed at the *SERPINA1* (3.53×10^{-13}; OR: 2.35) and *PTPN22* (1.77×10^{-6}; OR: 1.36) loci. Regarding ANCA specificity, the most significant signals were reported between rs141530233 (1.33×10^{-106}; OR: 6.19), rs1042169 (6.53×10^{-106}, OR: 6.09), and the rs62132293 *PRTN3* (3.59×10^{-13}, OR: 1.39) variants and PR3-ANCA positivity rather than MPO, confirming the findings of the two previous GWASs.

The first conclusion that can be drawn from these studies is that genetic associations are stronger with ANCA specificity rather than clinical syndrome: it was therefore proposed to classify AAV into PR3- and MPO-positive polyangiitis. This distinction already has a well-recognized clinical basis, as PR3- and MPO-ANCA-associated vasculitis often occurs in patient populations that differ on the basis of their age at presentation, cardiovascular risk, and relapse rates [58]. Moreover, the confirmation of the HLA system as a risk factor, together with the autoantigen PR3 and its main inhibitor α1-antitrypsin, confirmed the centrality of autoreactivity in the development of AAV. Further studies are required to better clarify the role of semaphorin 6A in AAV pathogenesis, which was not replicated in other populations.

In order to investigate the shared genetic component underlying predisposition to systemic vasculitis, a European group performed a cross-phenotype meta-analysis of genetic data from different clinically distinct patterns of vasculitis [59]. Immunochip genotyping data from 2465 patients diagnosed with giant cell arteritis, Takayasu's arteritis, AAV or IgA vasculitis, as well as 4632 unaffected controls were analyzed to identify common susceptibility loci for vasculitis development. The strongest association signal corresponded with an intergenic polymorphism located between HLA-DQB1 and HLA-DQA2 (rs6932517, P = 4.16E-14, OR = 0.74). This single-nucleotide polymorphism is in moderate linkage disequilibrium with the disease-specific human leucocyte antigen (HLA) class II associations of each type of vasculitis and could mark them. Outside the HLA region, the group identified the *KDM4C* gene as a common risk locus for vasculitides (rs16925200, P = 6.23E-07, OR = 1.75). This gene encodes for a histone demethylase involved in the epigenetic control of gene expression, increasing the evidences of the crucial role that epigenetic mechanisms have in the development of complex immune-mediated conditions.

One interesting question that still needs to be addressed is why, although the genetic background differs between PR3 and MPO AAV, the clinical phenotypes significantly overlap. One hypothesis is that ANCA, once developed, may generate inflammation through similar mechanisms and that currently unrecognized shared genetic associations, environmental factors, and chronic infections may contribute significantly to the final clinical phenotype [60].

6.4 Genetics of EGPA

Fewer genetic association studies were performed in EGPA than in GPA and MPA, mainly due to the lower frequency of the disease as well as the difficulties in disease classification. ANCA-positive EGPA is more often characterized by vasculitic manifestations, such as lung hemorrhage, peripheral neuropathy, glomerulonephritis, and purpura, and is the subset of EGPA easier to diagnose having a clear-cut clinical presentation and frequently relying on a biomarker such as ANCA [61]. In ANCA-negative cases (about 60% of EGPA patients), the diagnosis is significantly more difficult, as it overlaps with other immune-mediated diseases such as allergy/atopy or hypereosinophilic syndromes [62]. These difficulties have constituted the major obstacles in genetic studies in EGPA; in fact, to date, no GWAS has been published in this disease and the information about genetics of EGPA comes from relatively small candidate-gene studies.

The first set of candidate genes that were chosen to be explored were within the HLA locus: in 2007, an Italian study of 48 EGPA patients showed an association with *HLA-DRB4* [63], which was confirmed in a subsequent study of 102 German patients [64]. Interestingly, the Italian study showed that *HLA-DRB4* was particularly enriched in patients with "vasculitic" manifestations of EGPA, such as glomerulonephritis, mononeuritis multiplex, and purpura. The identification of an association in the HLA locus suggested that EGPA is characterized by an autoimmune nature. These findings are the most suggestive in EGPA, while other small studies have been performed with no replicated data.

Copy number variations (CNV) represent a significant source of genetic heterogeneity in addition to single-nucleotide variants; in fact, they could induce phenotypic heterogeneity influencing protein expression [65]. CNVs of Fcγ receptors (FcγRs) genes have been reported in association with autoimmune diseases such as systemic lupus erythematosus [66]. The role of CNVs of *FCGR3B* was investigated also in EGPA, and it was postulated that patients with only one copy of *FCGR3B* have an increased risk to develop the disease [67]. Again, this association was stronger in the subgroup of patients showing vasculitic manifestations, the subgroup more likely to be ANCA positive, suggesting that in some way an altered interaction between FcGR3B and ANCA might be the explanation for this association.

Data on genetics in EGPA are still poor; we may so far conclude that it is characterized by a likely autoimmune nature and that there is a possibly different genetic background between subsets of the disease with and without vasculitic manifestations; these conclusions are however preliminary, and the results of the ongoing GWAS run by the EVGC might be able to provide further insights.

6.5 Pharmacogenetics

Pharmacogenetics is the study of the role of genetic determinants in the variable response to therapy in terms of therapeutic efficacy as well as adverse effects [68]. Such studies are based on the analysis of candidate markers of individuals characterized by a different drug-response phenotype, with tests for association that compare genetic variation in a case-control study. Pharmacogenetics has ability to better predict response and/or toxicity based on a patient's genotype. Discoveries in these areas may lead to personalized therapies that enhance therapeutic response and minimize the adverse effects of a given therapy [69].

In the last years, the development of monoclonal antibodies directed against a particular immunological protein has permitted the treatment of several autoimmune disorders (i.e., RA and AAV, autoimmune hemolytic anemia, type 1 diabetes, and Sjogren's syndrome) [70–74]. One of these most used drugs is rituximab (RTX), a chimeric monoclonal antibody against the protein CD20. RTX is able to destroy both normal and malignant B cells that express CD20 (which is primarily found on the surface of B cells) and is therefore used to treat diseases which are characterized by having too many, overactive, or dysfunctional B cells [75]. Unfortunately, RTX has adverse effects, which can cause disability, such as tumor lysis syndrome (causing acute renal failure), infections (e.g., hepatitis B reactivation), progressive multifocal leukoencephalopathy, and pulmonary toxicity [76]. The mechanisms of action for RTX, mediated by its Fc portion, include apoptosis of CD20-positive cells, complement-dependent cytotoxicity (CDC), Fcg receptor (FcgR)-mediated mechanisms, antibody-dependent cellular cytotoxicity (ADCC), and phagocytosis. The combined effects result in the elimination of B cells from the body, allowing a new population of healthy B cells to develop from lymphoid stem cells [77].

Genetic variants that are functionally relevant to RTX action have already been identified. *FCGR3A* gene, which encodes the FcgRIIIa protein, displays a nucleotide polymorphism at position c.559 that results in an amino acid change at position p.158 of FcgRIIIa; this variation affects its affinity for human IgG1 [78, 79]; consequently to this change, human IgG1 binds more efficiently to NK cells homozygous for *FCGR3A*-158V than to NK cells homozygous for *FCGR3A*-158F.

Because FcgRIIIa is expressed only by monocytes/macrophages and NK cells (the main actors in ADCC), it has been postulated that patients homozygous for *FCGR3A*-158V show significantly better response to RTX because they have enhanced ADCC activity compared with *FCGR3A*-158F carriers. This was confirmed in other studies using RTX [80, 81]. In 2003, Weng and Levy [82] also showed that the FCGR2A-131H/R polymorphism significantly affects response and time to progression after RTX treatment, with better outcomes for *FCGR2A*-131H homozygous patients.

These results were not confirmed in other studies, founding no impact on RTX response [83], and by the suggestion that the association resulted from the strong linkage disequilibrium between *FCGR3A* and *FCGR2A* polymorphisms [84].

To date, there is no evidence that inherited mutations or polymorphisms of the CD20 gene (called MS4A1) influence the response to RTX [85].

Recently, a Spanish group selected 132 patients with systemic autoimmune diseases treated with RTX. Of these patients, 81 (61.4%) were patients with SLE; 16 (12.1%) presented different inflammatory myopathies such as polymyositis and dermatomyositis; 13 (9.8%) were AAV patients, including GPA, EGPA, and MPA; and the remaining 22 subjects had other systemic autoimmune diseases such as systemic sclerosis (SSc) or autoimmune hemolytic anemia. All patients were genotyped for *FCGR3A*-158F/V (rs396991) polymorphism using allelic discrimination technology, in order to determine whether the *FCGR3A* gene genetic variant contributes to the observed variation in response to RTX. Six months after RTX infusion, the response to the drug was evaluated: 61% of the patients showed a complete response, 27% a partial response, and 12% no response. A statistically significant difference was observed in 158V allele frequency between responders (38%) and nonresponders (16%) patients ($P = 0.01$; OR = 3.24, 95% confidence interval 1.17–11.1). RTX was also more effective in the 158V allele carriers (94%) than in homozygous 158FF patients (81%) ($P = 0.02$; OR = 3.96, 95% CI 1.10–17.68). This study suggested for the first time that *FCGR3A*-158F/V gene polymorphism plays a role in the response to RTX in autoimmune diseases, including AAV, even if with a small cohort; the results needed replication [86].

Another study identified a SNP in the regulatory region of the B-cell activating factor (BAFF) associated with a poor outcome after rituximab treatment; interestingly the carriers of the unfavorable genotype showed signs for increased B-cell activity such as a higher proportion of detectable B cells and a smaller IgM reduction 6 months after therapy [87]. BAFF has already been identified as central in AAV pathogenesis, and a rebound of its levels after rituximab treatment has been considered as a risk factor for treatment failures [19] at the point that trials exploring a combined approach of anti-CD20 and anti-BAFF drugs are ongoing; this genetic study provides a further rationale for identifying a potential biomarker.

Another drug used in the treatment of AAV is cyclophosphamide, a bifunctional DNA alkylating agent, which is incorporated in the treatment of most pediatric and adult malignancies and was one of the first nonhormonal agents to show antitumor activity in humans [88]. At lower doses, cyclophosphamide exerts a potent immunosuppressive effect [89]. Like all chemotherapies, variation in the efficacy and toxicity associated with cyclophosphamide has been described. Its adverse effects include cardiotoxicity, neurotoxicity, infertility, bladder toxicity, myelosuppression, and leukemogenesis [90]. Both toxicity and response to cyclophosphamide are quite variable. Several important pharmacogenetic discoveries of the cyclophosphamide effects have been performed using a candidate-gene approach focusing on known targets involved in CP bioactivation and/or detoxification; however, a whole-genome or a whole-exome approach may allow for a more comprehensive, unbiased approach for identifying important factors in cyclophosphamide clinical activity. Finally, genes involved in pharmacokinetic and pharmacodynamic effects of cyclophosphamide require discovery and validation in larger and more different patient cohorts.

All these studies, despite of interest, are characterized by several limitations and need further replication or follow-up studies in order to have their findings confirmed. However they represent good examples of what genetics can do in order to contribute to better defining disease prognosis.

6.6 Contribution of Genetics to AAV Classification

Significant overlap exists between GPA, MPA, and EGPA, leading to difficulties in clinical classification, which may impact on the therapeutic approach and disease monitoring with important consequences for the patients. Of interest, ANCA is a shared biomarker, and this, together with the important clinical overlap, may suggest a pathogenetic overlap between AAVs. Of note, only 40% of EGPA cases are ANCA positive, and the ANCA-negative subgroup is more frequently represented by a variant of the disease usually without vasculitic manifestations and more often characterized by clinical characteristics that arise as a consequence of hypereosinophilia. In this context of clinical uncertainty, genetics has played an important role in improving our understanding of AAV classification. In Table 6.2 the clinical and genetic characteristics supporting a reclassification of GPA and MPA according to ANCA specificity rather than the clinical characteristics are reported.

First of all, the GWASs in GPA and MPA provided the insight that the genetic background is more clearly associated with the ANCA specificity rather than the clinical diagnoses. The associations were in fact stronger when the population was stratified according to the ANCA specificity rather that the clinical phenotype. This provides the rationale for the suggestion of the probable need of re-think GPA and MPA more as PR3+ and MPO+ AAV. The idea that ANCA specificity might be more robustly able to differentiate disease subtypes rather than clinical syndrome was not new, and some clinical observations already pointed toward this direction.

Despite the lower prevalence of PR3 positivity, clinical phenotypes resembling GPA and the clinical characteristics of PR3+ AAV are indeed still detected also in

Table 6.2 Proposed reclassification of GPA and MPA in PR3+ and MPO+ AAV as supported by clinical phenotype and genetic evidence [58]

Variable	PR3+ AAV	MPO+ AAV
Mean age at onset	56–59	62–65
Male gender	66%	48%
ENT involvement	77%	23%
Eye involvement	40%	15%
Kidney-limited disease	2%	31%
Interstitial lung disease	0%	7.2%
Relapse (HR of PR3+ vs. MPO+)	1.89 (95% CI 1.33–2.69)	
Relapse-free patients 5 years after diagnoses	32%	60%
Cardiovascular risk (patients with at least 1 event over 5 years of follow-up)	6.6%	19.2%
Genetic associations	*HLA-DP* *PRTN3* *SERPINA1* *PTPN22*	*HLA-DQ*

ENT ear, nose, and throat involvement, *HR* hazard ratio

MPO-positive patients. This overlap suggests that, although convenient, the classification according to ANCA specificity has some limitations as well and there must therefore be also likely shared genetic variants associated with both syndromes; *PTPN22* is at the moment a strong candidate, but others may well be detected by better-powered studies. Future studies will need to be able to identify these associations in order to provide improvement in the understanding of disease pathogenesis as well as identifying new potential therapeutic targets.

6.7 Conclusions

Despite three GWASs in AAV have been performed so far and one in EGPA is currently ongoing, the field of genetics in AAV is still at an early stage of development. Few robust associations have been so far identified although the ones that have been found significantly contributed to our understanding of disease pathogenesis and classification. Some studies have also started to point their focus toward the role of genetics in defining prognosis.

References

1. Jennette JC, Falk RJ, Hu P, Xiao H. Pathogenesis of antineutrophil cytoplasmic autoantibody-associated small-vessel vasculitis. Annu Rev Pathol. 2013;8:139–60.
2. Jennette JC, Falk RJ, Andrassy K, et al. Nomenclature of systemic vasculitides. Proposal of an international consensus conference. Arthritis Rheum. 1994;37:187–92.

3. Ntatsaki E, Watts RA, Scott DG. Epidemiology of ANCA-associated vasculitis. Rheum Dis Clin N Am. 2010;36(3):447–61. https://doi.org/10.1016/j.rdc.2010.04.002. PubMed PMID: 20688243.
4. Jayne D, Rasmussen N, Andrassy K, et al. A randomized trial of maintenance therapy for vasculitis associated with antineutrophil cytoplasmic autoantibodies. N Engl J Med. 2003;349:36–44.
5. Mahr A, Katsahian S, Varet H, et al. Revisiting the classification of clinical phenotypes of anti-neutrophil cytoplasmic antibody-associated vasculitis: a cluster analysis. Ann Rheum Dis. 2013;72:1003–10.
6. Radice A, Sinico RA. Antineutrophil cytoplasmic antibodies (ANCA). Autoimmunity. 2005;38(1):93–103. Review. PubMed PMID: 15804710.
7. Sable-Fourtassou R, Cohen P, Mahr A, et al. Antineutrophil cytoplasmic antibodies and the Churg-Strauss syndrome. Ann Intern Med. 2005;143:632–8.
8. Chen M, Kallenberg CG. The environment, geoepidemiology and ANCA-associated vasculitides. Autoimmun Rev. 2010;9:A293–8.
9. Tanna A, Salama AD, Brookes P, Pusey CD. Familial granulomatosis with polyangiitis: three cases of this rare disorder in one Indoasian family carrying an identical HLA DPB1 allele. BMJ Case Rep. 2012;2012.
10. Knight A, Sandin S, Askling J. Risks and relative risks of Wegener's granulomatosis among close relatives of patients with the disease. Arthritis Rheum. 2008;58:302–7.
11. Alberici F, Martorana D, Bonatti F, Gioffredi A, Lyons PA, Vaglio A. Genetics of ANCA-associated vasculitides: HLA and beyond. Clin Exp Rheumatol. 2014;32(Suppl 82):90–7.
12. Furuta S, Jayne DR. Antineutrophil cytoplasm antibody-associated vasculitis: recent developments. Kidney Int. 2013;84:244–9.
13. Classen S, Staratschek-Jox A, Schultze JL. Use of genome-wide high-throughput technologies in biomarker development. Biomark Med. 2008;2(5):509–24. https://doi.org/10.2217/17520363.2.5.509. PubMed PMID: 20477427.
14. Hatemi G, Esatoglu SN, Yazici Y. Biomarkers in vasculitis. Curr Opin Rheumatol. 2018;30(1):30–5. https://doi.org/10.1097/BOR.0000000000000447. PubMed PMID: 28937415.
15. Bonatti F, Reina M, Neri TM, Martorana D. Genetic susceptibility to ANCA-associated vasculitis: state of the art. Front Immunol. 2014;5:577. https://doi.org/10.3389/fimmu.2014.00577. eCollection 2014. Review. PubMed PMID: 25452756; PubMed Central PMCID: PMC4233908.
16. Tabor HK, Risch NJ, Myers RM. Candidate-gene approaches for studying complex genetic traits: practical considerations. Nat Rev Genet. 2002;3(5):391–7. https://doi.org/10.1038/nrg796. Review. PubMed PMID: 11988764.
17. Dalca AV, Brudno M. Genome variation discovery with high-throughput sequencing data. Brief Bioinform. 2010;11(1):3–14. https://doi.org/10.1093/bib/bbp058. PubMed PMID: 20053733.
18. Wang WY, Barratt BJ, Clayton DG, Todd JA. Genome-wide association studies: theoretical and practical concerns. Nat Rev Genet. 2005;6(2):109–18. Review. PubMed PMID: 15716907.
19. Buzdugan L, Kalisch M, Navarro A, Schunk D, Fehr E, Bühlmann P. Assessing statistical significance in multivariable genome wide association analysis. Bioinformatics. 2016;32(13):1990–2000. https://doi.org/10.1093/bioinformatics/btw128. PubMed PMID: 27153677; PubMed Central PMCID: PMC4920127.
20. Johnson RC, Nelson GW, Troyer JL, Lautenberger JA, Kessing BD, Winkler CA, O'Brien SJ. Accounting for multiple comparisons in a genome-wide association study (GWAS). BMC Genomics. 2010;11:724. https://doi.org/10.1186/1471-2164-11-724. PubMed PMID: 21176216; PubMed Central PMCID: PMC3023815.
21. Kraft P, Zeggini E, Ioannidis JP. Replication in genome-wide association studies. Stat Sci. 2009;24(4):561–73. PubMed PMID: 20454541; PubMed Central PMCID: PMC2865141.
22. Cortes A, Brown MA. Promise and pitfalls of the Immunochip. Arthritis Res Ther. 2011;13(1):101. https://doi.org/10.1186/ar3204. Review. PubMed PMID: 21345260; PubMed Central PMCID: PMC3157635.

23. Kiezun A, Garimella K, Do R, Stitziel NO, Neale BM, McLaren PJ, Gupta N, Sklar P, Sullivan PF, Moran JL, Hultman CM, Lichtenstein P, Magnusson P, Lehner T, Shugart YY, Price AL, de Bakker PI, Purcell SM, Sunyaev SR. Exome sequencing and the genetic basis of complex traits. Nat Genet. 2012;44(6):623–30. https://doi.org/10.1038/ng.2303. PubMed PMID: 22641211; PubMed Central PMCID: PMC3727622.
24. Savage CO. Pathogenesis of anti-neutrophil cytoplasmic autoantibody (ANCA)-associated vasculitis. Clin Exp Immunol. 2011;164(Suppl 1):23–6. https://doi.org/10.1111/j.1365-2249.2011.04362.x. Review. PubMed PMID: 21447127; PubMed Central PMCID: PMC3095861.
25. Traherne JA. Human MHC architecture and evolution: implications for disease association studies. Int J Immunogenet. 2008;35(3):179–92. https://doi.org/10.1111/j.1744-313X.2008.00765.x. Review. PubMed PMID: 18397301; PubMed Central PMCID: PMC2408657.
26. Evseeva I, Nicodemus KK, Bonilla C, Tonks S, Bodmer WF. Linkage disequilibrium and age of HLA region SNPs in relation to classic HLA gene alleles within Europe. Eur J Hum Genet. 2010;18(8):924–32. https://doi.org/10.1038/ejhg.2010.32. PubMed PMID: 20354563; PubMed Central PMCID: PMC2987379.
27. Jagiello P, Gencik M, Arning L, et al. New genomic region for Wegener's granulomatosis as revealed by an extended association screen with 202 apoptosis-related genes. Hum Genet. 2004;114:468–77.
28. Cao Y, Scmitz JL, Yang J, et al. DRB1*15 allele is a risk factor for PR3-ANCA disease in African Americans. Clin J Am Soc Nephrol. 2011;22:1161–7.
29. Luo H, Chen M, Yang R, Xu PC, Zhao MH. The association of HLA-DRB1 alleles with antineutrophil cytoplasmic antibody-associated systemic vasculitis in Chinese patients. Hum Immunol. 2011;72:422–5.
30. Criswell LA, Pfeiffer KA, Lum RF, et al. Analysis of families in the multiple autoimmune disease genetics consortium (MADGC) collection: the PTPN22 620W allele associates with multiple autoimmune phenotypes. Am J Hum Genet. 2005;76:561–71.
31. Chelala C, Duchatelet S, Joffret ML, Bergholdt R, Dubois-Laforgue D, Ghandil P, Pociot F, Caillat-Zucman S, Timsit J, Julier C. PTPN22 R620W functional variant in type 1 diabetes and autoimmunity related traits. Diabetes. 2007;56(2):522–6. PubMed PMID: 17259401.
32. Hinks A, Barton A, John S, Bruce I, Hawkins C, Griffiths CE, Donn R, Thomson W, Silman A, Worthington J. Association between the PTPN22 gene and rheumatoid arthritis and juvenile idiopathic arthritis in a UK population: further support that PTPN22 is an autoimmunity gene. Arthritis Rheum. 2005;52(6):1694–9. PubMed PMID: 15934099.
33. Namjou B, Kim-Howard X, Sun C, Adler A, Chung SA, Kaufman KM, Kelly JA, Glenn SB, Guthridge JM, Scofield RH, Kimberly RP, Brown EE, Alarcón GS, Edberg JC, Kim JH, Choi J, Ramsey-Goldman R, Petri MA, Reveille JD, Vilá LM, Boackle SA, Freedman BI, Tsao BP, Langefeld CD, Vyse TJ, Jacob CO, Pons-Estel B, Argentine Collaborative Group, Niewold TB, Moser Sivils KL, Merrill JT, Anaya JM, Gilkeson GS, Gaffney PM, Bae SC, Alarcón-Riquelme ME, BIOLUPUS and GENLES Networks, Harley JB, Criswell LA, James JA, Nath SK. PTPN22 association in systemic lupus erythematosus (SLE) with respect to individual ancestry and clinical sub-phenotypes. PLoS One. 2013;8(8):e69404. https://doi.org/10.1371/journal.pone.0069404. eCollection 2013. PubMed PMID: 23950893; PubMed Central PMCID: PMC3737240.
34. Maine CJ, Hamilton-Williams EE, Cheung J, et al. PTPN22 alters the development of regulatory T cells in the thymus. J Immunol. 2012;188:5267–75.
35. JAGIELLO P, ARIES P, ARNING L, et al. The PTPN22 620W allele is a risk factor for Wegener's granulomatosis. Arthritis Rheum. 2005;52:4039–43.
36. Carr EJ, Niederer HA, Williams J, et al. Confirmation of the genetic association of CTLA4 and PTPN22 with ANCA-associated vasculitis. BMC Med Genet. 2009;10:121.
37. Martorana D, Maritati F, Malerba G, et al. PTPN22 R620W polymorphism in the ANCA-associated vasculitides. Rheumatology (Oxford). 2012;51:805–12.

38. Noel PJ, Boise LH, Green JM, et al. CD28 costimulation prevents cell death during primary T cell activation. J Immunol. 1996;157:636–42.
39. Giscombe R, Wang X, Huang D, et al. Coding sequence 1 and promoter single nucleotide polymorphisms in the CTLA-4 gene in Wegener's granulomatosis. J Rheumatol. 2002;29:950–3.
40. Langford CA, Monach PA, Specks U, et al. An open-label trial of abatacept (CTLA4-IG) in non-severe relapsing granulomatosis with polyangiitis (Wegener's). Ann Rheum Dis. 2014;73:1376–9.
41. Netea MG, Wijmenga C, O'Neill LA. Genetic variation in Toll-like receptors and disease susceptibility. Nat Immunol. 2012;13(6):535–42. https://doi.org/10.1038/ni.2284. Review. PubMed PMID: 22610250.
42. Holle JU, Windmöller M, Lange C, Gross WL, Herlyn K, Csernok E. Toll-like receptor TLR2 and TLR9 ligation triggers neutrophil activation in granulomatosis with polyangiitis. Rheumatology (Oxford). 2013;52(7):1183–9. https://doi.org/10.1093/rheumatology/kes415. PubMed PMID: 23407387.
43. Husmann CA, Holle JU, Moosig F, et al. Genetics of toll like receptor 9 in ANCA associated vasculitides. Ann Rheum Dis. 2014;73:890–6.
44. Lyons PA, Rayner TF, Trivedi S, Holle JU, Watts RA, Jayne DR, et al. Genetically distinct subsets within anca-associated vasculitis. N Engl J Med. 2012;367:214–23. https://doi.org/10.1056/NEJMoa1108735.
45. Xie G, Roshandel D, Sherva R, Monach PA, Lu EY, Kung T, et al. Association of granulomatosis with polyangiitis (Wegener's) with HLA-DBP1*04 and SEMA6A gene variants: evidence from genome-wide analysis. Arthritis Rheum. 2013;65:2457–68. https://doi.org/10.1002/art.38036.
46. Merkel PA, Xie G, Monach PA, Ji X, Ciavatta DJ, Byun J, Pinder BD, Zhao A, Zhang J, Tadesse Y, Qian D, Weirauch M, Nair R, Tsoi A, Pagnoux C, Carette S, Chung S, Cuthbertson D, Davis JC Jr, Dellaripa PF, Forbess L, Gewurz-Singer O, Hoffman GS, Khalidi N, Koening C, Langford CA, Mahr AD, McAlear C, Moreland L, Seo EP, Specks U, Spiera RF, Sreih A, St Clair EW, Stone JH, Ytterberg SR, Elder JT, Qu J, Ochi T, Hirano N, Edberg JC, Falk RJ, Amos CI, Siminovitch KA, Vasculitis Clinical Research Consortium. Identification of functional and expression polymorphisms associated with risk for antineutrophil cytoplasmic autoantibody-associated vasculitis. Arthritis Rheumatol. 2017;69(5):1054–66. https://doi.org/10.1002/art.40034. PubMed PMID: 28029757; PubMed Central PMCID: PMC5434905.
47. Jiang L, Jiang D, Han Y, Shi X, Ren C. Association of HLA-DPB1 polymorphisms with rheumatoid arthritis: a systemic review and meta-analysis. Int J Surg. 2018;52:98–104. https://doi.org/10.1016/j.ijsu.2018.01.046. Review. PubMed PMID: 29425827.
48. Lee JS, Park JK, Kim HJ, Lee HK, Song YW, Lee EB. Negatively-charged amino acids at the peptide-binding pocket of HLA-DPB1 alleles are associated with susceptibility to antitopoisomerase I-positive systemic sclerosis. Hum Immunol. 2016;77(7):550–4. https://doi.org/10.1016/j.humimm.2016.05.012. PubMed PMID: 27208855.
49. Furukawa H, Oka S, Kawasaki A, Shimada K, Sugii S, Matsushita T, Hashimoto A, Komiya A, Fukui N, Kobayashi K, Osada A, Ihata A, Kondo Y, Nagai T, Setoguchi K, Okamoto A, Okamoto A, Chiba N, Suematsu E, Kono H, Katayama M, Hirohata S, Sumida T, Migita K, Hasegawa M, Fujimoto M, Sato S, Nagaoka S, Takehara K, Tohma S, Tsuchiya N. Human leukocyte antigen and systemic sclerosis in Japanese: the sign of the four independent protective alleles, DRB1*13:02, DRB1*14:06, DQB1*03:01, and DPB1*02:01. PLoS One. 2016;11(4):e0154255. https://doi.org/10.1371/journal.pone.0154255. eCollection 2016. PubMed PMID: 27116456; PubMed Central PMCID: PMC4846066.
50. Jung SH, Yim SH, Hu HJ, Lee KH, Lee JH, Sheen DH, Lim MK, Kim SY, Park SW, Kim SH, Han K, Kim TH, Shim SC, Chung YJ. Genome-wide copy number variation analysis identifies deletion variants associated with ankylosing spondylitis. Arthritis Rheumatol. 2014;66(8):2103–12. https://doi.org/10.1002/art.38650. PubMed PMID: 24692264.

51. Fregonese L, Stolk J. Hereditary alpha-1-antitrypsin deficiency and its clinical consequences. Orphanet J Rare Dis. 2008;19(3):16. https://doi.org/10.1186/1750-1172-3-16. Review. PubMed PMID: 18565211; PubMed Central PMCID: PMC2441617.
52. Mahr AD, Edberg JC, Stone JH, et al. Alpha(1)-antitrypsin deficiency-related alleles Z and S and the risk of Wegener's granulomatosis. Arthritis Rheum. 2010;62:3760–7.
53. Pagnoux C. Updates in ANCA-associated vasculitis. Eur J Rheumatol. 2016;3(3):122–33. Epub 2016 Jan 29. Review. PubMed PMID: 27733943; PubMed Central PMCID: PMC5058451.
54. Schreiber A, Luft FC, Kettritz R. Membrane proteinase 3 expression and ANCA-induced neutrophil activation. Kidney Int. 2004;65(6):2172–83. PubMed PMID: 15149330.
55. Campbell EJ, Campbell MA, Owen CA. Bioactive proteinase 3 on the cell surface of human neutrophils: quantification, catalytic activity, and susceptibility to inhibition. J Immunol. 2000;165(6):3366–74. PubMed PMID: 10975855.
56. von Borstel A, Sanders JS, Rutgers A, Stegeman CA, Heeringa P, Abdulahad WH. Cellular immune regulation in the pathogenesis of ANCA-associated vasculitides. Autoimmun Rev. 2018;17(4):413–21. https://doi.org/10.1016/j.autrev.2017.12.002. Epub 2018 Feb 9. Review. PubMed PMID: 29428808.
57. Xie G, Roshandel D, Sherva R, Monach PA, Lu EY, Kung T, Carrington K, Zhang SS, Pulit SL, Ripke S, Carette S, Dellaripa PF, Edberg JC, Hoffman GS, Khalidi N, Langford CA, Mahr AD, St Clair EW, Seo P, Specks U, Spiera RF, Stone JH, Ytterberg SR, Raychaudhuri S, de Bakker PI, Farrer LA, Amos CI, Merkel PA, Siminovitch KA. Association of granulomatosis with polyangiitis (Wegener's) with HLA-DPB1*04 and SEMA6A gene variants: evidence from genome-wide analysis. Arthritis Rheum. 2013;65(9):2457–68. https://doi.org/10.1002/art.38036. PubMed PMID: 23740775; PubMed Central PMCID: PMC4471994.
58. Alberici F, Martorana D, Vaglio A. Genetic aspects of anti-neutrophil cytoplasmic antibody-associated vasculitis. Nephrol Dial Transplant. 2015;30(Suppl 1):i37–45. https://doi.org/10.1093/ndt/gfu386. Epub 2014 Dec 18. Review. PubMed PMID: 25523449.
59. Ortiz-Fernández L, Carmona FD, López-Mejías R, González-Escribano MF, Lyons PA, Morgan AW, Sawalha AH, Smith KGC, González-Gay MA, Martín J, Spanish GCA Study Group, UK GCA Consortium, Turkish Takayasu Study Group, Vasculitis Clinical Research Consortium, IgAV Study Group, AAV Study group. Cross-phenotype analysis of Immunochip data identifies KDM4C as a relevant locus for the development of systemic vasculitis. Ann Rheum Dis. 2018;77(4):589–95. https://doi.org/10.1136/annrheumdis-2017-212372. Epub 2018 Jan 27. Erratum in: Ann Rheum Dis. 2018 Jun;77(6):950. PubMed PMID: 29374629; PubMed Central PMCID: PMC5849568.
60. Mahr A, Katsahian S, Varet H, Guillevin L, Hagen EC, Höglund P, Merkel PA, Pagnoux C, Rasmussen N, Westman K, Jayne DR. French Vasculitis Study Group (FVSG) and the European Vasculitis Society (EUVAS). Revisiting the classification of clinical phenotypes of anti-neutrophil cytoplasmic antibody-associated vasculitis: a cluster analysis. Ann Rheum Dis. 2013;72(6):1003–10. https://doi.org/10.1136/annrheumdis-2012-201750. Epub 2012 Sep 8. PubMed PMID: 22962314.
61. Groh M, Pagnoux C, Baldini C, Bel E, Bottero P, Cottin V, Dalhoff K, Dunogué B, Gross W, Holle J, Humbert M, Jayne D, Jennette JC, Lazor R, Mahr A, Merkel PA, Mouthon L, Sinico RA, Specks U, Vaglio A, Wechsler ME, Cordier JF, Guillevin L. Eosinophilic granulomatosis with polyangiitis (Churg-Strauss) (EGPA) Consensus Task Force recommendations for evaluation and management. Eur J Intern Med. 2015;26(7):545–53. https://doi.org/10.1016/j.ejim.2015.04.022. Epub 2015 May 9. PubMed PMID: 25971154.
62. Gioffredi A, Maritati F, Oliva E, Buzio C. Eosinophilic granulomatosis with polyangiitis: an overview. Front Immunol. 2014;5:549. https://doi.org/10.3389/fimmu.2014.00549. eCollection 2014. Review. PubMed PMID: 25404930; PubMed Central PMCID: PMC4217511.
63. Vaglio A, Martorana D, Maggiore U, Grasselli C, Zanetti A, Pesci A, Garini G, Manganelli P, Bottero P, Tumiati B, Sinico RA, Savi M, Buzio C, Neri TM, Secondary and Primary Vasculitis Study Group. HLA-DRB4 as a genetic risk factor for Churg-Strauss syndrome. Arthritis Rheum. 2007;56(9):3159–66. PubMed PMID: 17763415.

64. Wieczorek S, Hellmich B, Gross WL, Epplen JT. Associations of Churg-Strauss syndrome with the HLA-DRB1 locus, and relationship to the genetics of antineutrophil cytoplasmic antibody-associated vasculitides: comment on the article by Vaglio et al. Arthritis Rheum. 2008;58(1):329–30. https://doi.org/10.1002/art.23209. PubMed PMID: 18163478.
65. Ionita-Laza I, Rogers AJ, Lange C, Raby BA, Lee C. Genetic association analysis of copy-number variation (CNV) in human disease pathogenesis. Genomics. 2009;93(1):22–6. https://doi.org/10.1016/j.ygeno.2008.08.012. Epub 2008 Oct 19. Review. PubMed PMID: 18822366; PubMed Central PMCID: PMC2631358.
66. Mueller M, Barros P, Witherden AS, Roberts AL, Zhang Z, Schaschl H, Yu CY, Hurles ME, Schaffner C, Floto RA, Game L, Steinberg KM, Wilson RK, Graves TA, Eichler EE, Cook HT, Vyse TJ, Aitman TJ. Genomic pathology of SLE-associated copy-number variation at the FCGR2C/FCGR3B/FCGR2B locus. Am J Hum Genet. 2013;92(1):28–40. https://doi.org/10.1016/j.ajhg.2012.11.013. Epub 2012 Dec 20. PubMed PMID: 23261299; PubMed Central PMCID: PMC3542466.
67. Martorana D, Bonatti F, Alberici F, Gioffredi A, Reina M, Urban ML, Maritati F, Adorni A, Radice A, Pizzolato S, Gregorini G, Jeannin G, Guida G, Boita M, Pesci A, Moroni G, Neri TM, Sinico RA, Vaglio A. Fcγ-receptor 3B (FCGR3B) copy number variations in patients with eosinophilic granulomatosis with polyangiitis. J Allergy Clin Immunol. 2016;137(5):1597–1599.e8. https://doi.org/10.1016/j.jaci.2015.09.053. Epub 2015 Dec 9. PubMed PMID: 26684293.
68. Ma Q, Lu AY. Pharmacogenetics, pharmacogenomics, and individualized medicine. Pharmacol Rev. 2011;63(2):437–59. https://doi.org/10.1124/pr.110.003533. Epub 2011 Mar 24. Review. PubMed PMID: 21436344.
69. Scott SA. Personalizing medicine with clinical pharmacogenetics. Genet Med. 2011;13(12):987–95. https://doi.org/10.1097/GIM.0b013e318238b38c. Review. PubMed PMID: 22095251; PubMed Central PMCID: PMC3290900.
70. Bossaller L, Rothe A. Monoclonal antibody treatments for rheumatoid arthritis. Expert Opin Biol Ther. 2013;13(9):1257–72. https://doi.org/10.1517/14712598.2013.811230. Epub 2013 Jun 21. Review. PubMed PMID: 23789825.
71. Lutalo PM, D'Cruz DP. Biological drugs in ANCA-associated vasculitis. Int Immunopharmacol. 2015;27(2):209–12. https://doi.org/10.1016/j.intimp.2015.04.023. Epub 2015 Apr 20. Review. PubMed PMID: 25907243.
72. D'Arena G, Taylor RP, Cascavilla N, Lindorfer MA. Monoclonal antibodies: new therapeutic agents for autoimmune hemolytic anemia? Endocr Metab Immune Disord Drug Targets. 2008;8(1):62–8. Review. PubMed PMID: 18393924.
73. Herold KC, Taylor L. Treatment of Type 1 diabetes with anti-CD3 monoclonal antibody: induction of immune regulation? Immunol Res. 2003;28(2):141–50. Review. PubMed PMID: 14610290.
74. Le Dantec C, Alonso R, Fali T, Montero E, Devauchelle V, Saraux A, Pers JO, Renaudineau Y. Rationale for treating primary Sjögren's syndrome patients with an anti-CD6 monoclonal antibody (Itolizumab). Immunol Res. 2013;56(2-3):341–7. https://doi.org/10.1007/s12026-013-8423-x. PubMed PMID: 23576060.
75. Taylor RP, Lindorfer MA. Drug insight: the mechanism of action of rituximab in autoimmune disease—the immune complex decoy hypothesis. Nat Clin Pract Rheumatol. 2007;3(2):86–95. Review. PubMed PMID: 17299446.
76. Kasi PM, Tawbi HA, Oddis CV, Kulkarni HS. Clinical review: serious adverse events associated with the use of rituximab—a critical care perspective. Crit Care. 2012;16(4):231. https://doi.org/10.1186/cc11304. Review. PubMed PMID: 22967460; PubMed Central PMCID: PMC3580676.
77. Pescovitz MD. Rituximab, an anti-cd20 monoclonal antibody: history and mechanism of action. Am J Transplant. 2006;6(5 Pt 1):859–66. Review. PubMed PMID: 16611321.
78. Kim SH, Jeong IH, Hyun JW, Joung A, Jo HJ, Hwang SH, Yun S, Joo J, Kim HJ. Treatment outcomes with rituximab in 100 patients with neuromyelitis optica: influence of FCGR3A polymorphisms on the therapeutic response to rituximab. JAMA Neurol. 2015;72(9):989–95. https://doi.org/10.1001/jamaneurol.2015.1276. PubMed PMID: 26167726.

79. Treon SP, Hansen M, Branagan AR, Verselis S, Emmanouilides C, Kimby E, Frankel SR, Touroutoglou N, Turnbull B, Anderson KC, Maloney DG, Fox EA. Polymorphisms in FcgammaRIIIA (CD16) receptor expression are associated with clinical response to rituximab in Waldenström's macroglobulinemia. J Clin Oncol. 2005;23(3):474–81. PubMed PMID: 15659493.
80. Moroi R, Endo K, Kinouchi Y, Shiga H, Kakuta Y, Kuroha M, Kanazawa Y, Shimodaira Y, Horiuchi T, Takahashi S, Shimosegawa T. FCGR3A-158 polymorphism influences the biological response to infliximab in Crohn's disease through affecting the ADCC activity. Immunogenetics. 2013;65(4):265–71. https://doi.org/10.1007/s00251-013-0679-8. Epub 2013 Jan 29. Erratum in: Immunogenetics. 2015 Sep;67(9):545. PubMed PMID: 23358932.
81. Burkhardt B, Yavuz D, Zimmermann M, Schieferstein J, Kabickova E, Attarbaschi A, Lisfeld J, Reiter A, Makarova O, Worch J, Bonn BR, Damm-Welk C. Impact of Fc gamma-receptor polymorphisms on the response to rituximab treatment in children and adolescents with mature B cell lymphoma/leukemia. Ann Hematol. 2016;95(9):1503–12. https://doi.org/10.1007/s00277-016-2731-x. Epub 2016 Jul 4. PubMed PMID: 27376362.
82. Weng WK, Levy R. Two immunoglobulin G fragment C receptor polymorphisms independently predict response to rituximab in patients with follicular lymphoma. J Clin Oncol. 2003;21(21):3940–7. Epub 2003 Sep 15. PubMed PMID: 12975461.
83. Kenkre VP, Hong F, Cerhan JR, Lewis M, Sullivan L, Williams ME, Gascoyne RD, Horning SJ, Kahl BS. Fc gamma receptor 3A and 2A polymorphisms do not predict response to rituximab in follicular lymphoma. Clin Cancer Res. 2016;22(4):821–6. https://doi.org/10.1158/1078-0432.CCR-15-1848. Epub 2015 Oct 28. PubMed PMID: 26510856; PubMed Central PMCID: PMC4755793.
84. Morgan AW, Robinson JI, Barrett JH, Martin J, Walker A, Babbage SJ, Ollier WE, Gonzalez-Gay MA, Isaacs JD. Association of FCGR2A and FCGR2A-FCGR3A haplotypes with susceptibility to giant cell arteritis. Arthritis Res Ther. 2006;8(4):R109. PubMed PMID: 16846526; PubMed Central PMCID: PMC1779375.
85. Sar A, Perizzolo M, Stewart D, Mansoor A, Difrancesco LM, Demetrick DJ. Mutation or polymorphism of the cd20 gene is not associated with the response to r-chop in diffuse large b cell lymphoma patients. Leuk Res. 2009;33:792–7.
86. Robledo G, Marquez A, Davila-Fajardo CL, et al. Association of the fcgr3a-158f/v gene polymorphism with the response to rituximab treatment in spanish systemic autoimmune disease patients. DNA Cell Biol. 2012;31:1671–7.
87. Alberici F, Smith RM, Fonseca M, et al. Association of a TNFSF13B (BAFF) regulatory region single nucleotide polymorphism with response to rituximab in antineutrophil cytoplasmic antibody-associated vasculitis. J Allergy Clin Immunol. 2017;139:1684–7.. e10.
88. Geetha D, Specks U, Stone JH, Merkel PA, Seo P, Spiera R, Langford CA, Hoffman GS, Kallenberg CG, St Clair EW, Fessler BJ, Ding L, Tchao NK, Ikle D, Jepson B, Brunetta P, Fervenza FC, Rituximab for ANCA-Associated Vasculitis Immune Tolerance Network Research Group. Rituximab versus cyclophosphamide for ANCA-associated vasculitis with renal involvement. J Am Soc Nephrol. 2015;26(4):976–85. https://doi.org/10.1681/ASN.2014010046. Epub 2014 Nov 7. PubMed PMID: 25381429; PubMed Central PMCID: PMC4378104.
89. Heijl C, Harper L, Flossmann O, Stücker I, Scott DG, Watts RA, Höglund P, Westman K, Mahr A, European Vasculitis Study Group (EUVAS). Incidence of malignancy in patients treated for antineutrophil cytoplasm antibody-associated vasculitis: follow-up data from European Vasculitis Study Group clinical trials. Ann Rheum Dis. 2011;70(8):1415–21. https://doi.org/10.1136/ard.2010.145250. Epub 2011 May 25. Review. PubMed PMID: 21616914.
90. Pinto N, Ludeman SM, Dolan ME. Drug focus: pharmacogenetic studies related to cyclophosphamide-based therapy. Pharmacogenomics. 2009;10(12):1897–903. https://doi.org/10.2217/pgs.09.134. Review. PubMed PMID: 19958089; PubMed Central PMCID: PMC2820268.

Giant Cell Arteritis

7

Francisco David Carmona, Javier Martín, and Miguel A. González-Gay

Contents

F. D. Carmona (✉)
Departamento de Genética e Instituto de Biotecnología, Universidad de Granada, Granada, Spain

Centro de Investigación Biomédica (CIBM), Universidad de Granada, Parque Tecnológico Ciencias de la Salud, Granada, Spain
e-mail: dcarmona@ugr.es

J. Martín
Instituto de Parasitología y Biomedicina 'López-Neyra', IPBLN-CSIC, Granada, Spain
e-mail: javiermartin@ipb.csic.es

M. A. González-Gay
Epidemiology, Genetics and Atherosclerosis Research Group on Systemic Inflammatory Diseases, Rheumatology Division, IDIVAL, Santander, Spain

School of Medicine, University of Cantabria, Santander, Spain

Cardiovascular Pathophysiology and Genomics Research Unit, Faculty of Health Sciences, School of Physiology, University of the Witwatersrand, Johannesburg, South Africa

J. Martín, F. D. Carmona (eds.), *Genetics of Rare Autoimmune Diseases*,
Rare Diseases of the Immune System, https://doi.org/10.1007/978-3-030-03934-9_7

7.1 Introduction

Giant cell arteritis (GCA), also known as temporal arteritis, cranial arteritis, and Horton's syndrome, is a granulomatous systemic vasculitis characterized by inflammatory damage of medium- and large-size blood vessels, particularly the aorta and its major branches, with a predisposition for the involvement of the extracranial branches of the carotid artery [1, 2]. GCA shows a complex etiology in which both environmental and genetic factors are involved in disease predisposition and progression [3]. It represents the most common type of vasculitis in Western countries after the fifth decade of life, affecting mostly women with a sex ratio around 3:1 [4, 5]. A North to South gradient in GCA prevalence has been described, with Scandinavian ethnic groups and North American populations of the same descent showing the highest rates (annual incidence higher than 17/100,000 persons per population age >50 years, compared to <12/100,000 persons per population age >50 years in Southern European countries) [5].

The clinical manifestations of GCA are the consequence of the chronic inflammatory process within the arterial walls. They include headache, transient or permanent blindness, jaw claudication, tongue necrosis, and central nervous system ischemic complications including stroke in some cases [6]. Up to half of GCA patients may also develop polymyalgia rheumatica (PMR), an inflammatory disorder characterized by severe pain and stiffness involving the shoulders, the pelvic girdle, and the neck, usually in individuals older than 50 years [7].

There are currently no biological markers of disease predisposition or progression for GCA, and, therefore, biopsy of the temporal artery showing disruption of the internal elastic laminae with infiltration of mononuclear cells is widely accepted as the gold standard to confirm diagnosis [8]. Likewise, no specific treatments have been developed for this disease either, being the glucocorticoid-mediated immunosuppression the common strategy used as soon as a diagnosis is suspected [9].

During the last decade, many studies have been performed to elucidate the genetic component of GCA. In this regard, the establishment of large international consortia and the use of the novel technologies for large-scale genotyping have allowed a big leap in the understanding of the molecular pathways involved in GCA development [10]. In this chapter, we will provide an overview of the current knowledge on the genetic background of GCA. Recent insights into the influence of epigenetics on disease predisposition and the possible common pathogenic pathways between GCA and other forms of vasculitis will be also discussed.

7.2 Immunopathological Mechanisms of GCA

Different lines of evidence suggest that GCA is an antigen-driven autoinflammatory and autoimmune condition mediated by different populations of T cells, including T helper (Th) 1 cells (Th1), Th17 cells, regulatory T (Treg) cells, and Th9 cells [11]. As described below, this assumption is consistent with the reported genetic associations, and it supports the hypothesis that an infectious agent could trigger the disease in genetically predisposed individuals [12, 13]. In this regard, different viruses and bacteria have been proposed as candidate pathogens involved in the initial activation of the inflammatory process within the vessel wall. These include parvovirus B19, herpes simplex virus, cytomegalovirus, varicella zoster virus, human parainfluenzae, and *Chlamydia pneumoniae*, among others [11]. Consistent with this idea, rhythmic fluctuations of GCA annual incidence with peaks overlapping seasons of higher incidence of airway infections have been described [14, 15]. However, most of those observations have not been replicated in independent studies, and definitive evidence is still to be provided. For instance, no single pathogen was detected in the temporal artery biopsy from 12 GCA patients using sequencing-based techniques [16].

Whatever the cause, the first pathological process observed in GCA patients corresponds with a loss of tolerance to the wall components leading to activation and expansion of resident dendritic cells (DC) of the adventitia. These cells act as sentinels that alert $CD4^+$ T cells and macrophages after detecting pathogen-associated molecular patterns (PPR) by means of Toll-like receptors (TLR) and production of pro-inflammatory cytokines and chemoattractant molecules. The involvement of TLRs is in agreement with the proposed idea of GCA triggered by infection [17–19]. As a consequence, immune cells infiltrate at the adventitia-media border from the vasa vasorum, and CD4+ T cells differentiate into interferon gamma (IFN-γ)-producing Th1 cells that induce subsequent activation of human leukocyte antigen (HLA)-DR-expressing macrophages. Finally, activated macrophages end up forming multinucleated giant cells and granulomas in the media, which promote chronic inflammation and arterial occlusion, which is responsible for the main clinical complications [19].

As discussed in the following section, GCA is mostly associated with HLA class II molecules, which is consistent with the proposed immunopathological mechanisms influencing GCA development and emphasizing the autoimmune nature of this condition.

7.3 Candidate Gene Studies

Many genetic studies on GCA have been performed during the past two decades following the candidate gene approach [3]. Despite lacking most of them an adequate statistical power to detect low to modest effect sizes, they have been of great help to better understand the pathophysiological mechanisms involved in disease risk and relevant outcomes.

7.3.1 Early HLA Associations

In humans, the HLA region is located at the short arm of the chromosome six (6p21.3) spanning approximately from 29,000,000 bp to 33,000,000 bp. This region contains more than 400 genes and pseudogenes, some of them encoding cell-surface antigen-presenting proteins with a central role in the immune response. Because of it, there is a considerable high sequence variation within the region, with more than

8000 annotated alleles for the classical HLA genes with an extensive linkage disequilibrium (LD) between them [20].

As in most immune-mediated diseases, the HLA system represents the most relevant susceptibility region for GCA susceptibility. This was something evident back in the 1980s, even considering the limitations in terms of statistical power that the genetic studies had at that time. As described below, the great efforts made by several research groups allowed the identification of different class I and II haplotypes consistently associated with GCA risk [3]. Most of these associations were subsequently confirmed by comprehensive analyses of the HLA region using large-scale genotyping and imputation methods [21].

7.3.1.1 HLA Class II Associations

Early studies highlighted that GCA is predominantly a HLA class II disease. Different HLA classical alleles of this subregion were associated with disease predisposition in independent populations of European ancestry from Spain, Italy, the USA, France, and Denmark. Associated haplotypes included *HLA-DR3*, *HLA-DR4*, *HLA-DR5*, and *HLA-DRB1*, with the latter showing the strongest evidence of association (specifically carriage of *DRB1*0401* and *DRB1*0404*) [22–33]. Some of those studies also reported that presence of the *HLA-DRB1*04* allele may correlate with corticosteroid resistance and increased predisposition to visual complications in GCA patients [31, 34, 35].

Besides, *HLA-DRB1*04* haplotypes carrying the "shared epitope" (SE) were also related to GCA development, which suggested that this form of vasculitis could share part of its genetic background with RA [26, 36]. As discussed later on in this chapter, this observation was confirmed in subsequent studies using deep screening of the HLA region and genome-wide genotyping [21].

7.3.1.2 HLA Class I Associations

Some haplotypes of the HLA class I subregion were also described as possible GCA markers, including *HLA-A*31*, *HLA-B*8*, *HLA-Cw3*, *HLA-Cw6*, *HLA-B*15*, and MHC class I polypeptide-related sequence A (*MICA*). However, the associations were considerably less consistent than those of the class II, and attempts to replicate them failed in most cases [22, 27, 37, 38]. Indeed, as described in the following section, a recent fine-mapping of the region using large study cohorts and novel imputation methods only detected association signals at the *HLA-B* gene [21].

7.3.2 Associations with Non-HLA Candidate Genes

Thanks to the hard work of different research groups, especially those led by Drs. González-Gay and Salvarani from Spain and Italy, respectively, the genetic component of GCA outside the HLA region was thoroughly explored using the candidate gene approach since the beginning of the present century. Unfortunately, most of the studies published during the first decade were performed using reduced populations and lacked replication steps in independent cohorts. Nonetheless, some associations with genes encoding proteins with relevant roles in the pathological pathways involved in GCA were identified, including key components of the inflammation process like cytokines and cytokine receptors (e.g., *IL17A*, *IL33*, *IL10*, *IL6*, *IFGN*, and *IL12RB2*), immunomodulatory proteins of the adaptive and innate immunity (e.g., *PTPN22*, *TLR4*, and *FCGR2A/3A*), proteins with endothelial functions (e.g., *ICAM1*, *VEGF*, and *NOS2A*), and molecules involved in apoptotic processes (e.g., *NLRP1*) [39–54]. Some of these genes seem to confer susceptibility also to other forms of vasculitis like Takayasu's arteritis (TAK), anti-neutrophil cytoplasmic antibodies (ANCA)-associated vasculitis (AAV), Behçet's disease (BD), immunoglobulin A vasculitis (IgAV), and Kawasaki disease, which suggest a common genetic component in vasculitides [55].

Among them, *PTPN22* represented the most consistent risk *loci* because of its high effect size (OR ~ 1.3) and validation in subsequent multicenter meta-analyses with data from several populations of European origin (including Spain, UK, Germany, and Norway) [42, 56]. *PTPN22* is an archetypal autoimmunity gene, as it is involved in the pathogenic mechanisms leading to a wide range of immune-mediated conditions, including type 1 diabetes, rheumatoid arthritis (RA), systemic lupus erythematosus, juvenile idiopathic arthritis, Graves' disease, vitiligo, Hashimoto's thyroiditis, myasthenia gravis, alopecia areata, Addison's disease, idiopathic thrombocytopenic purpura, psoriatic arthritis, granulomatosis with polyangiitis, polymyositis, and systemic sclerosis [57].

In humans this gene is located on chromosome 1p13.3-p13.1 and encodes a non-receptor protein tyrosine kinase named LYP that is expressed mainly in lymphoid tissues. LYP modulate the signal transduction in different immune cell types by modifying the phosphorylation state of its target proteins. In particular, it has a central role in the negative regulation of both the T-cell receptor (TCR) and B-cell receptor (BCR) signaling pathways after engagement of the antigen, by acting in a cooperative manner with the protein kinase CSK [58]. It seems that the effect on disease predisposition is mainly caused by a non-synonymous polymorphism located in the exon 14 of the gene (C1858T, rs2476601), which implies an arginine (R) to tryptophan (W) substitution in a protein-protein interaction domain of LYP (R620W). The presence of tryptophan at such position may interfere with the ability of LYP to bind CSK, preventing the formation of the complex and, therefore, affecting its down-regulatory function on the TCR and BCR signaling. Whether R620W is a gain- or loss-of-function variant remains controversial, although most evidences point to the first option [58]. Because of that, attempts to develop efficient LYP inhibitors for the treatment of *PTPN22*-associated diseases are currently being made [59].

Another key risk factor for GCA identified through candidate gene studies was *IL17A*, as it supported the high relevance proposed for Th17 cells in the immunopathological mechanisms underlying this type of vasculitis [39]. For instance, presence of Th17 cells has been reported in the arterial lesions of GCA patients, consistent with the high expression levels of *IL17* and other Th17-specific pro-inflammatory cytokines detected in the biopsies of GCA-affected temporal arteries [60–62]. In this regard, it has been proposed that Th17 cells may influence the clinical phenotypes of GCA in an early state of the disease, whereas the development of the chronic symptoms are more likely to be related to the pathological pathways orchestrated by IFNγ-producing Th1 cells [19]. Considering that corticosteroid therapy seems to be more effective on Th17 cells than on Th1 cells, the Th17/Th1 ratio could represent a valuable prognostic marker in GCA [60, 61].

7.4 Insights from Large-Scale Genetic Analyses

An international collaborative effort, involving many hospitals and research groups from Europe and North America, including the Spanish GCA Study Group, the European Vasculitis Genetics Consortium (EVGC), the Vasculitis Clinical Research Consortium (VCRC), and the UKGCA Consortium, has allowed the ambitious goal of conducting the first large-scale genetic studies in GCA by taking advantage of the high-throughput genotyping technology and the high statistical power of the large case series gathered (Fig. 7.1). This exciting achievement has represented a turning point in the understanding of the genetic component of the disease, and the insights gained may definitively help to lay down the foundations for future studies aimed at developing more efficient therapeutic strategies.

7.4.1 Use of the Immunochip to Fine-Map Immune-Related *Loci*

The first large-scale genetic analysis on GCA was published on 2015 using the Immunochip, a custom high-density array designed by the Immunochip Consortium (composed by the Wellcome Trust Case Control Consortium in collaboration with several leading groups focused on the investigation of the genetics of major autoimmune and autoinflammatory conditions) for immunogenetics gene mapping. This genotyping platform contained probes to type 196,524 polymorphisms, including single-nucleotide polymorphisms (SNPs), rare variants, and small insertion/deletion (INDEL) polymorphisms, as well as a dense HLA set and a large panel of ancestry markers [63]. The Immunochip has proven to be one of the most successful platforms to identify specific and common association signals in a wide spectrum of immune-mediated diseases [64], including the vasculitides TAK, BD, ANCA, and IgAV [65–67].

Seven countries participated in the Immunochip study on GCA (i.e., Spain, Italy, UK, USA, Canada, Norway, and Germany), which resulted in the largest case-control cohort included in a study of this form of vasculitis by far (1651 GCA patients diagnosed either by a biopsy of the temporal artery or by imaging techniques and 15,306 unaffected controls) [21]. The results obtained made evident the considerable high contribution of the HLA region to the disease susceptibility in comparison with the risk conferred by non-HLA *loci* (Fig. 7.1). Indeed, most of the genetic predispositions to GCA seemed to be driven by HLA class II molecules, specifically *HLA-DRB1* and *HLA-DQA1*, consistent with the pathogen infection triggering hypothesis described above. Interestingly, the dense SNP coverage of the Immunochip within the HLA region allowed a deep interrogation at the amino acid level by means of an imputation method that infers SNPs, two- and four-digit classical HLA alleles, and polymorphic amino acid positions at class I and II regions, using a reference panel of

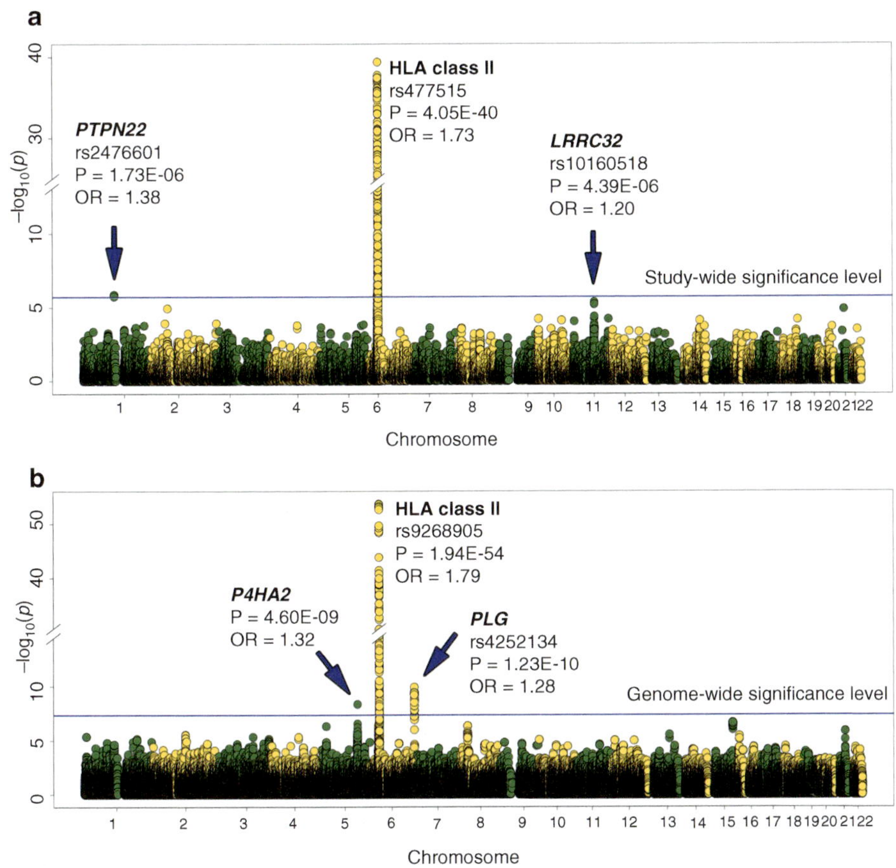

Fig. 7.1 Manhattan plot representation of the results of the (**a**) Immunochip and (**b**) genome-wide association studies of giant cell arteritis. The -log10 of the *P*-values are plotted against their physical chromosomal position. The blue line represents the study-wide level of significance in **a** ($P < 1.77 \times 10^{-6}$) and the genome-wide level of significance in **b** ($P < 5 \times 10^{-8}$). The most relevant associations are highlighted. The data were obtained from Carmona et al. 2015 and 2017 [21, 75]

European origin [68, 69]. The use of this bioinformatic tool allowed the authors to propose a model of three amino acid positions that explained most of the statistical significance observed in the HLA region. The major influence to disease risk of the model was conferred by the class II positions 13 of HLA-DRβ1 and 56 of HLA-DQα1 (Fig. 7.2), with position 45 of the class I molecule HLA-B exerting a significant but considerably lower contribution. The fact that these positions were located in the binding pocket of their corresponding HLA molecules, and that all three have been described to be directly involved in the peptide binding [70–72], gave a functional relevance to the model. Moreover, histidine at position 13 of HLA-DRβ1 represented the most significant signal not only of the amino acids included in the 3 amino acid model but also of all the polymorphisms analyzed in the Immunochip.

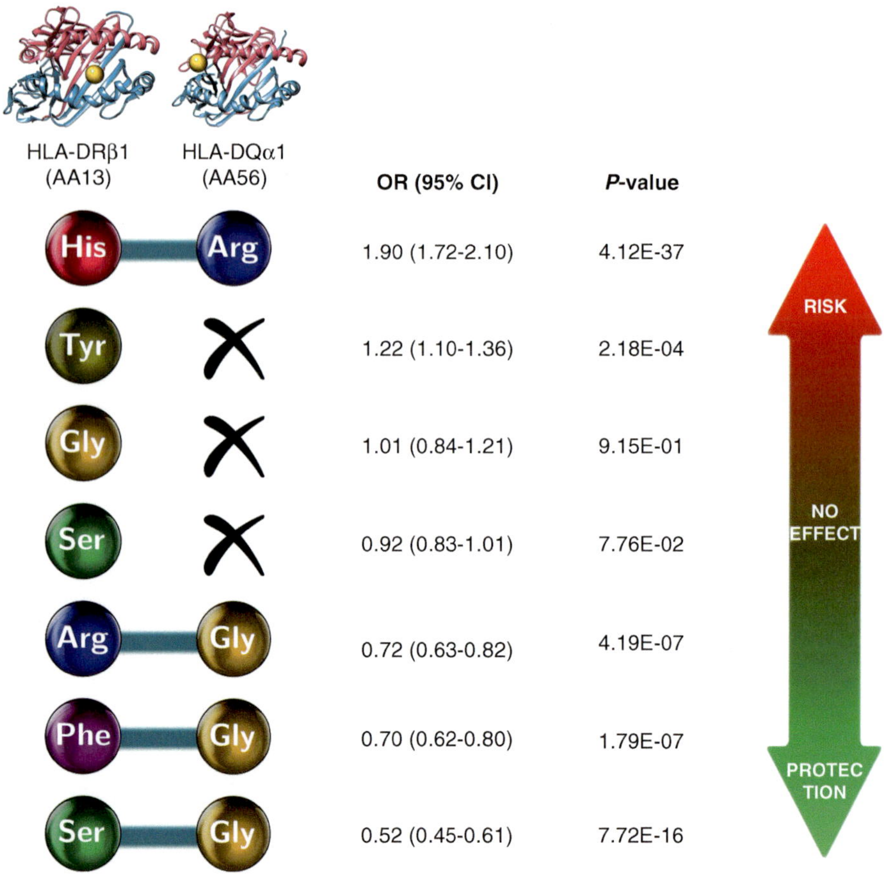

Fig. 7.2 Combinations of the amino acids included in the model that best explained the association of the HLA class II genomic region with giant cell arteritis in the Immunochip study [21]. The model included the position 13 of HLA-DRβ1 and the position 56 of DQα1. Odds ratios (OR), 95% confidence intervals (CI), and *P*-values are shown for each combination. *AA* amino acid. The "X" symbol represents absence of residue at the corresponding position

Again, this is in agreement with the early associations between GCA and HLA-DRB1*04 classical alleles, as HLA-DRβ1 His13 is one of the polymorphic residues that defines the associated haplotypes and suggests that this position is crucial for the loss of tolerance against vascular wall self-antigens in GCA.

Regarding the non-HLA hits of the Immunochip, the only marker that surpassed the study-wide significance level was *PTPN22* R620W, which was definitively confirmed as a relevant GCA gene. Considering that this genetic variant is the most important non-HLA genetic factor for RA, together with the fact that HLA-DRβ1 His13 is also one of the amino acids with strongest effect on RA risk, the authors decided to test a polygenic risk score model predictive of RA risk in GCA patients and controls using the Immunochip data. Remarkably, GCA patients showed significantly higher scores than controls, especially when considering the HLA region alone. This is consistent with the observations in the 1990s suggesting that the SE may have some influence in GCA predisposition [26, 36]. As these two diseases do not use to be comorbidities one to another and their clinical phenotypes clearly differ, it is likely that the shared genetic component between them influences early steps of both diseases related to the loss of tolerance against similar self-peptides [10].

On the other hand, *LRRC32* represented the second non-HLA hit of the GCA Immunochip, very close to the statistical significance. This gene encodes a type I membrane glycoprotein containing 20 leucine-rich repeats that has been implicated in the development and function of FOXP3+ Tregs [73]. Hence, the genetic insights obtained in the Immunochip also supported the previously proposed implication of this cell type in the cellular events leading to GCA phenotypes [74].

7.4.2 Unbiased Genome-Wide Screening

The publication of the first genome-wide association study (GWAS) of GCA in 2017 provided a wider overview of the genetic landscape of the disease. The study was performed on the initial seven cohorts included in the Immunochip and three additional ones from France, the Netherlands, and Ireland, comprising a total of 2134 GCA patients and 9125 unaffected individuals [75]. Whole-genome SNP genotype imputation was performed with the GWAS data using the 1000 Genome Project Phase III (1KGPh3) population as reference panel, resulting in 1,844,133 SNPs for the analysis.

The study confirmed once again HLA class II as the most relevant risk genomic region for GCA. As expected, two SNPs within the region showed independent effects, one located nearby *HLA-DRB1* (rs9268905) and the other close to *HLA-DQA1* (rs9275592). However, the most striking finding of the GWAS was the identification of plasminogen (*PLG*) and prolyl 4-hydroxylase subunit alpha 2 (*P4HA2*), which are involved in angiogenesis and vascular remodeling, as the major non-HLA genetic factors in GCA.

PLG encodes a blood zymogen that is the precursor of the plasmin and angiostatin proteins [76]. The plasminogen system is crucial in several processes that are of special relevance in GCA development, including angiogenesis, recruitment of immune cells, and inflammation, through stimulation of cytokine production and oxidative stress [77, 78]. Taking this into account, the authors hypothesized that the GCA-associated *PLG* variants' risk alleles could affect the balance of the plasminogen system by altering gene expression, which would end up favoring the typical pro-inflammatory environment of affected vessels [75].

Regarding *P4HA2*, this is an important hypoxia-responsive gene that encodes the α subunit of the collagen prolyl 4-hydroxylase, a key enzyme in collagen biosynthesis [79]. Interestingly, one of the alleles associated with GCA (rs101194) was annotated as cis eQTL in public databases altering *P4HA2* expression in both lymphoblastoid cell lines and the aorta, which is one of the most affected vessels in this form of vasculitis [75].

7.5 Epigenetic Mechanisms in GCA

Epigenetics refers to the heritable changes in gene expression without modification of the DNA sequence [80]. In complex diseases, epigenetic mechanisms represent the cross talk between environmental and genetic cues. In GCA, the aging process can be considered the single factor with highest impact on disease risk, as the disease incidence increases considerably from the seventh decade of life [5]. In this sense, it is likely that progressive age may promote GCA onset by remodeling of the immune system and restructuring of the blood vessel wall [81]. Besides aging, other possible factors proposed as environmental causal agents of GCA include microbial pathogens, light sensitivity, altitude and latitude, solar cycle, and geomagnetic activity [5, 82, 83].

To shed light into the epigenetic mechanisms implicated in GCA predisposition, Coit and colleagues performed a genome-wide DNA methylome analysis of temporal artery biopsies (TAB) from 12 GCA patients and 12 matched controls [84]. More than 800 genes showed hypomethylation (i.e., upregulation of gene expression) in TAB from GCA patients compared to controls. Hypomethylated *loci* included proinflammatory genes (e.g., *CD6*, *CD40LG*, *CCR7*, *IFNG*, *IL1B*, *IL2*, *IL6*, *IL18*, *IL21*, *IL23R*, *LTA*, *LTB*, *NLRP1*, *RUNX3*, and *TNF*), genes encoding proteins of the TCR complex (e.g., CD3D, CD3E, CD3G, and CD3Z), and genes involved in T-cell activation (e.g., *NFATC1*, *NFATC2*, *PPP3CC*, and *PTPN22*). As stated previously in this chapter, some of them (i.e., *IFNG*, *IL2*, *IL6*, *IL18*, *IL21*, *IL23R*, *NLRP1*, *PTPN22*, and *TNF*) were described as genetic risk factors for GCA in candidate gene studies [3, 42]. But most strikingly, gene ontology enrichment analysis of the hypomethylated genes showed overrepresentation in biological pathways involving Th1- and Th17-cell activation and differentiation, specifically in TCR/CD28 signaling and calcineurin (Ca)/NFAT-regulatory pathways. In fact, the highest hypomethylated state in GCA TABs was observed in *RUNX3*, which is involved in the maturation of IFN-γ-producing Th1 cells [85]. Therefore, epigenetic modifications on immune-related genes in the arterial microenvironment might influence the characteristic T-cell activation and Th1/Th17 polarization during GCA development [86]. Consistent with this idea, age-related DNA methylation changes in naïve CD4+ T have been described to alter regulatory mechanisms and signaling pathways involved in the development of autoimmune processes [87].

7.6 Shared Genetic Component with Other Forms of Vasculitis

One of the advantages of using the Immunochip platform is that it facilitates the comparison of the genetic component between the studied diseases, as the markers analyzed are the same and the SNP coverage in genes of the immune system is considerably high [64]. Taking into consideration that Immunochip data was available for GCA and TAK [21, 65], which is another granulomatous large-vessel vasculitis (LVV) that shares many common clinical, histopathologic, and radiographic features with GCA [19, 88], a combined meta-analysis of such data was performed in order to elucidate possible overlapping immunopathogenic pathways [89]. The results of the study evidenced that no genetic correlation between both forms of LVV was evident within the HLA region, which is due to the fact that GCA is mostly a HLA class II-associated disease (with weaker effects of class I markers), whereas the opposite occurs in TAK (i.e., class I harbors the strongest effect sizes with lower contribution of class II markers, as described in the next chapter). The distinct pattern of associated HLA haplotypes could be related to early disease-specific mechanisms of each form of vasculitis.

On the contrary, a significant shared heritability was observed outside the HLA region, either by using a bivariate restricted maximum likelihood (RML) method to calculate the genetic pleiotropy or by analyzing polygenic risk scores on one disease calculated with the susceptibility signals of the other disease. In this regard, *IL12B* represented the most relevant common gene predisposing both types of vasculitis. This gene encodes the P40 subunit that is present in both IL-12 and IL-23, which promote Th1 and Th17 cell differentiation, respectively (the latter along with IL-1β) [90]. Consistent with this association, it has been described that blocking of the p40 subunit with ustekinumab leads to a better prognosis in patients with refractory GCA [91]. Other suggestive common markers identified in this study included *NOS2*, *ERAP1*, *REL*, and *PRKQC* [89].

Finally, in a recent study, Ortiz-Fernández and collaborators extended the GCA-TAK cross-disease meta-analysis by adding Immunochip data from two additional vasculitides, AAV and IgAV [66]. In total, Immunochip data from 2465 patients diagnosed with any of these four types of vasculitis and 4632 unaffected controls were tested for common associations. This study described lysine demethylase (*KDM4C*) as a novel common susceptibility gene for the vasculitides analyzed and also for BD [66]. Interestingly, its encoded protein is a histone demethylase with a relevant function in the epigenetic regulation of gene expression and chromatin conformation [92].

7.7 Conclusions

During the last years, we have substantially increased the knowledge of the pathological mechanisms behind GCA (Table 7.1 and Fig. 7.3). This qualitative and quantitative leap has been possible due to the establishment of international collaborative consortia and the emergence of the new technologies for the genetic studies. We know now that GCA is a complex and polygenic condition in which environmental factors may trigger the disease in genetically predisposed individuals via epigenetic modifications in hematopoietic and vascular tissues [11]. The use of high-throughput genotyping platforms in large case-control cohorts has generated very valuable data that strongly support the notion of GCA as an antigen-driven immune-mediated disorder in which most of the genetic risk is carried by HLA class II molecules (specifically amino acids 13 and 56 of HLA-DRβ1 and HLA-DQα1, respectively) [21]. Indeed, GCA can be considered an archetypal HLA class

Table 7.1 Recent genetic associations with giant cell arteritis in well-powered studies outside the HLA region

Year	Gene	Variant	Location	Populations	*N* (case/control)	Strategy	OR (95% CI)	*P*-value (allele test)	Ref.
2013	*NLRP1*	rs8182352	Intergenic	Spain, Italy	685/2898	Candidate gene	1.20 (1.06–1.35)	2.62E-03	[41]
2013	*PTPN22*	rs2476601	Coding region	Spain, UK, Germany, Norway	911/8136	Candidate gene	1.62 (1.29–2.04)	1.06E-04	[42]
2014	*IL17A*	rs2275913	Intergenic	Spain, Italy, Germany, Norway	1266/3779	Candidate gene	1.17 (1.06–1.29)	1.85E-03	[39]
2014	*IL17A*	rs7747909	3′-UTR	Spain, Italy, Germany, Norway	1266/3779	Candidate gene	1.15 (1.04–1.27)	8.49E-03	[39]
2014	*IL33*	rs7025417	Intronic	Spain, Italy, Germany, Norway	1363/3908	Candidate gene	0.88 (0.78–0.99)	4.10E-02	[40]
2015	*LRRC32*	rs10160518	Intergenic	Spain, UK, USA, Canada, Italy, Germany, Norway	1651/15,306	Immunochip	1.20 (1.11–1.29)	4.39E-06	[21]
2017	*PLG*	rs4252134	Intronic	Spain, UK, USA, Canada, Italy, Germany, Norway, France, Netherlands, Switzerland, Ireland	2134/9125	GWAS	1.28 (1.19–1.39)	1.23E-10	[75]
2017	*P4HA2*	rs128738	Intronic	Spain, UK, USA, Canada, Italy, Germany, Norway, France, Netherlands, Switzerland, Ireland	2134/9125	GWAS	1.32 (1.20–1.45)	4.60E-09	[75]
2017	*IL12B*	rs755374	Intergenic	Spain, Italy, USA, Canada, Turkey	1434/3814	Meta-Immunochip[a]	1.19 (1.06–1.33)	7.54E-07	[89]
2018	*KDM4C*	rs16925200	Intronic	Spain, UK, USA, Canada, Turkey	2465/4632	Meta-Immunochip[b]	1.75 (1.41–2.18)	6.23E-07	[66]

SNP single-nucleotide polymorphism, *OR* odds ratio for the minor allele, *CI* confidence interval
[a]Cross-disease meta-analysis including GCA and TAK
[b]Cross-disease meta-analysis including GCA, TAK, AAV, and IgAV

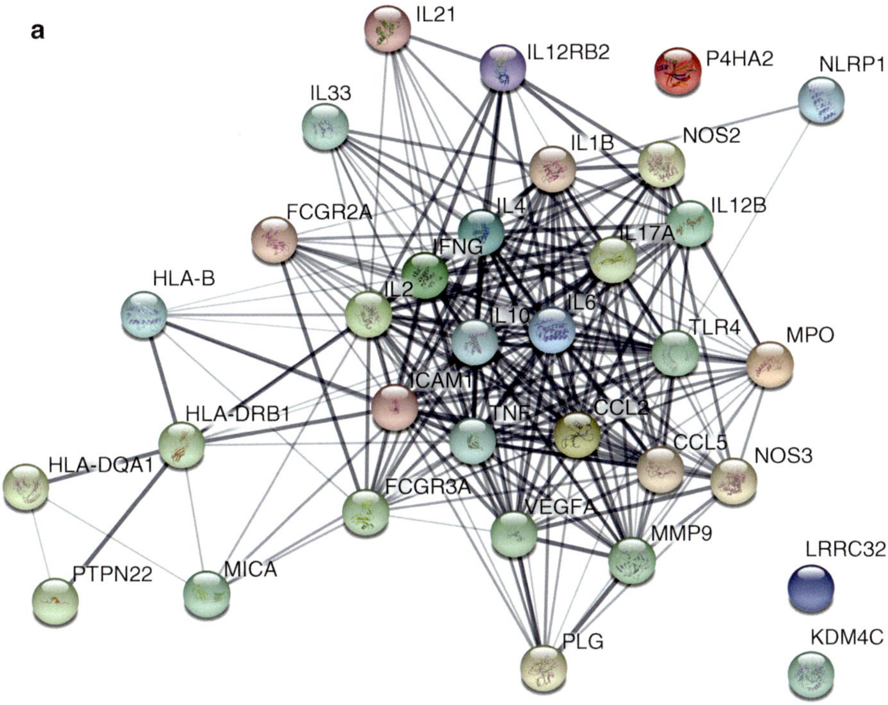

Fig. 7.3 (**a**) Interaction network and (**b**) functional enrichments of the genes showing evidence of association with GCA risk either by candidate gene studies or by large-scale approaches. STRING database was used to search for both direct and indirect interactions among selected genes. The width of the blue lines indicates the reliability of each interaction

b

Biological Process (GO)			
pathway ID	*pathway description*	*count in gene set*	*false discovery rate*
GO:0001817	regulation of cytokine production	17	2.1e-15
GO:0071222	cellular response to lipopolysaccharide	12	3.13e-15
GO:0051239	regulation of multicellular organismal process	25	5.14e-15
GO:0051240	positive regulation of multicellular organismal process	21	8.6e-15
GO:0001819	positive regulation of cytokine production	14	8.98e-14

Molecular Function (GO)			
pathway ID	*pathway description*	*count in gene set*	*false discovery rate*
GO:0005125	cytokine activity	11	1.25e-12
GO:0005102	receptor binding	18	4.46e-12
GO:0005126	cytokine receptor binding	10	8.51e-10
GO:0070851	growth factor receptor binding	7	7.27e-08
GO:0005515	protein binding	23	1.84e-06

Cellular Component (GO)			
pathway ID	*pathway description*	*count in gene set*	*false discovery rate*
GO:0005615	extracellular space	17	7.42e-10
GO:0098552	side of membrane	11	9.67e-09
GO:0009897	external side of plasma membrane	9	2.43e-08
GO:0044421	extracellular region part	21	1.08e-06
GO:0005576	extracellular region	21	1.68e-05
GO:0009986	cell surface	10	1.68e-05

KEGG Pathways			
pathway ID	*pathway description*	*count in gene set*	*false discovery rate*
05321	Inflammatory bowel disease (IBD)	14	2.55e-25
05323	Rheumatoid arthritis	12	5.59e-19
05140	Leishmaniasis	11	4.86e-18
05164	Influenza A	13	1.47e-17
04060	Cytokine-cytokine receptor interaction	14	6.38e-17

Fig. 7.3 (continued)

II disease in which non-HLA genes may have a lower but still essential contribution to the disease development. Among them, genes encoding regulatory molecules of the immune system (e.g., *IL17A*, *IL33*, *PTPN22*, or *LRRC32*) as well as proteins involved in angiogenesis and vascular remodeling (e.g., *PLG* and *P4HA2*) seem to play the most relevant roles [10, 75]. Interestingly, some of them have been described to show specific signatures of DNA methylation marks in cells located at the sites of inflammation [84].

However, there is still a long way ahead before reaching a complete understanding of the disease etiology. Common and specific pathological pathways between the different clinical outcomes of GCA and between GCA and other forms of vasculitis may be elucidated to better explain the phenotypic variance. It is also especially true for the frequent overlap between GCA and PMR [93]. In this regard, patients with clinically isolated ("pure") PMR were found to have lower degree of inflammatory response when compared to those with PMR associated with typical cranial GCA [94]. Moreover, at least a third of the patients considered as having isolated PMR have large-vessel involvement when imaging techniques, such as 18F-fluorodeoxyglucosepositron emission tomography (PET) with an integrated computed tomography (CT) imaging system, are performed [7]. Therefore, this is a necessary step that may definitively help us in the ambitious endeavor of developing efficient diagnostic and prognostic markers in parallel with personalized therapeutic strategies that can be implemented in the clinical practice in a near future.

References

1. Jennette JC, Falk RJ, Bacon PA, Basu N, Cid MC, Ferrario F, et al. 2012 revised International Chapel Hill Consensus Conference Nomenclature of Vasculitides. Arthritis Rheum. 2013;65(1):1–11. https://doi.org/10.1002/art.37715. PubMed PMID: 23045170.
2. Salvarani C, Cantini F, Boiardi L, Hunder GG. Polymyalgia rheumatica and giant-cell arteritis. N Engl J Med. 2002;347(4):261–71. https://doi.org/10.1056/NEJMra011913. PubMed PMID: 12140303.
3. Carmona FD, Gonzalez-Gay MA, Martin J. Genetic component of giant cell arteritis. Rheumatology (Oxford). 2014;53(1):6–18. https://doi.org/10.1093/rheumatology/ket231. Epub 2013/07/12. PubMed PMID: 23843109.
4. Borchers AT, Gershwin ME. Giant cell arteritis: a review of classification, pathophysiology, geoepidemiology and treatment. Autoimmun Rev. 2012;11(6–7):A544–54. https://doi.org/10.1016/j.autrev.2012.01.003. PubMed PMID: 22285588.
5. Gonzalez-Gay MA, Vazquez-Rodriguez TR, Lopez-Diaz MJ, Miranda-Filloy JA, Gonzalez-Juanatey C, Martin J, et al. Epidemiology of giant cell arteritis and polymyalgia rheumatica. Arthritis Rheum. 2009;61(10):1454–61. https://doi.org/10.1002/art.24459. PubMed PMID: 19790127.
6. Gonzalez-Gay MA, Martinez-Dubois C, Agudo M, Pompei O, Blanco R, Llorca J. Giant cell arteritis: epidemiology, diagnosis, and management. Curr Rheumatol Rep. 2010;12(6):436–42. https://doi.org/10.1007/s11926-010-0135-9. PubMed PMID: 20857242.
7. Gonzalez-Gay MA, Matteson EL, Castaneda S. Polymyalgia rheumatica. Lancet. 2017;390(10103):1700–12. https://doi.org/10.1016/S0140-6736(17)31825-1. PubMed PMID: 28774422.
8. Gonzalez-Gay MA, Garcia-Porrua C, Miranda-Filloy JA. Giant cell arteritis: diagnosis and therapeutic management. Curr Rheumatol Rep. 2006;8(4):299–302. PubMed PMID: 16839509.
9. Gonzalez-Gay MA, Miranda-Filloy JA, Lopez-Diaz MJ, Perez-Alvarez R, Gonzalez-Juanatey C, Sanchez-Andrade A, et al. Giant cell arteritis in northwestern Spain: a 25-year epidemiologic study. Medicine. 2007;86(2):61–8. https://doi.org/10.1097/md.0b013e31803d1764. PubMed PMID: 17435586.
10. Carmona FD, Martin J, Gonzalez-Gay MA. New insights into the pathogenesis of giant cell arteritis and hopes for the clinic. Expert Rev Clin Immunol. 2016;12(1):57–66. https://doi.org/10.1586/1744666X.2016.1089173. PubMed PMID: 26367100.
11. Samson M, Corbera-Bellalta M, Audia S, Planas-Rigol E, Martin L, Cid MC, et al. Recent advances in our understanding of giant cell arteritis pathogenesis. Autoimmun Rev. 2017;16(8):833–44. https://doi.org/10.1016/j.autrev.2017.05.014. PubMed PMID: 28564617.
12. Duhaut P, Bosshard S, Ducroix JP. Is giant cell arteritis an infectious disease? Biological and epidemiological evidence. Presse Med. 2004;33(19 Pt 2):1403–8. PubMed PMID: 15615251.

13. Salvarani C, Cantini F, Hunder GG. Polymyalgia rheumatica and giant-cell arteritis. Lancet. 2008;372(9634):234–45. https://doi.org/10.1016/S0140-6736(08)61077-6. PubMed PMID: 18640460.
14. Salvarani C, Gabriel SE, O'Fallon WM, Hunder GG. The incidence of giant cell arteritis in Olmsted County, Minnesota: apparent fluctuations in a cyclic pattern. Ann Intern Med. 1995;123(3):192–4. PubMed PMID: 7598301.
15. Petursdottir V, Johansson H, Nordborg E, Nordborg C. The epidemiology of biopsy-positive giant cell arteritis: special reference to cyclic fluctuations. Rheumatology (Oxford). 1999;38(12):1208–12. PubMed PMID: 10587547.
16. Bhatt AS, Manzo VE, Pedamallu CS, Duke F, Cai D, Bienfang DC, et al. In search of a candidate pathogen for giant cell arteritis: sequencing-based characterization of the giant cell arteritis microbiome. Arthritis Rheumatol. 2014;66(7):1939–44. https://doi.org/10.1002/art.38631. PubMed PMID: 24644069; PubMed Central PMCID: PMC4113339.
17. Krupa WM, Dewan M, Jeon MS, Kurtin PJ, Younge BR, Goronzy JJ, et al. Trapping of misdirected dendritic cells in the granulomatous lesions of giant cell arteritis. Am J Pathol. 2002;161(5):1815–23. https://doi.org/10.1016/S0002-9440(10)64458-6. PubMed PMID: 12414528; PubMed Central PMCID: PMC1850804.
18. Ma-Krupa W, Jeon MS, Spoerl S, Tedder TF, Goronzy JJ, Weyand CM. Activation of arterial wall dendritic cells and breakdown of self-tolerance in giant cell arteritis. J Exp Med. 2004;199(2):173–83. https://doi.org/10.1084/jem.20030850. PubMed PMID: 14734523; PubMed Central PMCID: PMC2211768.
19. Weyand CM, Goronzy JJ. Immune mechanisms in medium and large-vessel vasculitis. Nat Rev Rheumatol. 2013;9(12):731–40. https://doi.org/10.1038/nrrheum.2013.161. PubMed PMID: 24189842; PubMed Central PMCID: PMC4277683.
20. Horton R, Wilming L, Rand V, Lovering RC, Bruford EA, Khodiyar VK, et al. Gene map of the extended human MHC. Nat Rev Genet. 2004;5(12):889–99. https://doi.org/10.1038/nrg1489. PubMed PMID: 15573121.
21. Carmona FD, Mackie SL, Martin JE, Taylor JC, Vaglio A, Eyre S, et al. A large-scale genetic analysis reveals a strong contribution of the HLA class II region to giant cell arteritis susceptibility. Am J Hum Genet. 2015;96(4):565–80. https://doi.org/10.1016/j.ajhg.2015.02.009. PubMed PMID: 25817017; PubMed Central PMCID: PMC4385191.
22. Armstrong RD, Behn A, Myles A, Panayi GS, Welsh KI. Histocompatibility antigens in polymyalgia rheumatica and giant cell arteritis. J Rheumatol. 1983;10(4):659–61. PubMed PMID: 6413689.
23. Bignon JD, Barrier J, Soulillou JP, Martin P, Grolleau JY. HLA DR4 and giant cell arteritis. Tissue Antigens. 1984;24(1):60–2. PubMed PMID: 6333090.
24. Cid MC, Ercilla G, Vilaseca J, Sanmarti R, Villalta J, Ingelmo M, et al. Polymyalgia rheumatica: a syndrome associated with HLA-DR4 antigen. Arthritis Rheum. 1988;31(5):678–82. PubMed PMID: 3259885.
25. Combe B, Sany J, Le Quellec A, Clot J, Eliaou JF. Distribution of HLA-DRB1 alleles of patients with polymyalgia rheumatica and giant cell arteritis in a Mediterranean population. J Rheumatol. 1998;25(1):94–8. PubMed PMID: 9458210.
26. Dababneh A, Gonzalez-Gay MA, Garcia-Porrua C, Hajeer A, Thomson W, Ollier W. Giant cell arteritis and polymyalgia rheumatica can be differentiated by distinct patterns of HLA class II association. J Rheumatol. 1998;25(11):2140–5. PubMed PMID: 9818656.
27. Hansen JA, Healey LA, Wilske KR. Association between giant cell (temporal) arteritis and HLA-Cw3. Hum Immunol. 1985;13(3):193–8. PubMed PMID: 4008284.
28. Jacobsen S, Baslund B, Madsen HO, Tvede N, Svejgaard A, Garred P. Mannose-binding lectin variant alleles and HLA-DR4 alleles are associated with giant cell arteritis. J Rheumatol. 2002;29(10):2148–53. PubMed PMID: 12375325.
29. Lowenstein MB, Bridgeford PH, Vasey FB, Germain BF, Espinoza LR. Increased frequency of HLA-DR3 and DR4 in polymyalgia rheumatica-giant cell arteritis. Arthritis Rheum. 1983;26(7):925–7. PubMed PMID: 6603224.

30. Martinez-Taboda VM, Bartolome MJ, Lopez-Hoyos M, Blanco R, Mata C, Calvo J, et al. HLA-DRB1 allele distribution in polymyalgia rheumatica and giant cell arteritis: influence on clinical subgroups and prognosis. Semin Arthritis Rheum. 2004;34(1):454–64. PubMed PMID: 15305244.
31. Rauzy O, Fort M, Nourhashemi F, Alric L, Juchet H, Ecoiffier M, et al. Relation between HLA DRB1 alleles and corticosteroid resistance in giant cell arteritis. Ann Rheum Dis. 1998;57(6):380–2. PubMed PMID: 9771216; PubMed Central PMCID: PMC1752615.
32. Richardson JE, Gladman DD, Fam A, Keystone EC. HLA-DR4 in giant cell arteritis: association with polymyalgia rheumatica syndrome. Arthritis Rheum. 1987;30(11):1293–7. PubMed PMID: 3500727.
33. Weyand CM, Hicok KC, Hunder GG, Goronzy JJ. The HLA-DRB1 locus as a genetic component in giant cell arteritis. Mapping of a disease-linked sequence motif to the antigen binding site of the HLA-DR molecule. J Clin Invest. 1992;90(6):2355–61. https://doi.org/10.1172/JCI116125. PubMed PMID: 1469092; PubMed Central PMCID: PMC443390.
34. Gonzalez-Gay MA, Garcia-Porrua C, Llorca J, Hajeer AH, Branas F, Dababneh A, et al. Visual manifestations of giant cell arteritis. Trends and clinical spectrum in 161 patients. Medicine. 2000;79(5):283–92. PubMed PMID: 11039076.
35. Gonzalez-Gay MA, Garcia-Porrua C, Hajeer AH, Dababneh A, Ollier WE. HLA-DRB1*04 may be a marker of severity in giant cell arteritis. Ann Rheum Dis. 2000;59(7):574–5. PubMed PMID: 10950753; PubMed Central PMCID: PMC1753189.
36. Weyand CM, Hunder NN, Hicok KC, Hunder GG, Goronzy JJ. HLA-DRB1 alleles in polymyalgia rheumatica, giant cell arteritis, and rheumatoid arthritis. Arthritis Rheum. 1994;37(4):514–20. PubMed PMID: 8147928.
37. Kemp A, Marner K, Nissen SH, Heyn J, Kissmeyer-Nielsen F. HLA antigens in cases of giant cell arteritis. Acta Ophthalmol. 1980;58(6):1000–4. PubMed PMID: 6174016.
38. Gonzalez-Gay MA, Rueda B, Vilchez JR, Lopez-Nevot MA, Robledo G, Ruiz MP, et al. Contribution of MHC class I region to genetic susceptibility for giant cell arteritis. Rheumatology (Oxford). 2007;46(3):431–4. https://doi.org/10.1093/rheumatology/kel324. PubMed PMID: 17003171.
39. Marquez A, Hernandez-Rodriguez J, Cid MC, Solans R, Castaneda S, Fernandez-Contreras ME, et al. Influence of the IL17A locus in giant cell arteritis susceptibility. Ann Rheum Dis. 2014;73(9):1742–5. https://doi.org/10.1136/annrheumdis-2014-205261. PubMed PMID: 24919468.
40. Marquez A, Solans R, Hernandez-Rodriguez J, Cid MC, Castaneda S, Ramentol M, et al. A candidate gene approach identifies an IL33 genetic variant as a novel genetic risk factor for GCA. PLoS One. 2014;9(11):e113476. https://doi.org/10.1371/journal.pone.0113476. PubMed PMID: 25409453; PubMed Central PMCID: PMC4237421.
41. Serrano A, Carmona FD, Castaneda S, Solans R, Hernandez-Rodriguez J, Cid MC, et al. Evidence of association of the NLRP1 gene with giant cell arteritis. Ann Rheum Dis. 2013;72(4):628–30. https://doi.org/10.1136/annrheumdis-2012-202609. PubMed PMID: 23253924.
42. Serrano A, Marquez A, Mackie SL, Carmona FD, Solans R, Miranda-Filloy JA, et al. Identification of the PTPN22 functional variant R620W as susceptibility genetic factor for giant cell arteritis. Ann Rheum Dis. 2013;72(11):1882–6. https://doi.org/10.1136/annrheumdis-2013-203641. PubMed PMID: 23946333; PubMed Central PMCID: PMC4053592.
43. Rueda B, Roibas B, Martin J, Gonzalez-Gay MA. Influence of interleukin 10 promoter polymorphisms in susceptibility to giant cell arteritis in Northwestern Spain. J Rheumatol. 2007;34(7):1535–9. PubMed PMID: 17552041.
44. Boiardi L, Casali B, Farnetti E, Pipitone N, Nicoli D, Macchioni P, et al. Interleukin-10 promoter polymorphisms in giant cell arteritis. Arthritis Rheum. 2006;54(12):4011–7. https://doi.org/10.1002/art.22218. PubMed PMID: 17133531.
45. Gonzalez-Gay MA, Hajeer AH, Dababneh A, Garcia-Porrua C, Mattey DL, Amoli MM, et al. IL-6 promoter polymorphism at position -174 modulates the phenotypic expression of polymy-

algia rheumatica in biopsy-proven giant cell arteritis. Clin Exp Rheumatol. 2002;20(2):179–84. PubMed PMID: 12051396.
46. Enjuanes A, Benavente Y, Hernandez-Rodriguez J, Queralt C, Yague J, Jares P, et al. Association of NOS2 and potential effect of VEGF, IL6, CCL2 and IL1RN polymorphisms and haplotypes on susceptibility to GCA—a simultaneous study of 130 potentially functional SNPs in 14 candidate genes. Rheumatology (Oxford). 2012;51(5):841–51. https://doi.org/10.1093/rheumatology/ker429. PubMed PMID: 22258388.
47. Gonzalez-Gay MA, Hajeer AH, Dababneh A, Garcia-Porrua C, Amoli MM, Llorca J, et al. Interferon-gamma gene microsatellite polymorphisms in patients with biopsy-proven giant cell arteritis and isolated polymyalgia rheumatica. Clin Exp Rheumatol. 2004;22(6 Suppl 36):S18–20. PubMed PMID: 15675129.
48. Rodriguez-Rodriguez L, Carmona FD, Castaneda S, Miranda-Filloy JA, Morado IC, Narvaez J, et al. Role of rs1343151 IL23R and rs3790567 IL12RB2 polymorphisms in biopsy-proven giant cell arteritis. J Rheumatol. 2011;38(5):889–92. https://doi.org/10.3899/jrheum.101046. PubMed PMID: 21285166.
49. Morgan AW, Robinson JI, Barrett JH, Martin J, Walker A, Babbage SJ, et al. Association of FCGR2A and FCGR2A-FCGR3A haplotypes with susceptibility to giant cell arteritis. Arthritis Res Ther. 2006;8(4):R109. https://doi.org/10.1186/ar1996. PubMed PMID: 16846526; PubMed Central PMCID: PMC1779375.
50. Palomino-Morales R, Torres O, Vazquez-Rodriguez TR, Morado IC, Castaneda S, Callejas-Rubio JL, et al. Association between toll-like receptor 4 gene polymorphism and biopsy-proven giant cell arteritis. J Rheumatol. 2009;36(7):1501–6. https://doi.org/10.3899/jrheum.081286. PubMed PMID: 19531762.
51. Salvarani C, Casali B, Boiardi L, Ranzi A, Macchioni P, Nicoli D, et al. Intercellular adhesion molecule 1 gene polymorphisms in polymyalgia rheumatica/giant cell arteritis: association with disease risk and severity. J Rheumatol. 2000;27(5):1215–21. PubMed PMID: 10813290.
52. Boiardi L, Casali B, Nicoli D, Farnetti E, Chen Q, Macchioni P, et al. Vascular endothelial growth factor gene polymorphisms in giant cell arteritis. J Rheumatol. 2003;30(10):2160–4. PubMed PMID: 14528511.
53. Rueda B, Lopez-Nevot MA, Lopez-Diaz MJ, Garcia-Porrua C, Martin J, Gonzalez-Gay MA. A functional variant of vascular endothelial growth factor is associated with severe ischemic complications in giant cell arteritis. J Rheumatol. 2005;32(9):1737–41. PubMed PMID: 16142870.
54. Gonzalez-Gay MA, Oliver J, Sanchez E, Garcia-Porrua C, Paco L, Lopez-Nevot MA, et al. Association of a functional inducible nitric oxide synthase promoter variant with susceptibility to biopsy-proven giant cell arteritis. J Rheumatol. 2005;32(11):2178–82. PubMed PMID: 16265698.
55. Carmona FD, Martin J, Gonzalez-Gay MA. Genetics of vasculitis. Curr Opin Rheumatol. 2015;27(1):10–7. https://doi.org/10.1097/BOR.0000000000000124. PubMed PMID: 25405820.
56. Lester S, Hewitt AW, Ruediger CD, Bradbury L, De Smit E, Wiese MD, et al. PTPN22 R620W minor allele is a genetic risk factor for giant cell arteritis. RMD Open. 2016;2(1):e000246. https://doi.org/10.1136/rmdopen-2016-000246. PubMed PMID: 27110387; PubMed Central PMCID: PMC4838769.
57. Stanford SM, Bottini N. PTPN22: the archetypal non-HLA autoimmunity gene. Nat Rev Rheumatol. 2014;10(10):602–11. https://doi.org/10.1038/nrrheum.2014.109. PubMed PMID: 25003765; PubMed Central PMCID: PMC4375551.
58. Bottini N, Peterson EJ. Tyrosine phosphatase PTPN22: multifunctional regulator of immune signaling, development, and disease. Annu Rev Immunol. 2014;32:83–119. https://doi.org/10.1146/annurev-immunol-032713-120249. PubMed PMID: 24364806.
59. Du J, Qiao Y, Sun L, Wang X. Lymphoid-specific tyrosine phosphatase (Lyp): a potential drug target for treatment of autoimmune diseases. Curr Drug Targets. 2014;15(3):335–46. PubMed PMID: 24188455.

60. Espigol-Frigole G, Corbera-Bellalta M, Planas-Rigol E, Lozano E, Segarra M, Garcia-Martinez A, et al. Increased IL-17A expression in temporal artery lesions is a predictor of sustained response to glucocorticoid treatment in patients with giant-cell arteritis. Ann Rheum Dis. 2013;72(9):1481–7. https://doi.org/10.1136/annrheumdis-2012-201836. PubMed PMID: 22993227.
61. Deng J, Younge BR, Olshen RA, Goronzy JJ, Weyand CM. Th17 and Th1 T-cell responses in giant cell arteritis. Circulation. 2010;121(7):906–15. https://doi.org/10.1161/CIRCULATIONAHA.109.872903. PubMed PMID: 20142449; PubMed Central PMCID: PMC2837465.
62. Hernandez-Rodriguez J, Segarra M, Vilardell C, Sanchez M, Garcia-Martinez A, Esteban MJ, et al. Tissue production of pro-inflammatory cytokines (IL-1beta, TNFalpha and IL-6) correlates with the intensity of the systemic inflammatory response and with corticosteroid requirements in giant-cell arteritis. Rheumatology (Oxford). 2004;43(3):294–301. https://doi.org/10.1093/rheumatology/keh058. PubMed PMID: 14679293.
63. Cortes A, Brown MA. Promise and pitfalls of the Immunochip. Arthritis Res Ther. 2011;13(1):101. https://doi.org/10.1186/ar3204. PubMed PMID: 21345260; PubMed Central PMCID: PMC3157635.
64. Parkes M, Cortes A, van Heel DA, Brown MA. Genetic insights into common pathways and complex relationships among immune-mediated diseases. Nat Rev Genet. 2013;14(9):661–73. https://doi.org/10.1038/nrg3502. PubMed PMID: 23917628.
65. Saruhan-Direskeneli G, Hughes T, Aksu K, Keser G, Coit P, Aydin SZ, et al. Identification of multiple genetic susceptibility loci in Takayasu arteritis. Am J Hum Genet. 2013;93(2):298–305. https://doi.org/10.1016/j.ajhg.2013.05.026. PubMed PMID: 23830517; PubMed Central PMCID: PMC3738826.
66. Ortiz-Fernandez L, Carmona FD, Lopez-Mejias R, Gonzalez-Escribano MF, Lyons PA, Morgan AW, et al. Cross-phenotype analysis of Immunochip data identifies KDM4C as a relevant locus for the development of systemic vasculitis. Ann Rheum Dis. 2018;77(4):589–95. https://doi.org/10.1136/annrheumdis-2017-212372. PubMed PMID: 29374629; PubMed Central PMCID: PMC5849568.
67. Ortiz-Fernandez L, Carmona FD, Montes-Cano MA, Garcia-Lozano JR, Conde-Jaldon M, Ortego-Centeno N, et al. Genetic analysis with the Immunochip platform in Behcet disease. Identification of residues associated in the HLA class I region and new susceptibility loci. PLoS One. 2016;11(8):e0161305. https://doi.org/10.1371/journal.pone.0161305. PubMed PMID: 27548383; PubMed Central PMCID: PMC4993481.
68. de Bakker PI, Raychaudhuri S. Interrogating the major histocompatibility complex with high-throughput genomics. Hum Mol Genet. 2012;21(R1):R29–36. https://doi.org/10.1093/hmg/dds384. PubMed PMID: 22976473; PubMed Central PMCID: PMC3459647.
69. Jia X, Han B, Onengut-Gumuscu S, Chen WM, Concannon PJ, Rich SS, et al. Imputing amino acid polymorphisms in human leukocyte antigens. PLoS One. 2013;8(6):e64683. https://doi.org/10.1371/journal.pone.0064683. PubMed PMID: 23762245; PubMed Central PMCID: PMC3675122.
70. Brown JH, Jardetzky TS, Gorga JC, Stern LJ, Urban RG, Strominger JL, et al. Three-dimensional structure of the human class II histocompatibility antigen HLA-DR1. Nature. 1993;364(6432):33–9. https://doi.org/10.1038/364033a0. PubMed PMID: 8316295.
71. Tollefsen S, Hotta K, Chen X, Simonsen B, Swaminathan K, Mathews II, et al. Structural and functional studies of trans-encoded HLA-DQ2.3 (DQA1*03:01/DQB1*02:01) protein molecule. J Biol Chem. 2012;287(17):13611–9. https://doi.org/10.1074/jbc.M111.320374. PubMed PMID: 22362761; PubMed Central PMCID: PMC3340161.
72. Badrinath S, Huyton T, Schumacher H, Blasczyk R, Bade-Doeding C. Position 45 influences the peptide binding motif of HLA-B*44:08. Immunogenetics. 2012;64(3):245–9. https://doi.org/10.1007/s00251-011-0583-z. PubMed PMID: 22009320.
73. Wang R, Kozhaya L, Mercer F, Khaitan A, Fujii H, Unutmaz D. Expression of GARP selectively identifies activated human FOXP3+ regulatory T cells. Proc Natl Acad Sci U S

A. 2009;106(32):13439–44. https://doi.org/10.1073/pnas.0901965106. PubMed PMID: 19666573; PubMed Central PMCID: PMC2726405.
74. Samson M, Audia S, Fraszczak J, Trad M, Ornetti P, Lakomy D, et al. Th1 and Th17 lymphocytes expressing CD161 are implicated in giant cell arteritis and polymyalgia rheumatica pathogenesis. Arthritis Rheum. 2012;64(11):3788–98. https://doi.org/10.1002/art.34647. PubMed PMID: 22833233.
75. Carmona FD, Vaglio A, Mackie SL, Hernandez-Rodriguez J, Monach PA, Castaneda S, et al. A genome-wide association study identifies risk alleles in plasminogen and P4HA2 associated with giant cell arteritis. Am J Hum Genet. 2017;100(1):64–74. https://doi.org/10.1016/j.ajhg.2016.11.013. PubMed PMID: 28041642; PubMed Central PMCID: PMC5223025.
76. Law RH, Abu-Ssaydeh D, Whisstock JC. New insights into the structure and function of the plasminogen/plasmin system. Curr Opin Struct Biol. 2013;23(6):836–41. https://doi.org/10.1016/j.sbi.2013.10.006. PubMed PMID: 24252474.
77. Moser TL, Stack MS, Asplin I, Enghild JJ, Hojrup P, Everitt L, et al. Angiostatin binds ATP synthase on the surface of human endothelial cells. Proc Natl Acad Sci U S A. 1999;96(6):2811–6. PubMed PMID: 10077593; PubMed Central PMCID: PMC15851.
78. Miles LA, Parmer RJ. Plasminogen receptors: the first quarter century. Semin Thromb Hemost. 2013;39(4):329–37. https://doi.org/10.1055/s-0033-1334483. PubMed PMID: 23532575; PubMed Central PMCID: PMC3938387.
79. Myllyharju J. Prolyl 4-hydroxylases, the key enzymes of collagen biosynthesis. Matrix Biol. 2003;22(1):15–24. PubMed PMID: 12714038.
80. Dupont C, Armant DR, Brenner CA. Epigenetics: definition, mechanisms and clinical perspective. Semin Reprod Med. 2009;27(5):351–7. https://doi.org/10.1055/s-0029-1237423. PubMed PMID: 19711245; PubMed Central PMCID: PMC2791696.
81. Mohan SV, Liao YJ, Kim JW, Goronzy JJ, Weyand CM. Giant cell arteritis: immune and vascular aging as disease risk factors. Arthritis Res Ther. 2011;13(4):231. https://doi.org/10.1186/ar3358. PubMed PMID: 21861860; PubMed Central PMCID: PMC3239337.
82. Wing S, Rider LG, Johnson JR, Miller FW, Matteson EL, Crowson CS, et al. Do solar cycles influence giant cell arteritis and rheumatoid arthritis incidence? BMJ Open. 2015;5(5):e006636. https://doi.org/10.1136/bmjopen-2014-006636. PubMed PMID: 25979866; PubMed Central PMCID: PMC4442155.
83. Lee JL, Naguwa SM, Cheema GS, Gershwin ME. The geo-epidemiology of temporal (giant cell) arteritis. Clin Rev Allergy Immunol. 2008;35(1–2):88–95. https://doi.org/10.1007/s12016-008-8075-0. PubMed PMID: 18286386.
84. Coit P, De Lott LB, Nan B, Elner VM, Sawalha AH. DNA methylation analysis of the temporal artery microenvironment in giant cell arteritis. Ann Rheum Dis. 2016;75(6):1196–202. https://doi.org/10.1136/annrheumdis-2014-207116. PubMed PMID: 26038090.
85. Djuretic IM, Levanon D, Negreanu V, Groner Y, Rao A, Ansel KM. Transcription factors T-bet and Runx3 cooperate to activate Ifng and silence Il4 in T helper type 1 cells. Nat Immunol. 2007;8(2):145–53. https://doi.org/10.1038/ni1424. PubMed PMID: 17195845.
86. Coit P, Direskeneli H, Sawalha AH. An update on the role of epigenetics in systemic vasculitis. Curr Opin Rheumatol. 2018;30(1):4–15. https://doi.org/10.1097/BOR.0000000000000451. PubMed PMID: 28957963; PubMed Central PMCID: PMC5805392.
87. Dozmorov MG, Coit P, Maksimowicz-McKinnon K, Sawalha AH. Age-associated DNA methylation changes in naive CD4(+) T cells suggest an evolving autoimmune epigenotype in aging T cells. Epigenomics. 2017;9(4):429–45. https://doi.org/10.2217/epi-2016-0143. PubMed PMID: 28322571; PubMed Central PMCID: PMC5549647.
88. Kermani TA. Takayasu arteritis and giant cell arteritis: are they a spectrum of the same disease? Int J Rheum Dis. 2018;22(Suppl 1):41–8. https://doi.org/10.1111/1756-185X.13288. PubMed PMID: 29624864.
89. Carmona FD, Coit P, Saruhan-Direskeneli G, Hernandez-Rodriguez J, Cid MC, Solans R, et al. Analysis of the common genetic component of large-vessel vasculitides through a meta-Immunochip strategy. Sci Rep. 2017;7:43953. https://doi.org/10.1038/srep43953. PubMed PMID: 28277489; PubMed Central PMCID: PMC5344032.

90. Goriely S, Neurath MF, Goldman M. How microorganisms tip the balance between interleukin-12 family members. Nat Rev Immunol. 2008;8(1):81–6. https://doi.org/10.1038/nri2225. PubMed PMID: 18084185.
91. Conway R, O'Neill L, O'Flynn E, Gallagher P, McCarthy GM, Murphy CC, et al. Ustekinumab for the treatment of refractory giant cell arteritis. Ann Rheum Dis. 2016;75(8):1578–9. https://doi.org/10.1136/annrheumdis-2016-209351. PubMed PMID: 27143653.
92. Berry WL, Janknecht R. KDM4/JMJD2 histone demethylases: epigenetic regulators in cancer cells. Cancer Res. 2013;73(10):2936–42. https://doi.org/10.1158/0008-5472.CAN-12-4300. PubMed PMID: 23644528; PubMed Central PMCID: PMC3655154.
93. Gonzalez-Gay MA. Giant cell arteritis and polymyalgia rheumatica: two different but often overlapping conditions. Semin Arthritis Rheum. 2004;33(5):289–93. PubMed PMID: 15079759.
94. Gonzalez-Gay MA, Garcia-Porrua C, Vazquez-Caruncho M. Polymyalgia rheumatica in biopsy proven giant cell arteritis does not constitute a different subset but differs from isolated polymyalgia rheumatica. J Rheumatol. 1998;25(9):1750–5. PubMed PMID: 9733456.

Takayasu Arteritis

8

Elizabeth Gensterblum and Amr H. Sawalha

Contents

8.1 Introduction

Takayasu arteritis (TA) is an immune-mediated disease that predominately affects the aorta and its major branches. In 1990 the American College of Rheumatology proposed the presence of three of the following disease criteria for classification of TA: decreased brachial artery pulse, claudication of an extremity, blood pressure

E. Gensterblum
Division of Rheumatology, Department of Internal Medicine, University of Michigan, Ann Arbor, MI, USA
e-mail: gensterb@umich.edu

A. H. Sawalha (✉)
Division of Rheumatology, Department of Internal Medicine, University of Michigan, Ann Arbor, MI, USA

Center for Computational Medicine and Bioinformatics, University of Michigan, Ann Arbor, MI, USA
e-mail: asawalha@umich.edu

J. Martín, F. D. Carmona (eds.), *Genetics of Rare Autoimmune Diseases*, Rare Diseases of the Immune System, https://doi.org/10.1007/978-3-030-03934-9_8

discrepancy between arms, subclavian arterial bruit, narrowing of the aorta or its major branches or proximal arteries, and an age of onset less than or equal to 40 years of age [1]. TA has been sometimes referred to as pulseless disease, due to this decrease of brachial artery pulse. Other manifestations of TA may include aortic regurgitation, hypertension, and arterial lesions, specifically in the pulmonary, left mid-common carotid, distal brachiocephalic, and thoracic arteries, as well as the abdominal aorta [1]. The specific etiology of TA is not known, though it has been shown to have a genetic component, based on geographic and familial clustering, immunogenetic analysis, candidate gene studies, and three published large genotyping array experiments.

The pathophysiology of TA is incompletely understood, but the role of infiltrating immune cells, specifically T cells, has been described. The aortic tissues of TA patients are infiltrated with CD4+ T cells, CD8+ T cells, macrophages, natural killer cells, and γδ T cells [2] (Fig. 8.1). Specifically, the infiltrating CD4+ T cells demonstrate a T_H1/T_H17 phenotype. Compared to healthy controls, TA patients show increased concentrations of IL-2, IL-2R, IL-12, IL-23, IFNγ, TNFα, IL-1RA, and IL-17A. Moreover, CD4+ T cells that produce either IL-17A or IFNγ are increased in active TA patients compared to both TA in remission and healthy controls [3]. Interactions between CD4+ T cells and dendritic cells have also been implicated, as co-localized CD4+ T

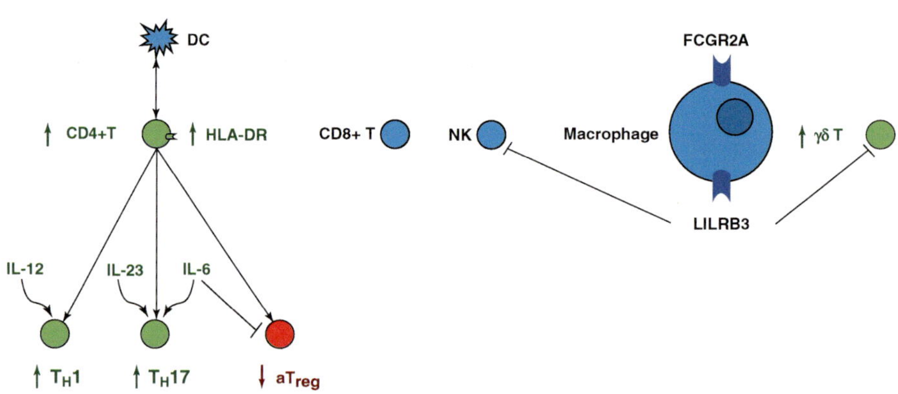

Fig. 8.1 Summary of immunologic roles of susceptibility genes associated with TA. Immune cells that have been found infiltrated in aortic tissue of TA patients are depicted. Only genes that have been identified in genotyping array studies are included in this summary. All genes that are demonstrably upregulated and all cell populations increased in PBMCs in TA are shown in green, all that are downregulated or decreased are shown in red, and all cells that have no altered prevalence are shown in blue. IL-12B, a component of both IL-23 and IL-12, is involved in T_H1/T_H17 cell differentiation. IL-6 is required for T_H17 differentiation. HLA-DRB1 is a late activation marker of CD4+ T cells, and HLA-DRB1 expressing CD4+ T cells are increased in TA. HLA-B can be expressed by all shown cells and targeted for apoptosis by NK cells. FCGR2A and LILRB3 are both found on the surface of macrophages. LILRB3 binds to MHC class I proteins, and inhibits apoptotic activity of NK cells and γδ T cells. While decreased expression of LILRB3 has not been demonstrated in TA patients, the variant that is associated with TA is correlated to decreased LILRB3 expression in healthy controls. Abbreviations: *T_H1* T helper 1 cell, *T_H17* T helper 17 cell, *aT_{reg}* activated regulatory T cell, *DC* dendritic cell, *NK* natural killer cell, *T* T cell, *IL* interleukin, *CD* cluster of differentiation

cells and dendritic cells have been found in inflamed arteries [4]. In addition, the leukocyte adhesion molecules VCAM-1 and ICAM-1 are increased in TA patients [5]. The peripheral blood mononuclear cells (PBMCs) of patients with active TA contain a higher proportion of γδ T cells than healthy controls and a higher proportion of γδ T cells that produce IFNγ [6]. Increased apoptosis of arterial cells has been described in TA, potentially mediated by perforin, which is released by infiltrating CD8+ T cells, γδ T cells, and natural killer cells [2]. Moreover, other costimulatory molecules that enhance natural killer cell-mediated apoptosis, such as 4-1bb, 4-1 bbl, and Fas, are increased in TA patients [7]. To summarize, while inflammation in TA is predominately CD4+ T-cell mediated, CD8+ T cells, γδ T cells, natural killer cells, dendritic cells, and macrophages have been shown to also play a role in the disease etiology.

8.2 Geographic and Familial Localization

Evidence of a genetic component to TA stems from the varying disease prevalence in different racial and ethnic groups. TA is most commonly described in Asian and South American populations [8]. Females are more likely to develop the disease than males across all ethnicities, and it is most commonly diagnosed between the age of 25 and 30 years [9, 10]. However, the exact proportion of female TA patients varies between countries; the highest proportion is in Japan, reporting an 8:1 female to male ratio [9]. Moreover, the prevalence of specific disease manifestations varies across geographic regions. For example, ascending aorta, aortic arch, and ocular involvement is more common among Japanese patients than in the rest of the world. Meanwhile, abdominal arterial involvement, as well as secondary hypertension, is more common in Indian, Chinese, and Thai populations [8]. The geographic localization of disease incidence, as well as the distribution of specific manifestations, suggest that genetic factors contribute to disease pathogenesis and progression.

In addition to patterns in geographic localization, familial aggregation of TA has been well documented. Several studies have shown TA aggregated within families [11–16]. Moreover, TA has been reported in monozygotic twins [17, 18]. Each of these family and twin studies suggests a potential genetic association with TA. Determining the genetic differences in these families has focused on human leukocyte antigen (HLA) typing in affected patients and their families. Of the HLA alleles found in affected, but not unaffected, siblings, the HLA-B*52 and HLA-A*24 alleles have been repeatedly described [12]. However, not all family studies show consistent and unique similarities between affected siblings compared to unaffected siblings [14, 18]. This suggests a role for both non-HLA polymorphisms and environmental factors in disease progression.

8.3 Associations Within the HLA Region

Research focused on identifying specific genetic components of TA initially focused on HLA types. An association between HLA-B*52 and TA was first documented in

1978, in a Japanese population [19]. This association has since been robustly described in other ethnicities, including in northern Indian [20], Thai [21], Mexican [22], Turkish [23], European-American [24], Greek [25], and Korean [26] cohorts, in addition to other Japanese cohorts [27–29] (Table 8.1). Variable prevalence of these HLA allelotypes throughout the world has been repeatedly put forward as an explanation for the geographic localization of TA patients, as the HLA-B*52 allele is more common in Japan compared to the rest of the world. In more recent studies, the allelotype HLA-B*52-01 has been specifically implicated. Large population studies have also identified other associated alleles. In Japanese cohorts, HLA-B*39, HLA-DRB1*15-02, HLA-DQA1*01-03, HLA-DQB1*06-01, HLA-B*67-01, and HLA-DPB1*09-01 have also been associated with TA [30–34]. In a Han Chinese cohort, HLA-DRB1*07 was associated with TA, as well as a DQA1*03-01-DQB1*03-01-DRB1*07 haplotype [35]. Additional associated HLA alleles have been described in multiple ethnicities (Table 8.1). In a Korean cohort, HLA-A*30-01 and HLA-DRB1*15-02 were associated with disease risk, while HLA-A*26-02 was found to be protective [26]. In Mexican patients, HLA-B*15 was associated with TA alongside HLA-B*52 [22]. In multiple populations, HLA-DPB1*09-01 has been found to be more common in TA patients [33, 34, 36]. In Han Chinese patients, this allele and the HLA-DPB1*17-01 allele have been correlated with an earlier age of onset [36]. However, the HLA-DPB1*09-01 allele is

Table 8.1 List of all HLA alleles associated with TA, including the ethnicity in which the effect has been described

Gene	Allelotype	Ethnicity	Reference
HLA-A	*30-01	Korean	[26]
HLA-B	*15	Mexican	[22]
HLA-B	*52	Japanese, Indian, Thai, Mexican, Turkish, European-American, Greek, Korean	[19–29, 32–34]
HLA-B	*39	Japanese	[33]
HLA-B	*67-01	Japanese	[31, 32]
HLA-DPB1	*09-01	Japanese, Han Chinese	[33, 34, 36]
HLA-DPB1	*17-01	Han Chinese	[36]
HLA-DQA1	*0103	Japanese	[34]
HLA-DQB1	*0601	Japanese	[34]
HLA-DRB1	*15-02	Japanese	[33, 34]
HLA-DRB1	*07	Han Chinese	[35]
HLA-DRB1	*15-02	Korean	[26]

Each of these allelotypes was identified using HLA allelotyping experiments, and only statistically significant ($p < 0.05$) allelotypes are included

commonly found alongside HLA-B*52, so this association may be due to a linkage disequilibrium effect and may not have an independent effect on disease etiology [36]. Because concurrent associations of allelotypes of separate genes may be due to linkage disequilibrium, the exact HLA variation that directly influences the mechanism of disease can be difficult to elucidate.

8.4 Non-HLA Candidate Gene Studies

Candidate gene studies targeting non-HLA loci have been used to identify additional genetic risk loci in TA (Table 8.2). Genes were selected for study based on the potential functional relevance of the proteins they code to disease etiology. The serum concentrations of the cytokines IL-12 and IL-6 have been shown to be increased in TA patients compared to healthy controls, while expression of IL-2 has been implicated in TA pathogenesis [3, 37]. As genetic polymorphisms can affect the rate of transcription of genes, as well as alter the activity of the translated proteins, these genes have been selected for a candidate gene study in a Turkish cohort. It was found that certain genotypes of *IL12B* (rs3213113, CC), *IL6* (rs1800795, GG), and *IL2* (rs2069762 TT) were more common in TA patients compared to healthy controls [37]. Other candidate genes that were selected based on their pro-inflammatory activity or role in other autoimmune diseases have been shown to be associated with TA. The cytokine IL-1 plays a role both in pro-inflammatory response and in vascular smooth muscle proliferation, so *IL1* and *IL1RN* polymorphisms were analyzed in a Mexican cohort [38]. Significant associations between TA and multiple genotypes within *IL1* and *IL1RN* were described (rs3811058 C, rs315952 C, and rs315951 G alleles; rs3811058 TC, rs419598 TT, and rs315952 TC genotypes). Another Mexican cohort demonstrated a preponderance of polymorphisms in *PON1* (rs854560 and

Table 8.2 List of all single-SNP alleles and genotypes with statistically significant associations ($p < 0.05$) with TA, which have been identified in candidate gene association studies

Gene	Variant	Risk allele/ genotype	Ethnicity	Study type	Reference
IL1	rs3811058	C	Mexican	Candidate gene	[38]
IL1	rs3811058	TC	Mexican	Candidate gene	[38]
IL1RN	rs315952	C	Mexican	Candidate gene	[38]
IL1RN	rs315951	G	Mexican	Candidate gene	[38]
IL1RN	rs419598	TT	Mexican	Candidate gene	[38]
IL1RN	rs315952	TC	Mexican	Candidate gene	[38]
IL2	rs2069762	TT	Turkish	Candidate gene	[37]
IL6	rs1800795	GG	Turkish	Candidate gene	[37]
IL12B	rs3213113	CC	Turkish	Candidate gene	[37]
PON1	rs854560	A	Mexican	Candidate gene	[39]
PON1	rs705379	T	Mexican	Candidate gene	[39]
FCGR2A/ FCGR3A	rs10919543	G	Han Chinese	Candidate gene	[48]

rs705379) in TA patients [39]. Furthermore, a PON1 enzyme with these polymorphisms was shown to be less active than the wild-type PON1. Nevertheless, polymorphisms in promising candidate genes are not always found to be relevant to the disease. In two studies focused on Turkish cohorts, polymorphisms around the genes *PDCD1* (PD-1.3, PD-1.5, PD-1.6) [40] and *PTPN22* (rs2476601) [41] were equally frequent in TA patients and healthy controls. This series of studies in Turkish and Mexican cohorts has identified several genetic polymorphisms within proteins that could be directly involved with TA etiology.

8.5 Insights from Genotyping Array Experiments

Large-scale genotyping array experiments have been used to identify novel genetic susceptibility loci in TA. One genome-wide association study (GWAS) has been performed comparing TA patients to healthy controls, using both a Turkish and a European-American cohort (Figs. 8.1 and 8.2). In a meta-analysis

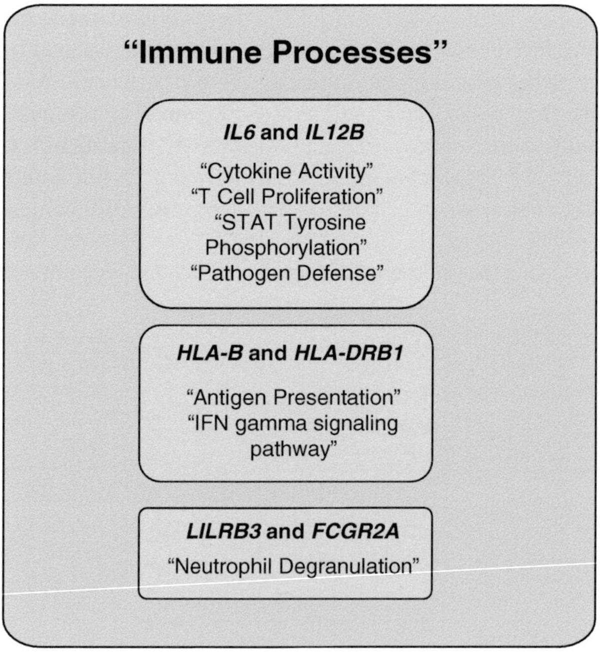

Fig. 8.2 Overlapping ontologies of genes with variants associated with TA, as identified by genotyping array studies. Listed are gene ontology (GO) terms shared between both genes in each cluster, identified using the UniProt-GOA database [57]. Every gene identified is annotated with the GO term "Immune System Processes" (GO:0002376) or "Immune Response" (GO:0006955). *IL12B* and *IL6* are both annotated with multiple pathogen defense GO terms; the overlapping terms are defense response to gram-negative bacteria, defense response to virus, and defense response to protozoan. Each gene with variants associated with TA in a large genotyping study has an immune-related function, with specific ontologies shared between genes listed

of both cohorts, this study found significant associations between TA and three loci: *IL6* (rs2069837, meta-analysis OR, 2.1; p, 6.7 × 10^{-9}), *RPS9/LILRB3* (rs11666453, OR, 1.6; p, 2.34 × 10^{-8}), and a locus on chromosome 21q22, near *PSMG1* (rs2836878, OR, 1.8; p, 3.62 × 10^{-10}) (Table 8.3) [42]. The cytokine IL-6 plays a role in T-cell differentiation. It is required for T_H17 differentiation, and also inhibits T_{reg} differentiation, which may play a role in the increased T_H17 and decreased T_{reg} populations seen in active TA [3, 43]. Because the associated SNP rs2069837 is found within an enhancer region of *IL6*, it may prove to play a role in the dysregulation of IL-6 shown in TA. Variation in *LILRB3* may also directly affect pathogenesis. While LILRB3 is involved in repression of the anti-MHC class 1 immune response, the variant rs11666453 is associated with a decrease in *LILRB3* expression [42]. As *HLA-B*, an MHC class I gene, has been repeatedly implicated in TA, this suggests that variation negatively affecting the expression of *LILRB3* may play a role in this same disease pathway. Variations affecting the function of *LILRB3* and *IL6* may directly affect the pathways involved in disease etiology.

Two targeted arrays have been performed to identify additional genetic associations with TA. A Turkish cohort and a European-American cohort were also fine mapped using an Immuno BeadChip Microarray (ImmunoChip), which targets immune-related genes and genes that have been previously associated with immune-mediated diseases (Figs. 8.1 and 8.2). Genetic associations with a GWAS level of significance were established in *FCGR2A/FCGR3A* (rs10919543, meta-analysis OR, 1.81; p, 5.89 × 10^{-12}) and *IL12B* (rs56167332, meta-analysis OR, 1.54; p, 2.18 × 10^{-8}) [24]. The *FCGR2A/FCGR3A*

Table 8.3 List of variants associated with TA, identified by genotyping array

Gene	Variant	Risk allele	Ethnicity	Study type	Reference
IL6	rs2069837	A	Turkish/European American	GWAS	[42]
RPS9/LILRB3	rs11666543	G	Turkish/European American	GWAS	[42]
Chr.21q22	rs2836878	G	Turkish/European American	GWAS	[42]
FCGR2A/ FCGR3A	rs10919543	G	Turkish/European American	ImmunoChip Array	[24]
HLA-DRB1/ HLA-DQA1	rs113452171	C	Turkish/European American	ImmunoChip Array	[24]
HLA-B/MICA	rs12524487	T	Turkish/European American	ImmunoChip Array	[24]
IL12B	rs56167332	A	Turkish/European American	ImmunoChip Array	[24]
IL12B	rs6871626	A	Japanese	Exome Array	[27]

Only variants identified with a genome-wide level of significance are included ($p < 5 \times 10^{-8}$). In scenarios where multiple variants within the same locus within the same study were statistically significant only the index variant, the variant with the lowest p value, was included

polymorphism is associated with increased *FCGR2A* expression in lymphoblastoid cells. Typically, *FCGR2A* is expressed on macrophages and neutrophils, and is involved in phagocytosis, so this variant may affect the activity of the infiltrating macrophages found in TA [44]. In the HLA region, a novel association with the *HLADRB1/HLADQA1* locus (rs113452171, OR, 2.34; *p*, 3.74×10^{-9}; rs189754752, OR, 2.47; *p*, 4.22×10^{-9}) was independent of a HLA-B*52 effect. Along with HLA-B*52-01, TA patients demonstrated an increased frequency of HLA-Cw*12-02 and rs12524487, an intergenic SNP near *HLA-B* not associated with an HLA allelotype. However, because HLA-Cw*12-02 and rs12524487 are in linkage disequilibrium with HLA-B*52-01, these could all be part of the same genetic effect.

Genetic effects have been also described via genotyping arrays in two Japanese cohorts. Using an Exome BeadChip, an array targeting exonic variants, a polymorphism within the *IL12B* (rs6871626, meta-analysis OR, 1.76; *p*, 1.7×10^{-13}) locus was described [27]. This genetic variant is in strong linkage disequilibrium with rs56167332, the index SNP in *IL12B* associated with TA in the ImmunoChip study described above [24] (Figs. 8.1 and 8.2). In Japanese patients, the *IL12B* locus was also found to be associated with aortic regurgitation (*p*, 0.0046). In addition, in these Japanese cohorts, a suggestive association with the transcription factor gene *MLX* was described, but this did not reach a genome level of significance (rs665268, *p*, 5.2×10^{-7}). This same study validated the well-described association with HLA-B*52 (OR, 2.44; *p*, 2.8×10^{-21}).

Both of these genotyping studies identified polymorphisms in *IL12B* that contribute to genetic risk for TA. There are multiple mechanisms by which differences of the expression of IL-12B may contribute to disease progression. The IL-12B subunit, p40, is common to both IL-12 and IL-23, and increased levels of both cytokines have been reported in TA patients [3]. IL-12 is involved in T_H1 differentiation, and IL-23 is important for T_H17 cell maintenance; furthermore, both cell types are increased in active TA [45, 46]. As part of the T_H1 response, IL-12 activates IFNγ production and related signaling cascades; moreover, IL-12-stimulated PBMCs have been shown to inhibit angiogenesis by inhibiting endothelial cell growth in an IFNγ-dependent manner [47]. It has been suggested that this inhibition of angiogenesis leads to slower healing of aortic lesions that form during active TA [44].

The genetic variants identified from these array-based genotyping studies were subsequently examined with a candidate gene association study in Han Chinese patients and controls. The *FCGR2A/FCG3A* variant (rs10919543), previously identified in Turkish and European-American populations, was replicated (Table 8.3) [48]. However, this same study found no effect in the variants previously described in the *MLX*, *HLA-B/MICA*, and *IL12B* (rs665268, rs12524487, and rs56167332, respectively). This suggests the presence of ethnicity-specific genetic loci in TA. The genetic association between TA and the *FCGR2A/FCGR3A* locus was further validated in Han Chinese patients in a larger subsequent study [49].

8.6 Similarities with Other Diseases

Some of the genetic associations described in TA are shared by other immune-mediated diseases. TA and ulcerative colitis (UC) have both been associated with a risk locus in *FCGR2A*/*FCGR3A* and the locus on chromosome 21q22 [24]. In a study of 470 TA patients, concurrent UC was found to be significantly higher than the prevalence of UC in Japan (6.4% vs. 0.11%; p, 1.0×10^{-10}) [50], confirming earlier observations [51]. It was also found that UC patients develop TA earlier than patients with only a TA diagnosis, though there is no evidence that one disease usually precedes the other. Genetically, HLA-B*52 frequency, but not rs6871626 (*IL12B*) allele frequency, was increased in patients with both diseases, compared to patients with only TA (OR,12.14; p, 1.0×10^{-5}) [50]. This enforces the observation that UC and TA share genetic risk loci [24], leading to the increased comorbidity of both diseases. Furthermore, TA has been shown to be genetically distinct from other diseases. The *HLA-B* alleles associated with TA and tuberculosis have been shown to be genetically distinct, despite the occurrence of arterial lesions in both diseases [52].

Genetic similarities between TA and giant cell arteritis (GCA) have been evaluated on a large scale using the ImmunoChip platform [53]. GCA is another large-vessel vasculitis, which similar to TA can also affect the aorta, but unlike TA, generally affects older patients. After comparing variant genotypes through a meta-analysis using ImmunoChip genetic data in both diseases, it was found that both TA and GCA share the *IL12B* risk locus (rs755374, p, 7.54×10^{-7}). Moreover, GCA was found to be predominantly HLA class II mediated, significantly associated with the *HLA-DRB1*/*HLA-DQA1* locus, while the HLA class I effect focused around *HLA-B*/*MICA* was again validated in TA (most significant variants, rs9405038 and rs12524487, respectively) [53].

8.7 Conclusions and Future Implications

Until very recently, the genetic association with HLA-B*52 was the only genetic risk locus confirmed for TA in multiple ethnicities. Progress in the last few years has led to the discovery and replication of several additional genetic risk loci with a GWAS level of significance for this complex disease. These findings shed light into the disease pathogenesis and implicate key immune-related mechanisms that can be potentially targeted for therapy. However, despite this progress, the functional consequences for the genetic risk variants identified in TA are still largely unknown, and the limited sample size for studies performed to date precluded from the identification of the complete genetic makeup underlying this disease.

Very little is known about how the genetic risk variants for TA contribute to disease severity or other clinical characteristics. There is some evidence that both the HLA-B*52 allele and the *IL12B* risk locus are associated with disease severity. HLA-B*52 has been associated with use of higher prednisone doses, higher

C-reactive protein levels, early disease onset, more extensive aortic involvement, left ventricular dysfunction, and aortic regurgitation in TA [23, 54, 55]. In a Japanese cohort, individuals with the risk allele in *IL12B* (rs6871626-A) had a higher probability for disease relapse [56]. These observations suggest that genetic information could be developed to help in better assessing disease prognosis and outcome in TA in the future. Further, as the functional mechanisms impacted by each genetic susceptibility variant are more thoroughly understood, novel therapeutic options and individualized treatment plans for TA patients could become available.

References

1. Arend WP, Michel BA, Bloch DA, Hunder GG, Calabrese LH, Edworthy SM, Fauci AS, Leavitt RY, Lie JT, Lightfoot RW Jr, et al. The American College of Rheumatology 1990 criteria for the classification of Takayasu arteritis. Arthritis Rheum. 1990;33:1129–34.
2. Seko Y, Minota S, Kawasaki A, Shinkai Y, Maeda K, Yagita H, Okumura K, Sato O, Takagi A, Tada Y, et al. Perforin-secreting killer cell infiltration and expression of a 65-kD heat-shock protein in aortic tissue of patients with Takayasu's arteritis. J Clin Invest. 1994;93:750–8.
3. Saadoun D, Garrido M, Comarmond C, Desbois AC, Domont F, Savey L, Terrier B, Geri G, Rosenzwajg M, Klatzmann D, et al. Th1 and Th17 cytokines drive inflammation in Takayasu arteritis. Arthritis Rheumatol. 2015;67:1353–60.
4. Inder SJ, Bobryshev YV, Cherian SM, Wang AY, Lord RS, Masuda K, Yutani C. Immunophenotypic analysis of the aortic wall in Takayasu's arteritis: involvement of lymphocytes, dendritic cells and granulocytes in immuno-inflammatory reactions. Cardiovasc Surg. 2000;8:141–8.
5. Noguchi S, Numano F, Gravanis MB, Wilcox JN. Increased levels of soluble forms of adhesion molecules in Takayasu arteritis. Int J Cardiol. 1998;66(Suppl 1):S23–33; discussion S35-26.
6. Chauhan SK, Tripathy NK, Sinha N, Nityanand S. T-cell receptor repertoire of circulating gamma delta T-cells in Takayasu's arteritis. Clin Immunol. 2006;118:243–9.
7. Seko Y, Sugishita K, Sato O, Takagi A, Tada Y, Matsuo H, Yagita H, Okumura K, Nagai R. Expression of costimulatory molecules (4-1BBL and Fas) and major histocompatibility class I chain-related A (MICA) in aortic tissue with Takayasu's arteritis. J Vasc Res. 2004;41:84–90.
8. Numano F. Differences in clinical presentation and outcome in different countries for Takayasu's arteritis. Curr Opin Rheumatol. 1997;9:12–5.
9. Numano F, Okawara M, Inomata H, Kobayashi Y. Takayasu's arteritis. Lancet. 2000;356:1023–5.
10. Phillip R, Luqmani R. Mortality in systemic vasculitis: a systematic review. Clin Exp Rheumatol. 2008;26:S94–104.
11. Jeeva I, Sajid J, Ali O, Bonthron DT, Frossard PM. Atypical Takayasu arteritis: a family with five affected siblings. Med Sci Monit. 2007;13:CS101–5.
12. Morishita KA, Rosendahl K, Brogan PA. Familial Takayasu arteritis—a pediatric case and a review of the literature. Pediatr Rheumatol Online J. 2011;9:6.
13. Numano F. Hereditary factors of Takayasu arteritis. Heart Vessels Suppl. 1992;7:68–72.
14. Makino N, Senda Y, Yamaguchi Y. Takayasu's disease in two brothers. Analysis of HLA types. Br Heart J. 1981;46:446–8.
15. Kodama K, Kida O, Morotomi Y, Tanaka K. Male siblings with Takayasu's arteritis suggest genetic etiology. Heart Vessel. 1986;2:51–4.
16. Heo JH, Kim M. Familial Takayasu's arteritis in female siblings. Rheumatol Int. 2011;31:815–8.
17. Numano F, Isohisa I, Kishi U, Arita M, Maezawa H. Takayasu's disease in twin sisters. Possible genetic factors. Circulation. 1978;58:173–7.
18. Enomoto S, Iwasaki Y, Bannai S, Nara Y, Matsuoka A, Aizawa Y, Shibata A. Takayasu's disease in twin sisters. Jpn Heart J. 1984;25:147–52.

19. Isohisa I, Numano F, Maezawa H, Sasazuki T. HLA-Bw52 in Takayasu disease. Tissue Antigens. 1978;12:246–8.
20. Mehra NK, Jaini R, Balamurugan A, Kanga U, Prabhakaran D, Jain S, Talwar KK, Sharma BK. Immunogenetic analysis of Takayasu arteritis in Indian patients. Int J Cardiol. 1998;66(Suppl 1):S127–32; discussion S133.
21. Charoenwongse P, Kangwanshiratada O, Boonnam R, Hoomsindhu U. The association between the HLA antigens and Takayasu's arteritis in Thai patients. Int J Cardiol. 1998;66(Suppl 1):S117–20.
22. Vargas-Alarcon G, Flores-Dominguez C, Hernandez-Pacheco G, Zuniga J, Gamboa R, Soto ME, Granados J, Reyes PA. Immunogenetics and clinical aspects of Takayasu's arteritis patients in a Mexican Mestizo population. Clin Exp Rheumatol. 2001;19:439–43.
23. Sahin Z, Bicakcigil M, Aksu K, Kamali S, Akar S, Onen F, Karadag O, Ozbalkan Z, Ates A, Ozer HT, et al. Takayasu's arteritis is associated with HLA-B*52, but not with HLA-B*51, in Turkey. Arthritis Res Ther. 2012;14:R27.
24. Saruhan-Direskeneli G, Hughes T, Aksu K, Keser G, Coit P, Aydin SZ, Alibaz-Oner F, Kamali S, Inanc M, Carette S, et al. Identification of multiple genetic susceptibility loci in Takayasu arteritis. Am J Hum Genet. 2013;93:298–305.
25. Karageorgaki ZT, Bertsias GK, Mavragani CP, Kritikos HD, Spyropoulou-Vlachou M, Drosos AA, Boumpas DT, Moutsopoulos HM. Takayasu arteritis: epidemiological, clinical, and immunogenetic features in Greece. Clin Exp Rheumatol. 2009;27:S33–9.
26. Lee SW, Kwon OJ, Park MC, Oh HB, Park YB, Lee SK. HLA alleles in Korean patients with Takayasu arteritis. Clin Exp Rheumatol. 2007;25:S18–22.
27. Terao C, Yoshifuji H, Kimura A, Matsumura T, Ohmura K, Takahashi M, Shimizu M, Kawaguchi T, Chen Z, Naruse TK, et al. Two susceptibility loci to Takayasu arteritis reveal a synergistic role of the IL12B and HLA-B regions in a Japanese population. Am J Hum Genet. 2013;93:289–97.
28. Yajima M, Numano F, Park YB, Sagar S. Comparative studies of patients with Takayasu arteritis in Japan, Korea and India—comparison of clinical manifestations, angiography and HLA-B antigen. Jpn Circ J. 1994;58:9–14.
29. Yoshida M, Kimura A, Katsuragi K, Numano F, Sasazuki T. DNA typing of HLA-B gene in Takayasu's arteritis. Tissue Antigens. 1993;42:87–90.
30. Kobayashi Y, Numano F. 3. Takayasu arteritis. Intern Med. 2002;41:44–6.
31. Terao C, Yoshifuji H, Ohmura K, Murakami K, Kawabata D, Yurugi K, Tazaki J, Kinoshita H, Kimura A, Akizuki M, et al. Association of Takayasu arteritis with HLA-B 67:01 and two amino acids in HLA-B protein. Rheumatology (Oxford). 2013;52:1769–74.
32. Takamura C, Ohhigashi H, Ebana Y, Isobe M. New human leukocyte antigen risk allele in Japanese patients with Takayasu arteritis. Circ J. 2012;76:1697–702.
33. Kimura A, Kitamura H, Date Y, Numano F. Comprehensive analysis of HLA genes in Takayasu arteritis in Japan. Int J Cardiol. 1996;54(Suppl):S61–9.
34. Dong RP, Kimura A, Numano F, Yajima M, Hashimoto Y, Kishi Y, Nishimura Y, Sasazuki T. HLA-DP antigen and Takayasu arteritis. Tissue Antigens. 1992;39:106–10.
35. Lv N, Wang Z, Dang A, Zhu X, Liu Y, Zheng D, Liu G. HLA-DQA1, DQB1 and DRB1 alleles associated with Takayasu arteritis in the Chinese Han population. Hum Immunol. 2015;76:241–4.
36. Lv N, Dang A, Wang Z, Zheng D, Liu G. Association of susceptibility to Takayasu arteritis in Chinese Han patients with HLA-DPB1. Hum Immunol. 2011;72:893–6.
37. Saruhan-Direskeneli G, Bicakcigil M, Yilmaz V, Kamali S, Aksu K, Fresko I, Akkoc N, Kiraz S, Ozer HT, Tunc E, et al. Interleukin (IL)-12, IL-2, and IL-6 gene polymorphisms in Takayasu's arteritis from Turkey. Hum Immunol. 2006;67:735–40.
38. Soto Lopez ME, Gamboa Avila R, Hernandez E, Huesca-Gomez C, Castrejon-Tellez V, Perez-Mendez O, Reyes PA, Fragoso-Lona JM, Vargas-Alarcon G, Cruz-Robles D. The interleukin-1 gene cluster polymorphisms are associated with Takayasu's arteritis in Mexican patients. J Interf Cytokine Res. 2013;33:369–75.

39. Huesca-Gomez C, Soto ME, Castrejon-Tellez V, Perez-Mendez O, Gamboa R. PON1 gene polymorphisms and plasma PON1 activities in Takayasu's arteritis disease. Immunol Lett. 2013;152:77–82.
40. Direskeneli H, Tuna-Erdogan E, Gunduz F, Bandurska-Luque A, Alparslan B, Kebe M, Uyar FA, Bicakcigil M, Aksu K, Kamali S, et al. PDCD1 polymorphisms are not associated with Takayasu's arteritis in Turkey. Clin Exp Rheumatol. 2012;30:S11–4.
41. Sahin N, Aksu K, Kamali S, Bicakcigil M, Ozbalkan Z, Fresko I, Ozer H, Akar S, Onat AM, Cobankara V, et al. PTPN22 gene polymorphism in Takayasu's arteritis. Rheumatology (Oxford). 2008;47:634–5.
42. Renauer PA, Saruhan-Direskeneli G, Coit P, Adler A, Aksu K, Keser G, Alibaz-Oner F, Aydin SZ, Kamali S, Inanc M, et al. Identification of Susceptibility Loci in IL6, RPS9/LILRB3, and an Intergenic Locus on Chromosome 21q22 in Takayasu Arteritis in a Genome-Wide Association Study. Arthritis Rheumatol. 2015;67:1361–8.
43. Tanaka T, Narazaki M, Kishimoto T. IL-6 in inflammation, immunity, and disease. Cold Spring Harb Perspect Biol. 2014;6:a016295.
44. Terao C, Yoshifuji H, Mimori T. Recent advances in Takayasu arteritis. Int J Rheum Dis. 2014;17:238–47.
45. Bettelli E, Carrier Y, Gao W, Korn T, Strom TB, Oukka M, Weiner HL, Kuchroo VK. Reciprocal developmental pathways for the generation of pathogenic effector TH17 and regulatory T cells. Nature. 2006;441:235–8.
46. Murphy KM, Reiner SL. The lineage decisions of helper T cells. Nat Rev Immunol. 2002;2:933–44.
47. Strasly M, Cavallo F, Geuna M, Mitola S, Colombo MP, Forni G, Bussolino F. IL-12 inhibition of endothelial cell functions and angiogenesis depends on lymphocyte-endothelial cell cross-talk. J Immunol. 2001;166:3890–9.
48. Qin F, Wang H, Song L, Lu XL, Yang LR, Liang EP, Wang W, Zou YB, Bian J, Wu HY, et al. Single nucleotide polymorphism rs10919543 in FCGR2A/FCGR3A region confers susceptibility to Takayasu arteritis in Chinese population. Chin Med J. 2016;129:854–9.
49. Chen S, Wen X, Li J, Li Y, Li L, Tian X, Yuan H, Zhang F, Li Y. Association of FCGR2A/FCGR3A variant rs2099684 with Takayasu arteritis in the Han Chinese population. Oncotarget. 2017;8:17239–45.
50. Terao C, Matsumura T, Yoshifuji H, Kirino Y, Maejima Y, Nakaoka Y, Takahashi M, Amiya E, Tamura N, Nakajima T, et al. Takayasu arteritis and ulcerative colitis: high rate of co-occurrence and genetic overlap. Arthritis Rheumatol. 2015;67:2226–32.
51. Watanabe R, Ishii T, Nakamura K, Shirai T, Fujii H, Saito S, Harigae H. Ulcerative colitis is not a rare complication of Takayasu arteritis. Mod Rheumatol. 2014;24:372–3.
52. Soto ME, Vargas-Alarcon G, Cicero-Sabido R, Ramirez E, Alvarez-Leon E, Reyes PA. Comparison distribution of HLA-B alleles in mexican patients with takayasu arteritis and tuberculosis. Hum Immunol. 2007;68:449–53.
53. Carmona FD, Coit P, Saruhan-Direskeneli G, Hernandez-Rodriguez J, Cid MC, Solans R, Castaneda S, Vaglio A, Direskeneli H, Merkel PA, et al. Analysis of the common genetic component of large-vessel vasculitides through a meta-Immunochip strategy. Sci Rep. 2017;7:43953.
54. Origuchi T, Fukui S, Umeda M, Nishino A, Nakashima Y, Koga T, Kawashiri SY, Iwamoto N, Ichinose K, Tamai M, et al. The severity of Takayasu arteritis is associated with the HLA-B52 allele in Japanese patients. Tohoku J Exp Med. 2016;239:67–72.
55. Renauer P, Sawalha AH. The genetics of Takayasu arteritis. Presse Med. 2017;46(7–8 Pt 2):e179–87.
56. Matsumura T, Amiya E, Tamura N, Maejima Y, Komuro I, Isobe M. A novel susceptibility locus for Takayasu arteritis in the IL12B region can be a genetic marker of disease severity. Heart Vessel. 2016;31:1016–9.
57. Huntley RP, Sawford T, Mutowo-Meullenet P, Shypitsyna A, Bonilla C, Martin MJ, O'Donovan C. The GOA database: gene Ontology annotation updates for 2015. Nucleic Acids Res. 2015;43:D1057–63.

Primary Biliary Cirrhosis, Primary Sclerosing Cholangitis, and Autoimmune Hepatitis

9

David González-Serna, Martin Kerick, and Javier Martín

Contents

9.1 Introduction

The three major Autoimmune liver diseases (AILDs), comprising primary biliary cirrhosis (PBC; also referred to as primary biliary cholangitis) [1], primary sclerosing cholangitis (PSC) [2], and autoimmune hepatitis (AIH) [3], are principal causes for last-stage liver disease. AILDs are complex conditions encompassing a range of

D. González-Serna (✉) · M. Kerick · J. Martín
Instituto de Parasitología y Biomedicina 'López-Neyra', IPBLN-CSIC, Parque Tecnológico Ciencias de la Salud, Granada, Spain
e-mail: sna.david@ipb.csic.es; mkerick@ipb.csic.es; javiermartin@ipb.csic.es

J. Martín, F. D. Carmona (eds.), *Genetics of Rare Autoimmune Diseases*, Rare Diseases of the Immune System, https://doi.org/10.1007/978-3-030-03934-9_9

disorders affecting the hepatobiliary system, which arise from the interaction between genetic susceptibility and unknown environmental factors that affect disease predisposition and progression [4]. Support of an autoimmune cause is provided by strong genetic links with human leukocyte antigen (HLA), the presence of high circulating autoantibodies (which are different for each disease), and a higher probability of concomitant autoimmune disease affecting other organ systems. It is noteworthy the uncommon factor of these diseases, with a prevalence rate of 1.91 to 49.2 per 100,000 in the case of PBC, 0 to 16.2 per 100,000 in PSC, and 4 to 42.1 per 100,000 in AIH [5–7].

These diseases can impact people of all ages and persist as a chronic illness rather than acute illness. AILDs represent a relevant cause of liver failure and transplantation worldwide, in which treatments to disease progression are only available in PBC [8] and AIH [9], but not in PSC [2], being this liver transplantation the only curable treatment in all three diseases [10]. To date, liver biochemistry, liver histology, autoantibody profile, and imaging are the main procedures in which management and treatment strategies have relied on regarding these three conditions. Nevertheless, recent research has led to improved knowledge of pathophysiology thanks to the development of large-scale AILDs patient cohorts and the implementation of high-throughput methods [11].

During the last years, more and more studies are shedding light on the genetic component of these three hepatic autoimmune conditions. The increasing number of international collaborative studies, together with the use of high-density genotyping platforms and the performance of genome-wide association studies (GWAS), represent a powerful strategy for exploring the genetic landscape of AILDs. From the classical HLA alleles to the most recently discovered genetic associations, in this chapter we will provide an overview of the current knowledge on the genetic background, considering the individual and shared genetic component of PBC, PSC, and AIH with other autoimmune diseases.

9.2 Primary Biliary Cirrhosis

9.2.1 Immunopathology of PBC

PBC is an idiopathic autoimmune chronic liver disease characterized by progressive loss of intrahepatic bile ducts, resulting in progressive fibrosis and cholestasis [1]. Most of the patients present autoantibodies against the E2 component of pyruvate dehydrogenase enzyme present on the inner mitochondrial membrane [12], which are usually called “anti-mitochondrial antibodies” (AMA). Additionally, the majority of the patients also present at least one concomitant autoimmune condition [13]. AMA detection is the principal diagnostic and predictive method for the disease, being present at elevated titer in most of the patients. Furthermore, different PBC-specific antinuclear autoantibodies (ANA) can be observed in 30% of patients [14].

Autoantibodies against mitochondria components show an intense linear staining pattern in the apical region of biliary epithelial cells (BEC) in patients.

Furthermore, AMA is associated with apoptosis [15]. PBC is a typical autoimmune disease with a T-cell signature, in which the principal cellular infiltrate is mainly comprised of CD4+ T cells, and lower increases in cytotoxic (CD8+) T cells. An increase in the number of CD4+ T cells is predominantly observed in the liver and the hilar lymph nodes [16]. It is noteworthy the presence of CD8+ and CD4+ T cells specific to mitochondrial autoantigens in livers and liver lymph nodes, as well as in peripheral blood of patients. Enhanced expression of class I and II major histocompatibility complex (MHC) proteins has been demonstrated at the surface of bile ducts of PBC patients, presenting antigen to cytotoxic (CD8+) and helper (CD4+) T cells, respectively [17].

The cytokine signature is another key factor in the PBC pathogenesis. Evidence sustain a model focused toward the effects of balancing immunoregulatory pathways, in particular, Th1 and Th17 cells. Elevated levels of interferon gamma (IFNγ) and IL-18 (considered activators of Th1 pathway) and reduced levels of IL-10 (predominantly Th2 cytokine) have been detected in PBC patients as compared to levels detected in healthy controls [18]. Immunohistochemical studies support these observations, with PBC liver samples showing IL-12/Th1 and IL-23/Th17 staining, showing Th17 skewing prominently in advanced PBC patients [19].

9.2.2 HLA Associations

The human leukocyte antigen (HLA) region, located on the most gene-dense genomic region on the short arm of chromosome 6, plays an essential role in many medically and biologically relevant processes, including most autoimmune diseases. The relevant genes encode cell surface proteins involved in the binding and presentation of self and non-self-peptides corresponding to HLA class I (A, B, and C) and class II (DR, DQ, and DP). Among the single nucleotide polymorphisms (SNPs) reported to be associated with PBC susceptibility in large-scale genetic studies, only HLA has been consistently linked to the disease between the different patient cohorts across ethnicities [20–29]. Particularly, these studies have shown that the peak association signal is between HLA *DQA1* and *DQB1*.

Initial studies linked *DR*08* allele group with susceptibility to suffer for PBC [30]. Subsequent cumulative studies of a much larger sample of PBC have demonstrated that the disease is associated with *DRB1*08* and *DRB1*02* as predisposing and *DRB1*11* and *DRB1*13* as protective alleles [31, 32]. A more recent meta-analysis performed with the aim to observe relationships between HLA class II and susceptibility to PBC found that *HLA DR*07* and *DR*08* alleles were risk factors, while *DR*11*, *DR*12*, *DR*13*, and *DR*15* alleles were protective [33]. Notably, most of the associated amino acids are almost unique to the specific HLA classical allele and correspond to crucial residues in the antigen-binding pocket.

Regarding the HLA haplotype association with susceptibility to PBC, it has been noticed in several studies across ethnicities that HLA *DR*08* alleles caused disease susceptibility, whereas *DRB1*11* and *DRB1*13* were protective alleles in haplotype analysis [31, 34–36]. Interestingly, both *DRB1*11* and *DRB1*13* have also been associated with different infectious diseases, such as hepatitis C [37], human immunodeficiency [38], and human papilloma [39] viruses. Thus, pathogenic mechanisms involved in PBC may be partially related to those of bacterial infection, as the mentioned HLA class II protective alleles play a critical role in blocking infectious pathogens. Nevertheless, the proportion of individuals carrying the mentioned haplotypes constitute only a minority of PBC patients, evidencing that many other non-HLA genes, as well as environmental factors, should play an important role in the pathogenesis of the disease.

9.2.3 Non-HLA Associations

The key fact that enforces the importance of non-HLA associations in genetic predisposition to PBC is that mainly between 80 and 90% of patients do not carry the most common HLA susceptibility alleles. In this regard, other genes are suggested to contribute to disease development. GWASs are the most common tool utilized to identify genetic susceptibility loci among different diseases. At the present time, six GWASs [20, 21, 23, 24, 28, 29], two Immunochip studies [25, 26], and two meta-analyses [22, 27] have successfully identified 44 non-HLA loci associated with PBC susceptibility. These investigations have been performed in subjects with PBC and controls from North American, European, and Japanese populations. Table 9.1 summarizes the main genetic associations outside the HLA region.

The first GWAS, performed in Canadian population, identified two principal susceptibility loci, *interleukin (IL)12A* and *IL12RB2*, which encode IL-12 p35 and IL-12 receptor β2, respectively [20]. Additional fine-mapping Immunochip studies identified a particular five-allele haplotype of the *IL12A* gene as a susceptibility factor for PBC [25]. These efforts started bringing to light the IL-12 signaling pathway, which is of key importance in the pathophysiology of PBC. Two subsequent GWAS, that used US, Italian, and Canadian subjects, confirmed the previous susceptibility loci and identified three additional associations, including *SPIB, IRF5-TNPO3, IKZF3, and MMEL1* [21, 22]. *IRF5,* an interferon regulatory factor induced by IFNγ, plays a particularly important role in generating Th1 type responses, while *SPIB* is involved in T-cell lineage decisions [21]. These three genes are directly involved with immunomodulation [22]. A larger GWAS including 1800 cases and 5000 controls from the UK identified 12 additional loci associated with PBC (being *DENND1B, STAT4, CD80, NFKB1, IL7R, CXCR5, TNFRSF1A, and CLEC16A* the most outstanding) at the genome-wide significance level ($p < 5 \times 10^{-8}$) as well as confirmed previous associations at least at the suggestive significance level ($p < 1 \times 10^{-5}$) [23]. Some interesting findings emerged from this study, as CD80 is an inducible co-stimulatory molecule on antigen-presenting cells, and a deficiency in this transmembrane glycoprotein results in reduced humoral response to immunization [40]. On the other hand, the activation of TNFRSF1A, which encodes a member of the tumor necrosis factor family of receptors, can cause apoptosis through activation of NF-κB [41]. Notably, apoptosis is one of the main traits related to AMA in PBC patients [15]. A subsequent GWAS performed in Japanese

Table 9.1 Main loci associated with susceptibility to primary biliary cirrhosis reaching genome-wide significance ($p < 5 \times 10^{-8}$) outside the HLA region

Chr	Candidate gene(s)	Lead SNP	Location	Populations	*N* (case/control)	OR (95% CI)	*P*-value (allele test)	Year	Ref.
1	*IL12RB2*	rs72678531	Intronic	UK	2861/8514	1.61 (1.49–1.73)	2.47×10^{-38}	2012	[26]
	DENND1B	rs12134279	Intergenic	UK	1840/5163	1.34 (1.25–1.45)	2.06×10^{-14}	2011	[23]
	MMEL1	rs3748816	Exonic	USA, Canada	1351/4700	1.33 (1.20–1.47)	3.15×10^{-8}	2010	[21]
	CD58	rs2300747	Intronic	Han Chinese	1122/4036	1.29 (1.15–1.43)	4.54×10^{-8}	2017	[29]
2	*STAT4, NAB1*	rs10931468	Intronic	UK	1840/5163	1.50 (1.37–1.64)	2.35×10^{-19}	2011	[23]
	CD28, CRLA4, ICOS	rs4675369	Intergenic	Han Chinese	1122/4036	1.37 (1.24–1.50)	6.56×10^{-11}	2017	[29]
	CCL20	rs4973341	Intergenic	USA, Canada, UK, Italy	2764/10,475	0.82 (0.74–0.90)	2.34×10^{-10}	2015	[27]
	IL1RL1, IL1RL2	rs12712133	Intergenic	USA, Canada, UK, Italy	2764/10,475	1.14 (1.07–1.21)	5.19×10^{-9}	2015	[27]
3	*IL12A*	rs2366643	Intergenic	UK	2861/8514	1.35 (1.27–1.44)	3.92×10^{-22}	2012	[26]
	CD80	rs2293370	Intronic	UK	2861/8514	1.39 (1.29–1.52)	6.84×10^{-16}	2012	[26]
	PLCL2	rs1372072	Intronic	UK	1840/5163	1.20 (1.12–1.27)	2.28×10^{-8}	2011	[23]
4	*DGKQ*	rs11724804	Intronic	USA, Canada, UK, Italy	2764/10,475	1.22 (1.12–1.33)	9.01×10^{-12}	2015	[27]
	NFKB1	rs7665090	Intergenic	UK	1840/5163	1.26 (1.18–1.34)	4.06×10^{-12}	2011	[23]
	C5orf30	rs526231	Intergenic	USA, Canada, UK, Italy	2764/10,475	0.87 (0.81–0.93)	1.14×10^{-8}	2015	[27]
5	*IL7R*	rs6871748	Intergenic	UK	2861/8514	1.30 (1.21–1.40)	2.26×10^{-13}	2012	[26]
6	*OLIG1, TNFAIP3*	rs6933404	Intergenic	USA, Canada, UK, Italy	2764/10,475	1.18 (1.09–1.27)	1.27×10^{-10}	2015	[27]
7	*IRF5, TNPO3*	rs35188261	Intronic	UK	2861/8514	1.52 (1.39–1.63)	6.52×10^{-22}	2012	[26]
9	*TNFSF15*	rs4979462	Intronic	Japan	1274/1091	1.56 (1.39–1.76)	2.84×10^{-14}	2012	[24]
	IL21R	rs2189521	Exonic	Han Chinese	1122/4036	0.73 (0.65–0.81)	5.40×10^{-9}	2017	[29]
11	*CXCR5, DDX6*	rs80065107	Intergenic	UK	2861/8514	1.39 (1.28–1.50)	7.20×10^{-16}	2012	[26]
	RPS6KA4	rs538147	Intronic	UK	1840/5163	1.37 (1.25–1.50)	2.69×10^{-12}	2011	[23]
	POU2AF1	rs4938534	Intergenic	Japan	1274/1091	1.39 (1.24–1.56)	2.38×10^{-8}	2012	[24]

(continued)

Table 9.1 (continued)

Chr	Candidate gene(s)	Lead SNP	Location	Populations	*N* (case/control)	OR (95% CI)	*P*-value (allele test)	Year	Ref.
12	*TNFRSF1A, LTBR*	rs1800693	Intronic	UK	2861/8514	1.27 (1.19–1.34)	1.18×10^{-14}	2012	[26]
	SH2B3	rs11065979	Intergenic	UK	2861/8514	1.20 (1.13–1.27)	2.87×10^{-9}	2012	[26]
14	*RAD51B*	rs911263	Intergenic	UK	2861/8514	1.26 (1.17–1.35)	9.95×10^{-11}	2012	[26]
16	*CLEC16A, SOCS1*	rs1646019	Intronic	UK	2861/8514	1.31 (1.23–1.41)	6.72×10^{-15}	2012	[26]
	IRF8	rs11117432	Intergenic	UK	1840/5163	1.31 (1.21–1.43)	4.66×10^{-11}	2011	[23]
	PRKCB	rs3785396	Intronic	Japan	894/1029	1.35 (1.20–1.48)	7.10×10^{-8}	2017	[28]
17	*GSDMB, IKZF3*	rs8067378	Intergenic	UK	2861/8514	1.26 (1.19–1.34)	6.05×10^{-14}	2012	[26]
	ZPBP2	rs11557467	Exonic	USA, Canada	1351/4700	0.72 (0.66–0.79)	3.50×10^{-13}	2010	[21]
	MAPT	rs17564829	Intronic	UK	2861/8514	1.25 (1.16–1.35)	2.15×10^{-9}	2012	[26]
19	*TYK2*	rs34536443	Exonic	UK	2861/8514	1.91 (1.59–2.28)	1.23×10^{-12}	2012	[26]
	SPIB	rs3745516	Intronic	Italy	945/4651	1.46 (1.29–1.63)	7.9×10^{-11}	2010	[22]
	ARID3A	rs10415976	Intronic	Han Chinese	1122/4036	0.75 (0.68–0.82)	1.06×10^{-9}	2017	[29]
22	*SYNGR1*	rs2267407	Intronic	UK	2861/8514	1.29 (1.21–1.38)	1.29×10^{-13}	2012	[26]

Chr chromosome; *SNP* single nucleotide polymorphism; *OR* odds ratio for the minor allele; *CI* confidence interval

population showed two novel risk loci associated with PBC, *TNFSF15*, and *POU2AF1* genes [24]. In addition, a GWAS recently performed in Chinese population confirmed a high association between *TNFSF15* and PBC [29]. Nevertheless, some discrepancies were found between non-HLA loci associated with PBC in European and Asian ancestry populations. In this respect, *IL12A* and *IL12RB2* loci were associated only in Caucasian population. These findings help to highlight the importance of ethnic differences in the pathogenesis of the complex disease and how common genetic variation can impact in a different way the susceptibility to PBC. Another critical point is the performance of stratified analysis attending to different clinical traits, which leads to the discovery of specific associations. In this regard, a recently published study performed in Japanese population found that *NELFCD* and *CTSZ* loci are associated with jaundice-stage progression, a trait that affects approximately 10–20% of PBC patients [42]. *CTSZ* is a cathepsin that regulates various cellular physiological functions, such as migration, invasion, and maturation of immune cells [43].

Additionally, two Immunochip studies found three new loci associated with PBC: *SH2B3*, *MAPT*, and *TYK2* [25, 26]. Interestingly, *SH2B3* represent a shared autoimmune disease locus, and the protein encoded, Lnk, is involved in many cytokine signaling pathways as well as in the negative regulation of T-cell activation [44]. In this line, in vivo studies performed in mice models showed that deficiency in SH2B3 resulted in higher levels of activated T cells and a tendency to autoimmunity [45].

It is of particular interest that many genes implicated in PBC pathogenesis have also been reported in many other autoimmune diseases, such as systemic sclerosis (SSc), systemic lupus erythematosus (SLE), or rheumatoid arthritis (RA) [46]. For example, SNPs within the STAT4 locus have been associated with increased risk of SLE and RA [47], among others. Another good example could be NF-κB, a transcription factor activated in several autoimmune diseases that coordinates the expression of a wide variety of genes involved in immune response [48]. Notably, one-third of patients with PBC are affected by another autoimmune disease [49]. Hence, we can conclude that the genetic overlap between PBC and other autoimmune diseases is evident and emphasizes that there are few disease-specific genetic associations in PBC. In this line, understanding the mechanisms underlying such diseases may unravel crucial information in the pathophysiology of PBC.

9.3 Primary Sclerosing Cholangitis

9.3.1 Immunopathology of PSC

PSC is a chronic liver disease marked by biliary infiltration leading to fibrosis of bile duct structures and recurrent cirrhosis and cholestasis [2]. One of the hallmarks of this condition is that PSC is closely associated with inflammatory bowel disease (PSC-IBD) in 50–80% of cases [50]. Biliary infiltrates are mostly composed of activated memory or effector T cells, but also B cells, macrophages, and natural killer cells are included [51]. In addition, these T cells and B cells can be detected in other tertiary lymphoid structures as PSC is associated with portal-associated lymphoid tissues, leading to portal inflammation and the development of neolymphoid tissue in the liver [52].

Effector lymphocytes activated during an inflammatory process in the colon can express homing receptors that may direct migration to the liver and gut [53]. In this line, after an inflammatory process, mucosal lymphocytes are recruited via the endothelial adhesion molecule MADCAM1 and the chemokine CCL25, which are mostly specific from colon [54–56]. This aberrant overexpression of MADCAM1 and CCL25 can result from the combination of hepatic inflammation, which course with high levels of tumor necrosis factor α (TNFα), and the activation of the vascular adhesion protein 1 (VAP1) by bacterial or dietary antigens. Activation of endothelial VAP1 in portal blood leads to activation of NF-κB, which is of key importance in autoimmune process, as well as an increased expression of MADCAM1 and recruitment of α4β7+ T cells [57, 58]. The implication of MADCAM1 and CCL25 in colon inflammatory processes set the basis for the recruitment of effector cells to the liver and bowel in PSC.

9.3.2 HLA Associations

HLA region is implicated in nearly every immune-mediated disorder. Early reports along with current large-scale association studies confirm that HLA region is the strongest genetic association reported in PSC-IBD patients [59, 60], together with PBC and many other autoimmune diseases. Subsequent fine-mappings of the HLA locus have identified *HLA B*08* (HLA class I) and *DRB1* (HLA class II) as the main risk alleles in PSC-IBD [61]. Both HLA *B*08* and *DRB1* are associated with many immunopathological diseases such as SLE, diabetes mellitus (DM), and common variable immunodeficiency (CVID) [62], supporting the fact that breakdown of immune tolerance could lead to autoimmune hepatobiliary destruction. However, despite these HLA alleles are shared between many immune conditions, most of the HLA associations found in PSC are different from those in IBD, with the exception of the *HLA DRB1*15:01* allele [63], evidencing genetic differences in HLA region among these two conditions.

Regarding HLA haplotypes associated with PSC, the *A*01:01-C*07:01-B*08:01-DRB3*01:01-DRB1*03:01-DQA1*05:01-DQB1*02:01* and the *DRB1*13:01-DQA1*01:03-DQB1*06:03* are the two most prominent risk HLA haplotypes [64, 65]. On the other hand, the *DRB1*04-DQA1*03-DQB1*03* haplotype represents the most consistently observed protective association with PSC [61, 64–67]. Nevertheless, a recently published study revealed different proportion in *HLA-DQB1*06:03* allele between European and admixed/non-European PSC population carrying haplotypes containing the *HLA-DRB1*13:01* allele [68]. Therefore, the study of multiethnic populations could lead to the identification of causative alleles in PSC-associated haplotypes. Further to this point, many challenges of interpreting the HLA findings in PSC must be overcome to obtain insights that point toward key antigenic triggers.

9.3.3 Non-HLA Associations

Over the last years, GWAS and high-throughput targeted genotyping arrays have identified a total of 23 non-HLA loci associated with susceptibility and progression of PSC-IBD reaching the genome-wide level of significance [65, 69–77] (Table 9.2). The majority of genes within these loci relate to immune pathways that have been previously identified as risk loci in other immune disorders [78].

MST1-BCL2L11 was one of the first observed loci associated with PSC susceptibility. Interestingly, the *MST1* gene encodes a macrophage-stimulating protein expressed at high levels in the gallbladder epithelium, being a candidate gene associated with both PSC and IBD [70]. On the other hand, *BCL2L11* encodes a protein that is crucial for maintaining immunological tolerance through T-cell apoptosis [79]. Subsequent fine-mapping studies confirmed previous associations and found one new risk locus reaching genome-wide significance level, the *IL2RA* locus [72]. Of note, genetic variants at *IL2RA* locus are associated with other autoimmune diseases, such as RA, DM, and psoriasis [80], and additionally, spontaneous mutation of this gene in human can cause systemic autoimmunity and multi-organ inflammation [81]. The *IL2-IL21* locus showed suggestive association with PSC [72]. However, it is considered a general autoimmune risk locus as the IL-2 cytokine plays a crucial role in modulating the immune response by promoting T-cell activation, as well as maintaining homeostasis of T regulatory cells [82]. A subsequent larger GWAS including 1900 PSC cases and 6400 controls identified one new susceptibility region reaching the genome-wide significance level, the *MMEL1-TNFRSF14* locus, representing the first genetic overlap between PSC and PBC [21]. It is noteworthy to mention that the SNP associated showed opposite effect sizes in PSC and PBC [21, 71], highlighting *MMEL1* as a relevant candidate gene in the immunopathology of AILDs.

Due to the high concomitance of IBD in PSC patients, as well as the shared genetic component of most autoimmune conditions, researchers started performing association studies including more than one trait, in order to identify shared susceptibility loci between different diseases. In this line, Ellinghaus and colleagues performed the first GWAS including PSC and ulcerative colitis (UC) patients, identifying *GPR35* and *TCF4* as risk loci independently associated with both diseases [73]. *TCF4* encodes a transcription factor involved in cell differentiation and growth; furthermore, its deficiency leads to a block in T-cell and B-cell development in mice model [83]. On the other hand, the exact functions of *GPR35,* which belongs to the G-protein-coupled receptor family, are not known. Nevertheless, it has been shown to function as a receptor of kynurenic acid, whose concentrations are high in bile and intestinal contents and increase during inflammation [84]. In addition, pathway analysis showed that the majority of loci shared between PSC and UC involve genomic regions that regulate innate and adaptive immune system [85]. Further dense genotyping of immune-related disease regions identified nine new risk loci for PSC, distinguishing *PRKD2*, *SIK2*, and *HDAC7* [74]. Particularly, the histone encoded by the *HDAC7* gene has been implicated in the negative selection of T cells in the thymus [86]. Notably, when T-cell receptors are engaged, the protein kinase PRKD2 phosphorylates HDAC7, leading to nuclear exclusion of HDAC7 and thus

Table 9.2 Loci associated with susceptibility to primary sclerosing cholangitis reaching genome-wide significance ($p < 5 \times 10^{-8}$) outside the HLA region

Chr	Candidate gene(s)	Lead SNP	Location	Populations	*N* (case/control)	OR (95% CI)	*P*-value (allele test)	Year	Ref.
1	*MMEL1, TNFRSF14*	rs3748816	Exonic	Scandinavia, Germany, Belgium, Netherlands, USA	1936/6470	0.79 (0.71–0.88)	2.11×10^{-8}	2012	[71]
2	*CD28*	rs7426056	Intronic	Pan-European, USA, Canada	3789/25,079	1.30 (1.23–1.37)	1.89×10^{-20}	2013	[74]
	GPR35	rs4676410	Intronic	Germany, Scandinavia, Belgium, Netherlands	1401/5530	1.38 (1.24–1.53)	2.43×10^{-9}	2013	[73]
	CCL20	rs7556897	Intergenic	Pan-European	3408/34,213	0.84 (0.80–0.89)	4.73×10^{-9}	2016	[75]
	BCL2L11	rs6720394	Intronic	Scandinavia, Germany, Belgium, Netherlands, USA	1740/5136	1.29 (1.10–1.51)	4.12×10^{-8}	2011	[70]
3	*MST1*	rs3197999	Exonic	Scandinavia, Germany, Belgium, Netherlands, USA	1740/5136	1.39 (1.24–1.56)	1.10×10^{-16}	2011	[70]
	FOXP1	rs80060485	Intronic	Scandinavia, Germany, USA, Canada, Africa, Han Chinese, Japan	4796/19,955	1.44 (1.32–1.58)	2.62×10^{-15}	2016	[76]
4	*IL2, IL21*	rs13140464	Intergenic	Pan-European, USA, Canada	3789/25,079	1.30 (1.21–1.40)	8.87×10^{-13}	2013	[74]
	NFKB1	rs17032705	Intronic	Pan-European	3408/34,213	1.17 (1.11–1.23)	3.82×10^{-10}	2016	[75]
6	*BACH2*	rs56258221	Intergenic	Pan-European, USA, Canada	3789/25,079	1.23 (1.16–1.31)	8.36×10^{-12}	2013	[74]
10	*IL2RA*	rs4147359	Intergenic	UK	992/5162	1.25 (1.16–1.36)	1.54×10^{-8}	2012	[72]
11	*CCDC88B*	rs663743	Exonic	Scandinavia, Germany, USA, Canada, Africa, Han Chinese, Japan	4796/19,955	1.20 (1.14–1.26)	2.24×10^{-13}	2016	[76]
	SIK2	rs7937682	Intronic	Pan-European, USA, Canada	3789/25,079	1.17 (1.11–1.24)	3.17×10^{-9}	2013	[74]

12	*SH2B3, ATXN2*	rs3184504	Exonic	Pan-European, USA, Canada	3789/25,079	1.18 (1.12–1.24)	5.91×10^{-11}	2013	[74]
	RIC8B	rs12369214	Intronic	Pan-European	3408/34,213	0.85 (0.80–0.89)	1.30×10^{-9}	2016	[75]
	HDAC7	rs11168249	Intronic	Pan-European, USA, Canada	3789/25,079	1.15 (1.10–1.21)	5.49×10^{-9}	2013	[74]
16	*CLEC16A, SOCS1*	rs11649613	Intronic	Pan-European	3408/34,213	1.19 (1.13–1.25)	1.08×10^{-11}	2016	[75]
18	*TCF4*	rs1452787	Intronic	Germany, Scandinavia, Belgium, Netherlands	1401/5530	0.75 (0.68–0.83)	2.61×10^{-8}	2013	[73]
	CD226	rs1788097	Intronic	Pan-European, USA, Canada	3789/25,079	1.15 (1.10–1.21)	3.06×10^{-8}	2013	[74]
19	*PRKD2*	rs60652743	Intronic	Pan-European, USA, Canada	3789/25,079	1.25 (1.16–1.34)	6.51×10^{-10}	2013	[74]
21	*PSMG1*	rs2836883	Intergenic	Pan-European, USA, Canada	3789/25,079	1.28 (1.21–1.36)	3.19×10^{-17}	2013	[74]
	UBASH3A	rs1893592	Intronic	Scandinavia, Germany, USA, Canada, Africa, Han Chinese, Japan	4796/19,955	1.22 (1.15–1.29)	2.19×10^{-12}	2016	[76]

Chr chromosome; *SNP* single nucleotide polymorphism; *OR* odds ratio for the minor allele; *CI* confidence interval

resulting in negative selection and apoptosis of T cells [87]. Furthermore, this negative selection involves Nur77, an important transcription factor in leukocytes that is regulated by SIK2 [88]. A posterior analysis of five chronic inflammatory diseases including PSC, UC, Crohn's disease (CD), psoriasis, and ankylosing spondylitis identified four new risk loci associated with PSC (*CCL20*, *NFKB1*, *RIC8B*, and *CLEC16A*) [75]. All of these four loci have been previously associated at least with one of the five diseases included in the meta-analysis, highlighting the profound pleiotropy shared between these chronic inflammatory conditions.

Finally, it is noteworthy to mention the importance of performing stratified analyses in order to identify genetic associations related to a specific feature. In this regard, one recently published study identified variants in the *RSPO3* loci associated with disease progression in PSC [77]. For liver transplant-free survival, authors demonstrated the differential expression of *RSPO3*, a member of the R-Spondin protein family, in key liver-resident effector cells.

9.4 Autoimmune Hepatitis

9.4.1 Immunopathology of AIH

AIH is a typical chronic autoimmune-mediated liver disease characterized by an increased serum IgG level and the emergence of autoantibodies, such as anti-smooth muscle antibodies (ASMA) and antinuclear antibodies (ANA) by chronic inflammation of the liver [89–91]. The presence of interface hepatitis with a marked infiltration of lymphocytes and plasma cells is typically observed in most of the cases [92]. This condition develops based on immune tolerance against hepatocytes and the consequent immune response [93]. In this regard, pathogenesis of AIH is mainly driven by activated autoreactive T cells [94]. Regulatory T cells suppress these autoreactive T cells under normal conditions; however, when this mechanism is disrupted, immune tolerance disturbances appear. The reduction of regulatory T cells and the subsequent TGF-β production in the setting of AIH lead to an increased production of IL-6. This IL-6 production results in Th17 induction; indeed, an increased number of intrahepatic Th17 cells and higher IL-17 levels have been reported in AIH patients [95]. Thus, this regulatory T/Th17 cells' balance emerges as a key factor in AIH pathogenesis [96].

On the other hand, innate immunity also plays an important role in AIH pathogenesis, as viral infection and drugs are the most common environmental factors associated with the onset of AIH [97, 98]. It has been suggested that these microorganisms and drug metabolites could disrupt immune tolerance to self-antigens through toll-like receptors (TLRs) expressed on hepatocytes [99].

9.4.2 HLA Associations

HLA serology was studied extensively in AIH patients since 1980. The first association observed was performed in northern European populations and corresponded to the A1-D8-DR3 haplotype [100]. Apart from the DR3 antigen, DR4 was found to be a secondary antigen and was linked to AIH onset in Japan [101].

A number of studies have been published on HLA risk alleles due to the advent of HLA typing by PCR methods. In this regard, AIH was associated with the *DRB1*04:04* and *DRB1*04:05* alleles in Japanese [102], Mexican [103], and Korean [104] populations. In European populations, the *DRB1*03:01* and *DRB1*04:01* alleles were the strongest associations reported in AIH [105, 106]. Furthermore, these two HLA associations were confirmed by the first and only GWAS performed in AIH patients to date, in which *DRB1*03:01* and *DRB1*04:01* alleles represented the strongest associations in northern Europeans [107]. In Latin American populations, the *DRB1*13:01* allele was associated with susceptibility to AIH [108, 109]. On the other hand, several investigations have also described protective alleles for AIH, highlighting the *DRB1*15:01* allele in Japanese and North American populations [102, 106]. Regarding the HLA haplotype analysis, *DRB1*04:05-DQB1*04:01* was associated with susceptibility to AIH in Japan [102] and Korea [104], while *DRB1*15:01-DQB1*06:02* conferred resistance in the Japanese population [102]. In Caucasian population, both *DRB1*03:01-DQB1*02:01* and *DRB1*04:01-DQB1*03:02* have been identified as risk haplotypes, while *DRB1*15:01-DQA1*01:02-DQB1*06:02* acts as a protective haplotype [106]. However, despite the number of HLA associations identified in AIH through different populations, the mechanism underlying these associations is not clearly elucidated. In this regard, the study of the amino acids that form the binding pockets in the HLA molecule could help interpreting the HLA findings in AIH. For example, the *DRB1* association with AIH could be explained by the amino acid motifs in the corresponding antigen-presenting grooves, and, in fact, a model based on lysine at position 71 of the DRβ polypeptide has been proposed in Caucasian patients with AIH [110].

9.4.3 Non-HLA Associations

Unlike PBC and PSC, in which many GWAS and fine-mapping studies have identified a number of associated genes, only one large-scale genetic study has been performed in AIH patients [107]. de Bore et al. performed the first multicenter GWAS on AIH predisposition in Dutch and German patients, identifying *SH2B3* and *CARD10* as susceptibility loci in AIH. As mentioned before, the gene product of *SH2B3*, also known as LNK, has a key role in many cytokine signaling pathways as well as in the inhibition of T-cell activation [44]. The association of this locus with AIH was recently confirmed in a candidate gene study performed in a Japanese cohort [111]. *SH2B3* also became the first locus associated with the three AILDs, representing a key target in the pathogenic process of liver autoimmunity. In addition, a suggestive associated variant was identified close to the *CARD10* gene, which encodes for a scaffold protein that induces proinflammatory NF-κB activation and, interestingly, is widely expressed in hepatocytes [112].

On the other hand, many candidate gene studies have successfully identified susceptibility loci in AIH. In this regard, a polymorphism of the *CTLA-4* gene was associated with increased incidence of AIH in Caucasian population [113]. This locus is of particular interest as the switching from immune activation to immune memory occurs through the upregulation of CTLA-4 on CD25+ T cells [114]. Polymorphisms of the tumor necrosis factor-receptor superfamily (*TNFRSF*) gene have also been associated with susceptibility to AIH onset in Japanese population [115]. Furthermore, *TNIP1* (TNFAIP3-interacting protein 1) locus was recently associated with AIH in a Japanese cohort [116], thus evidencing the importance of the TNF signaling pathway in the pathogenesis of AIH [117].

9.5 Conclusions

There is a clear genetic component to disease risk in each of the AILDs. These three conditions also have a critical environmental input, and the interaction between genetic and environmental component of AILDs is still unknown. Until recently, risk HLA haplotypes were the only genetic factor identified in these diseases, which were insufficient to explain most of the disease heritability. However, during the last years, we have considerably increased the knowledge of the immunopathological mechanisms behind AILDs. These developments were possible thanks to the appearance of the new technologies for the genetic analysis and establishment of large international consortia. In this line, GWAS and analogous chip-based studies, such as the Immunochip, as well as the performance of fine-mapping studies have increased our knowledge of a relatively large number of variants associated with susceptibility to PBC and PSC and are also starting to unravel the genetic component of AIH.

Nevertheless, despite the multiple genetic associations described to date, there is a long way ahead before reaching a complete knowledge of the genetic risk in hepatic autoimmunity. In this regard, deficiencies in GWAS methodology in detecting rare variants, along with the relative ignorance of the environmental and epigenetic component of these diseases, could be limiting our comprehension from the genetic point of view. Thus, further studies including larger samples sizes, sequencing-based approaches able to detect rare variants, as well as the investigation of epigenetic influence would be of great interest. In addition, future investigation of the shared genetic component could help to elucidate common pathways in the pathogenesis of the three AILDs. Thus, a cross-disease meta-analysis of GWAS data of PBC, PSC, and AIH could be a successful initial approach that overcomes the small sample size issue. Nevertheless, almost all genetic studies of AILDs are performed in Caucasian populations, which could be masking new specific genetic associations in other ethnicities. Therefore, future genetic studies will need to proceed with an accurate examination of environmental influences and epigenetics interactions, as well as considering genomes distinct from Caucasian populations.

References

1. Hirschfield GM, Gershwin ME. The immunobiology and pathophysiology of primary biliary cirrhosis. Annu Rev Pathol. 2013;8:303–30.
2. Hirschfield GM, Karlsen TH, Lindor KD, Adams DH. Primary sclerosing cholangitis. Lancet. 2013;382(9904):1587–99.
3. Corrigan M, Hirschfield GM, Oo YH, Adams DH. Autoimmune hepatitis: an approach to disease understanding and management. Br Med Bull. 2015;114(1):181–91.
4. Hirschfield GM, Chapman RW, Karlsen TH, Lammert F, Lazaridis KN, Mason AL. The genetics of complex cholestatic disorders. Gastroenterology. 2013;144(7):1357–74.
5. Boonstra K, Beuers U, Ponsioen CY. Epidemiology of primary sclerosing cholangitis and primary biliary cirrhosis: a systematic review. J Hepatol. 2012;56(5):1181–8.
6. Delgado JS, Vodonos A, Malnick S, Kriger O, Wilkof-Segev R, Delgado B, et al. Autoimmune hepatitis in southern Israel: a 15-year multicenter study. J Dig Dis. 2013;14(11):611–8.
7. Gronbaek L, Vilstrup H, Jepsen P. Autoimmune hepatitis in Denmark: incidence, prevalence, prognosis, and causes of death. A nationwide registry-based cohort study. J Hepatol. 2014;60(3):612–7.
8. Pares A, Caballeria L, Rodes J. Excellent long-term survival in patients with primary biliary cirrhosis and biochemical response to ursodeoxycholic acid. Gastroenterology. 2006;130(3):715–20.
9. European Association for the Study of the Liver. EASL Clinical Practice Guidelines: autoimmune hepatitis. J Hepatol. 2015;63(4):971–1004.
10. European Association for the Study of the Liver. EASL Clinical Practice Guidelines: liver transplantation. J Hepatol. 2016;64(2):433–85.
11. Bossen L, Gerussi A, Lygoura V, Mells GF, Carbone M, Invernizzi P. Support of precision medicine through risk-stratification in autoimmune liver diseases—histology, scoring systems, and non-invasive markers. Autoimmun Rev. 2018;17(9):854–65.
12. Gershwin ME, Mackay IR, Sturgess A, Coppel RL. Identification and specificity of a cDNA encoding the 70 kd mitochondrial antigen recognized in primary biliary cirrhosis. J Immunol. 1987;138:3525–31.
13. Somers EC, Thomas SL, Smeeth L, HalL AJ. Are individuals with an autoimmune disease at higher risk of a second autoimmune disorder? Am J Epidemiol. 2009;169(6):749–55.
14. Bogdanos DP, Komorowski L. Disease-specific autoantibodies in primary biliary cirrhosis. Clin Chim Acta. 2011;412(7):502–12.
15. Migliaccio C, Nishio A, de Water JV, Ansari AA, Leung PSC, Nakanuma Y, et al. Monoclonal antibodies to mitochondrial E2 components define autoepitopes in primary biliary cirrhosis. J Immunol. 1998;161:5157–63.
16. Hashimoto E, Lindor KD, Homburger HA, Dickson ER, Czaja AJ, Wiesner RH, et al. Immunohistochemical characterization of hepatic lymphocytes in primary biliary cirrhosis in comparison with primary sclerosing cholangitis and autoimmune chronic active hepatitis. Mayo Clin Proc. 1993;68(11):1049–55.
17. Van den Oord JJ, Sciot R, Desmet VJ. Expression of MHC products by normal and abnormal bile duct epithelium. J Hepatol. 1986;3:310–7.
18. Nagano T, Yamamoto K, Matsumoto S, Okamoto R, Tagashira M, Ibuki N, et al. Cytokine profile in the liver of primary biliary cirrhosis. J Clin Immunol. 1999;19:422–7.
19. Yang CY, Ma X, Tsuneyama K, Huang S, Takahashi T, Chalasani NP, et al. IL-12/Th1 and IL-23/Th17 biliary microenvironment in primary biliary cirrhosis: implications for therapy. Hepatology. 2014;59(5):1944–53.
20. Hirschfield GM, Liu X, Xu C, Lu Y, Xie G, Lu Y, et al. Primary biliary cirrhosis associated with HLA, IL12A, and IL12RB2 variants. N Engl J Med. 2009;360:2544–55.
21. Hirschfield GM, Liu X, Han Y, Gorlov IP, Lu Y, Xu C, et al. Variants at IRF5-TNPO3, 17q12-21 and MMEL1 are associated with primary biliary cirrhosis. Nat Genet. 2010;42(8):655–7.

22. Liu X, Invernizzi P, Lu Y, Kosoy R, Lu Y, Bianchi I, et al. Genome-wide meta-analyses identify three loci associated with primary biliary cirrhosis. Nat Genet. 2010;42(8):658–60.
23. Mells GF, Floyd JA, Morley KI, Cordell HJ, Franklin CS, Shin SY, et al. Genome-wide association study identifies 12 new susceptibility loci for primary biliary cirrhosis. Nat Genet. 2011;43(4):329–32.
24. Nakamura M, Nishida N, Kawashima M, Aiba Y, Tanaka A, Yasunami M, et al. Genome-wide association study identifies TNFSF15 and POU2AF1 as susceptibility loci for primary biliary cirrhosis in the Japanese population. Am J Hum Genet. 2012;91(4):721–8.
25. Juran BD, Hirschfield GM, Invernizzi P, Atkinson EJ, Li Y, Xie G, et al. Immunochip analyses identify a novel risk locus for primary biliary cirrhosis at 13q14, multiple independent associations at four established risk loci and epistasis between 1p31 and 7q32 risk variants. Hum Mol Genet. 2012;21(23):5209–21.
26. Liu JZ, Almarri MA, Gaffney DJ, Mells GF, Jostins L, Cordell HJ, et al. Dense fine-mapping study identifies new susceptibility loci for primary biliary cirrhosis. Nat Genet. 2012;44(10):1137–41.
27. Cordell HJ, Han Y, Mells GF, Li Y, Hirschfield GM, Greene CS, et al. International genome-wide meta-analysis identifies new primary biliary cirrhosis risk loci and targetable pathogenic pathways. Nat Commun. 2015;6:8019.
28. Kawashima M, Hitomi Y, Aiba Y, Nishida N, Kojima K, Kawai Y, et al. Genome-wide association studies identify PRKCB as a novel genetic susceptibility locus for primary biliary cholangitis in the Japanese population. Hum Mol Genet. 2017;26(3):650–9.
29. Qiu F, Tang R, Zuo X, Shi X, Wei Y, Zheng X, et al. A genome-wide association study identifies six novel risk loci for primary biliary cholangitis. Nat Commun. 2017;8:14828.
30. Manns MP, Bremm A, Schneider PM, Notghi A, Gerken G, Prager-Eberle M, et al. HLA DRw8 and complement C4 deficiency as risk factors in primary biliary cirrhosis. Gastroenterology. 1991;101(5):1367–73.
31. Donaldson PT, Baragiotta A, Heneghan MA, Floreani A, Venturi C, Underhill JA, et al. HLA class II alleles, genotypes, haplotypes, and amino acids in primary biliary cirrhosis: a large-scale study. Hepatology. 2006;44(3):667–74.
32. Invernizzi P, Selmi C, Poli F, Frison S, Floreani A, Alvaro D, et al. Human leukocyte antigen polymorphisms in Italian primary biliary cirrhosis: a multicenter study of 664 patients and 1992 healthy controls. Hepatology. 2008;48(6):1906–12.
33. Li M, Zheng H, Tian QB, Rui MN, Liu DW. HLA-DR polymorphism and primary biliary cirrhosis: evidence from a meta-analysis. Arch Med Res. 2014;45(3):270–9.
34. Umemura T, Joshita S, Ichijo T, Yoshizawa K, Katsuyama Y, Tanaka E, et al. Human leukocyte antigen class II molecules confer both susceptibility and progression in Japanese patients with primary biliary cirrhosis. Hepatology. 2012;55(2):506–11.
35. Zhao DT, Liao HY, Zhang X, Liu YM, Zhao Y, Zhang HP, et al. Human leucocyte antigen alleles and haplotypes and their associations with antinuclear antibodies features in Chinese patients with primary biliary cirrhosis. Liver Int. 2014;34(2):220–6.
36. Yasunami M, Nakamura H, Tokunaga K, Kawashima M, Nishida N, Hitomi Y, et al. Principal contribution of HLA-DQ alleles, DQB1*06:04 and DQB1*03:01, to disease resistance against primary biliary cholangitis in a Japanese population. Sci Rep. 2017;7(1):11093.
37. Alric L, Fort M, Izopet J, Vinel JP, Charlet JP, Selves J, et al. Genes of the major histocompatibility complex class II influence the outcome of hepatitis C virus infection. Gastroenterology. 1997;113:1675–81.
38. Hendel H, Caillat-Zucman S, Lebuanec H, Carrington M, O'Brien S, Andrieu JM, et al. New class I and II HLA alleles strongly associated with opposite patterns of progression to AIDS. J Immunol. 1999;162:6942–6.
39. de Gruijl TD, Bontkes HJ, Walboomers JM, Coursaget P, Stukart MJ, Dupuy C, et al. Immune responses against human papillomavirus (HPV) type 16 virus-like particles in a cohort study of women with cervical intraepithelial neoplasia. I. Differential T-helper and IgG responses in relation to HPV infection and disease outcome. J Gen Virol. 1999;80:399–408.

40. Good-Jacobson KL, Song E, Anderson S, Sharpe AH, Shlomchik MJ. CD80 expression on B cells regulates murine T follicular helper development, germinal center B cell survival, and plasma cell generation. J Immunol. 2012;188(9):4217–25.
41. Kumpfel T, Hohlfeld R. TNFRSF1A, TRAPS and multiple sclerosis. Nat Rev Neurol. 2009;5(10):528–9.
42. Nishida N, Aiba Y, Hitomi Y, Kawashima M, Kojima K, Kawai Y, et al. NELFCD and CTSZ loci are associated with jaundice-stage progression in primary biliary cholangitis in the Japanese population. Sci Rep. 2018;8(1):8071.
43. Kos J, Vizin T, Fonovic UP, Pislar A. Intracellular signaling by cathepsin X: molecular mechanisms and diagnostic and therapeutic opportunities in cancer. Semin Cancer Biol. 2015;31:76–83.
44. Li Y, He X, Schembri-King J, Jakes S, Hayashi J. Cloning and characterization of human Lnk, an adaptor protein with pleckstrin homology and Src homology 2 domains that can inhibit T cell activation. J Immunol. 2000;164(10):5199–206.
45. Katayama H, Mori T, Seki Y, Anraku M, Iseki M, Ikutani M, et al. Lnk prevents inflammatory CD8(+) T-cell proliferation and contributes to intestinal homeostasis. Eur J Immunol. 2014;44(6):1622–32.
46. Joshita S, Umemura T, Tanaka E, Ota M. Genetics and epigenetics in the pathogenesis of primary biliary cholangitis. Clin J Gastroenterol. 2018;11(1):11–8.
47. Remmers EF, Plenge RM, Lee AT, Graham RR, Hom G, Behrens TW, et al. STAT4 and the risk of rheumatoid arthritis and systemic lupus erythematosus. N Engl J Med. 2007;357(10):977–86.
48. Li Q, Verma IM. NF-kappaB regulation in the immune system. Nat Rev Immunol. 2002;2(10):725–34.
49. Gershwin ME, Selmi C, Worman HJ, Gold EB, Watnik M, Utts J, et al. Risk factors and comorbidities in primary biliary cirrhosis: a controlled interview-based study of 1032 patients. Hepatology. 2005;42(5):1194–202.
50. Loftus EV Jr, Harewood GC, Loftus CG, Tremaine WJ, Harmsen WS, Zinsmeister AR, et al. PSC-IBD: a unique form of inflammatory bowel disease associated with primary sclerosing cholangitis. Gut. 2005;54(1):91–6.
51. Borchers AT, Shimoda S, Bowlus C, Keen CL, Gershwin ME. Lymphocyte recruitment and homing to the liver in primary biliary cirrhosis and primary sclerosing cholangitis. Semin Immunopathol. 2009;31(3):309–22.
52. Grant AJ, Goddard S, Ahmed-Choudhury J, Reynolds G, Jackson DG, Briskin M, et al. Hepatic expression of secondary lymphoid chemokine (CCL21) promotes the development of portal-associated lymphoid tissue in chronic inflammatory liver disease. Am J Pathol. 2002;160:1445–55.
53. Grant AJ, Lalor PF, Salmi M, Jalkanen S, Adams DH. Homing of mucosal lymphocytes to the liver in the pathogenesis of hepatic complications of inflammatory bowel disease. Lancet. 2002;359(9301):150–7.
54. Grant AJ, Lalor PF, Hubscher SG, Briskin M, Adams DH. MAdCAM-1 expressed in chronic inflammatory liver disease supports mucosal lymphocyte adhesion to hepatic endothelium (MAdCAM-1 in chronic inflammatory liver disease). Hepatology. 2001;33(5):1065–72.
55. Eksteen B, Grant AJ, Miles A, Curbishley SM, Lalor PF, Hubscher SG, et al. Hepatic endothelial CCL25 mediates the recruitment of CCR9+ gut-homing lymphocytes to the liver in primary sclerosing cholangitis. J Exp Med. 2004;200(11):1511–7.
56. Eksteen B, Miles A, Curbishley SM, Tselepis C, Grant AJ, Walker LSK, et al. Epithelial inflammation is associated with CCL28 production and the recruitment of regulatory T cells expressing CCR10. J Immunol. 2006;177(1):593–603.
57. Miles A, Liaskou E, Eksteen B, Lalor PF, Adams DH. CCL25 and CCL28 promote alpha4 beta7-integrin-dependent adhesion of lymphocytes to MAdCAM-1 under shear flow. Am J Physiol Gastrointest Liver Physiol. 2008;294(5):G1257–67.
58. Aspinall AI, Curbishley SM, Lalor PF, Weston CJ, Blahova M, Liaskou E, et al. CX(3)CR1 and vascular adhesion protein-1-dependent recruitment of CD16(+) monocytes across human liver sinusoidal endothelium. Hepatology. 2010;51(6):2030–9.

59. Schrumpf E, Fausa O, Førre O, Dobloug JH, Ritland S, Thorsby E. HLA antigens and immunoregulatory T cells in ulcerative colitis associated with hepatobiliary disease. Scand J Gastroenterol. 1982;17:187–91.
60. Chapman RW, Varghese Z, Gaul R, Patel G, Kokinon N, Sherlock S. Association of primary sclerosing cholangitis with HLA-B8. Gut. 1983;24:38–41.
61. Naess S, Lie BA, Melum E, Olsson M, Hov JR, Croucher PJ, et al. Refinement of the MHC risk map in a scandinavian primary sclerosing cholangitis population. PLoS One. 2014;9(12):e114486.
62. Price P, Witt C, Allock R, Sayer D, Garlepp M, Kok CC, et al. The genetic basis for the association of the 8.1 ancestral haplotype (Al, B8, DR3) with multiple immunopathological diseases. Immunol Rev. 1999;167:257–74.
63. Okada Y, Yamazaki K, Umeno J, Takahashi A, Kumasaka N, Ashikawa K, et al. HLA-Cw*1202-B*5201-DRB1*1502 haplotype increases risk for ulcerative colitis but reduces risk for Crohn's disease. Gastroenterology. 2011;141(3):864–71 e1-5.
64. Donaldson PT, Norris S. Evaluation of the role of MHC Class II alleles, haplotypes and selected amino acid sequences in primary sclerosing cholangitis. Autoimmunity. 2002;35(8):555–64.
65. Mells GF, Kaser A, Karlsen TH. Novel insights into autoimmune liver diseases provided by genome-wide association studies. J Autoimmun. 2013;46:41–54.
66. Donaldson PT, Farrant JM, Wilkinson ML, Hayllar K, Portmann BC, Williams R. Dual association of HLA DR2 and DR3 with primary sclerosing cholangitis. Hepatology. 1991;13:129–33.
67. Wiencke K, Karlsen TH, Boberg KM, Thorsby E, Schrumpf E, Lie BA, et al. Primary sclerosing cholangitis is associated with extended HLA-DR3 and HLA-DR6 haplotypes. Tissue Antigens. 2007;69(2):161–9.
68. Henriksen EKK, Viken MK, Wittig M, Holm K, Folseraas T, Mucha S, et al. HLA haplotypes in primary sclerosing cholangitis patients of admixed and non-European ancestry. HLA. 2017;90(4):228–33.
69. Karlsen TH, Franke A, Melum E, Kaser A, Hov JR, Balschun T, et al. Genome-wide association analysis in primary sclerosing cholangitis. Gastroenterology. 2010;138(3):1102–11.
70. Melum E, Franke A, Schramm C, Weismuller TJ, Gotthardt DN, Offner FA, et al. Genome-wide association analysis in primary sclerosing cholangitis identifies two non-HLA susceptibility loci. Nat Genet. 2011;43(1):17–9.
71. Folseraas T, Melum E, Rausch P, Juran BD, Ellinghaus E, Shiryaev A, et al. Extended analysis of a genome-wide association study in primary sclerosing cholangitis detects multiple novel risk loci. J Hepatol. 2012;57(2):366–75.
72. Srivastava B, Mells GF, Cordell HJ, Muriithi A, Brown M, Ellinghaus E, et al. Fine mapping and replication of genetic risk loci in primary sclerosing cholangitis. Scand J Gastroenterol. 2012;47(7):820–6.
73. Ellinghaus D, Folseraas T, Holm K, Ellinghaus E, Melum E, Balschun T, et al. Genome-wide association analysis in primary sclerosing cholangitis and ulcerative colitis identifies risk loci at GPR35 and TCF4. Hepatology. 2013;58(3):1074–83.
74. Liu JZ, Hov JR, Folseraas T, Ellinghaus E, Rushbrook SM, Doncheva NT, et al. Dense genotyping of immune-related disease regions identifies nine new risk loci for primary sclerosing cholangitis. Nat Genet. 2013;45(6):670–5.
75. Ellinghaus D, Jostins L, Spain SL, Cortes A, Bethune J, Han B, et al. Analysis of five chronic inflammatory diseases identifies 27 new associations and highlights disease-specific patterns at shared loci. Nat Genet. 2016;48(5):510–8.
76. Ji SG, Juran BD, Mucha S, Folseraas T, Jostins L, Melum E, et al. Genome-wide association study of primary sclerosing cholangitis identifies new risk loci and quantifies the genetic relationship with inflammatory bowel disease. Nat Genet. 2017;49(2):269–73.
77. Alberts R, de Vries EMG, Goode EC, Jiang X, Sampaziotis F, Rombouts K, et al. Genetic association analysis identifies variants associated with disease progression in primary sclerosing cholangitis. Gut. 2018;67:1517–24.
78. Henriksen EK, Melum E, Karlsen TH. Update on primary sclerosing cholangitis genetics. Curr Opin Gastroenterol. 2014;30(3):310–9.

79. Strasser A. The role of BH3-only proteins in the immune system. Nat Rev Immunol. 2005;5(3):189–200.
80. Rai E, Wakeland EK. Genetic predisposition to autoimmunity—what have we learned? Semin Immunol. 2011;23(2):67–83.
81. Sharfe N, Dadi HK, Shahar M, Roifman CM. Human immune disorder arising from mutation of the a chain of the interleukin-2 receptor. Proc Natl Acad Sci U S A. 1997;94:3168–71.
82. Letourneau S, Krieg C, Pantaleo G, Boyman O. IL-2- and CD25-dependent immunoregulatory mechanisms in the homeostasis of T-cell subsets. J Allergy Clin Immunol. 2009;123(4):758–62.
83. Bergqvist I, Eriksson M, Saarikettu J, Eriksson B, Corneliussen B, Grundström T, et al. The basic helix-loop-helix transcription factor E2–2 is involved in T lymphocyte development. Eur J Immunol. 2000;30:2857–63.
84. Wang J, Simonavicius N, Wu X, Swaminath G, Reagan J, Tian H, et al. Kynurenic acid as a ligand for orphan G protein-coupled receptor GPR35. J Biol Chem. 2006;281(31):22021–8.
85. Karlsen TH, Kaser A. Deciphering the genetic predisposition to primary sclerosing cholangitis. Semin Liver Dis. 2011;31(2):188–207.
86. Kasler HG, Young BD, Mottet D, Lim HW, Collins AM, Olson EN, et al. Histone deacetylase 7 regulates cell survival and TCR signaling in CD4/CD8 double-positive thymocytes. J Immunol. 2011;186(8):4782–93.
87. Dequiedt F, Van Lint J, Lecomte E, Van Duppen V, Seufferlein T, Vandenheede JR, et al. Phosphorylation of histone deacetylase 7 by protein kinase D mediates T cell receptor-induced Nur77 expression and apoptosis. J Exp Med. 2005;201(5):793–804.
88. Clark K, MacKenzie KF, Petkevicius K, Kristariyanto Y, Zhang J, Choi HG, et al. Phosphorylation of CRTC3 by the salt inducible kinases controls the interconversion of classically activated and regulatory macrophages. Proc Natl Acad Sci U S A. 2012;109:16986–91.
89. Czaja AJ, Manns MP. Advances in the diagnosis, pathogenesis, and management of autoimmune hepatitis. Gastroenterology. 2010;139(1):58–72 e4.
90. Manns MP, Czaja AJ, Gorham JD, Krawitt EL, Mieli-Vergani G, Vergani D, et al. Diagnosis and management of autoimmune hepatitis. Hepatology. 2010;51(6):2193–213.
91. Heneghan MA, Yeoman AD, Verma S, Smith AD, Longhi MS. Autoimmune hepatitis. Lancet. 2013;382(9902):1433–44.
92. Czaja AJ. Autoimmune hepatitis. Part A: pathogenesis. Expert Rev Gastroenterol Hepatol. 2007;1:113–28.
93. Liberal R, Grant CR, Mieli-Vergani G, Vergani D. Autoimmune hepatitis: a comprehensive review. J Autoimmun. 2013;41:126–39.
94. Longhi MS, Ma Y, Mieli-Vergani G, Vergani D. Adaptive immunity in autoimmune hepatitis. Dig Dis. 2010;28(1):63–9.
95. Zhao L, Tang Y, You Z, Wang Q, Liang S, Han X, et al. Interleukin-17 contributes to the pathogenesis of autoimmune hepatitis through inducing hepatic interleukin-6 expression. PLoS One. 2011;6(4):e18909.
96. Zhao L, Qiu DK, Ma X. Th17 cells: the emerging reciprocal partner of regulatory T cells in the liver. J Dig Dis. 2010;11(3):126–33.
97. Vento S, Cainelli F. Is there a role for viruses in triggering autoimmune hepatitis? Autoimmun Rev. 2004;3(1):61–9.
98. Bjornsson E, Talwalkar J, Treeprasertsuk S, Kamath PS, Takahashi N, Sanderson S, et al. Drug-induced autoimmune hepatitis: clinical characteristics and prognosis. Hepatology. 2010;51(6):2040–8.
99. Wu J, Meng Z, Jiang M, Zhang E, Trippler M, Broering R, et al. Toll-like receptor-induced innate immune responses in non-parenchymal liver cells are cell type-specific. Immunology. 2010;129(3):363–74.
100. Krawitt EL, Kilby AE, Albertini RJ, Schanfield MS, Chastenay BF, Harper PC, et al. Immunogenetic studies of autoimmune chronic active hepatitis: HLA, immunoglobulin allotypes and autoantibodies. Hepatology. 1987;7:1305–10.

101. Seki T, Kiyosawa K, Inoko H, Ota M. Association of autoimmune hepatitis with HLA-Bw54 and DR4 in Japanese patients. Hepatology. 1990;12:1300–4.
102. Umemura T, Katsuyama Y, Yoshizawa K, Kimura T, Joshita S, Komatsu M, et al. Human leukocyte antigen class II haplotypes affect clinical characteristics and progression of type 1 autoimmune hepatitis in Japan. PLoS One. 2014;9(6):e100565.
103. Vázquez-García MN, Aláez C, Olivo A, Debaz H, Pérez-Luque E, Burguete A, et al. MHC class II sequences of susceptibility and protection in Mexicans with autoimmune hepatitis. J Hepatol. 1998;28:985–90.
104. Lim YS, Oh HB, Choi SE, Kwon OJ, Heo YS, Lee HC, et al. Susceptibility to type 1 autoimmune hepatitis is associated with shared amino acid sequences at positions 70-74 of the HLA-DRB1 molecule. J Hepatol. 2008;48(1):133–9.
105. Doherty DG, Donaldson PT, Underhill JA, Farrant JM, Duthie A, Mieli-Vergani G, et al. Allelic sequence variation in the HLA Class II genes and proteins in patients with autoimmune hepatitis. Hepatology. 1994;19:609–15.
106. Strettell M, Donaldson P, Thomson L, Santrach P, Moore S, Czaja A, et al. Allelic basis for HLA-encoded susceptibility to type 1 autoimmune hepatitis. Gastroenterology. 1997;112:2028–35.
107. de Boer YS, van Gerven NM, Zwiers A, Verwer BJ, van Hoek B, van Erpecum KJ, et al. Genome-wide association study identifies variants associated with autoimmune hepatitis type 1. Gastroenterology. 2014;147(2):443–52 e5.
108. Bittencourt PL, Goldberg AC, Cancado ELR, Porta G, Carrilho FJ, Farias AQ, et al. Genetic heterogeneity in susceptibility to autoimmune hepatitis types 1 and 2. Am J Gastroenterol. 1999;94:1906–13.
109. Fortes Mdel P, Machado IV, Gil G, Fernandez-Mestre M, Dagher L, Leon RV, et al. Genetic contribution of major histocompatibility complex class II region to type 1 autoimmune hepatitis susceptibility in Venezuela. Liver Int. 2007;27(10):1409–16.
110. Donaldson PT. Genetics of liver disease: immunogenetics and disease pathogenesis. Gut. 2004;53(4):599–608.
111. Umemura T, Joshita S, Hamano H, Yoshizawa K, Kawa S, Tanaka E, et al. Association of autoimmune hepatitis with Src homology 2 adaptor protein 3 gene polymorphisms in Japanese patients. J Hum Genet. 2017;62(11):963–7.
112. Blonska M, Lin X. NF-kappaB signaling pathways regulated by CARMA family of scaffold proteins. Cell Res. 2011;21(1):55–70.
113. Agarwal K, Czaja AJ, Jones DE, Donaldson PT. Cytotoxic T lymphocyte antigen-4 (CTLA-4) gene polymorphisms and susceptibility to type 1 autoimmune hepatitis. Hepatology. 2000;31:49–53.
114. McCoy KD, Le Gros G. The role of CTLA-4 in the regulation of T cell immune responses. Immunol Cell Biol. 1999;77:1–10.
115. Hiraide A, Imazeki F, Yokosuka O, Kanda T, Kojima H, Fukai K, et al. Fas polymorphisms influence susceptibility to autoimmune hepatitis. Am J Gastroenterol. 2005;100(6):1322–9.
116. Oka S, Higuchi T, Furukawa H, Nakamura M, Komori A, Abiru S, et al. Association of a single nucleotide polymorphism in TNIP1 with type-1 autoimmune hepatitis in the Japanese population. J Hum Genet. 2018;63(6):739–44.
117. Borman MA, Urbanski S, Swain MG. Anti-TNF-induced autoimmune hepatitis. J Hepatol. 2014;61(1):169–70.

Genetics of Multiple Sclerosis

10

Antonio Alcina, Maria Fedetz, and Fuencisla Matesanz

Contents

10.1 Introduction

Multiple sclerosis (MS) is a demyelinating disease of the central nervous system. It was defined for the first time as "la scléroseen plaques" by Jean-Martin Charcot in 1868, and in the 1960s it was called multiple sclerosis (MS), as we know it today [1]. The disease classically manifests in fully or partially reversible episodes of neurologic disability, and approximately 15% of patients have a progressive course from onset [2]. The clinical course of MS is highly variable, ranging from individuals showing occasional sensory nuisance to patients with fulminant course and death within months after disease onset [3]. It is diagnosed in most of the cases between 30 and 40 years of age, and it is almost three times more frequent in women than men.

A. Alcina · M. Fedetz · F. Matesanz (✉)
Instituto de Parasitología y Biomedicina 'López-Neyra', IPBLN-CSIC, Parque Tecnológico Ciencias de la Salud, Granada, Spain
e-mail: pulgoso@ipb.csic.es; mfedez@ipb.csic.es; lindo@ipb.csic.es

J. Martín, F. D. Carmona (eds.), *Genetics of Rare Autoimmune Diseases*,
Rare Diseases of the Immune System, https://doi.org/10.1007/978-3-030-03934-9_10

10.2 Epidemiology and Family Aggregation of MS

MS affects around 2.3 million people worldwide with very different incidence and prevalence among human populations [4]. MS risk varies within the same geographical region across racial and ethnic groups. The global median prevalence reported by World Health Organization (WHO) in 2013 was 33 per 100,000 [5]. The worldwide MS prevalence has increased in the last few years even in regions considered of low incidence. It is not clear if this increase can be due to better diagnosis and reporting, lifestyle changes, or environmental factors [6–8]. Familial contribution to MS etiology is recognized. Since the first systematic family study in MS in 1933 [9], many others have been performed. The familial recurrence rate is about 15% and is higher as it increases the closeness between relatives with around 35% in monozygotic twins [10]. The epidemiological studies have implicated an interplay between genetic and environmental factors in the etiology of MS and suggested that it is a complex trait in which susceptibility is determined by several genes [11].

10.3 Human Leukocyte Antigen

The fist genetic factors identified associated with MS were variants within the major histocompatibility complex (MHC). This region is located on the short arm of chromosome 6 and contains, among others, the human leukocyte antigen (*HLA*) genes [12]. The first studies that associated *HLA* variants with MS were published in 1972 [13, 14]. They localized these variants at HLA-class I region in A and B genes. Subsequently, it was determined that the class I alleles associated with MS were part of the extended class I and class II haplotypes and that the main signal was located at class II region where DR and DQ genes are encoded [14]. The specific haplotype associated with MS was determined as HLA-DRB1*15:01-DQB*06:02 and, at that time, it was estimated to explain about 25–35% of the genetic component of MS [15, 16]. Many studies using fine mapping techniques and large MS populations have identified the genes and alleles responsible for the MS association in the HLA locus. The more prominent risk allele in MS is HLA-DRB1*15:01, which, in addition, has been associated with disease severity [15]. Over 30 additional independent allelic and genetic associations within the extended MHC region have been identified as HLA-DRB1*03:01, HLA-DRB1*13:03, HLA-DRB1*08:01, and HLA-DQB1*03:02, at the class II DR and DQ loci or HLA-A*02:01, HLA-B*44:02, HLA-B*38:01, and HLA-B*55:01 at HLA-class I region [17–20]. Despite the significant effort made to understand the variation of HLA in MS cohorts comprising many thousands of individuals, the role of MHC in the pathogenesis of the disease is not fully understood.

10.4 History of the Search for the Genetic Basis of MS

Although the strongest genetic risk factor is within the HLA, it does not explain the totality of the genetic contribution to MS susceptibility. Important efforts have been made to determine additional loci. The identification of the risk loci in MS, as for other traits, has been conditioned to the development of new genotyping and sequencing techniques, as well as the advancement of knowledge of the human genome.

The success identifying variants at the MHC made believe that non-MHC loci would be easy to find. However, this led to decades of frustration in which many loci have been pinpointed using linkage or candidate gene approaches, but few of them have been undeniably established as susceptibility loci.

Whole-genome screens for linkage based on around 100 MS sib pairs using 300–400 microsatellites were published by independent groups from the UK, the USA, and Canada [21–23]. Posterior studies, in a total of nine populations, were performed in families, but none of them identified any statistically significant linkage. Meta-analysis combining all these studies confirmed genome-wide significance just in the HLA region [24].

In order to solve the design problems of the previous approaches, the International Multiple Sclerosis Genetics Consortium (IMSGC) performed a larger study with denser map of SNPs in 730 multiplex families from Australia, Scandinavia, the USA, and the UK [25]. However, once again, only MHC region reached statistical significance. Despite the apparent failure of these studies, they provide useful guidance concerning the size of effects of MS susceptibility loci as well as the size of the cohorts needed for this type of analysis.

Candidate gene approach was the most common strategy for identification of susceptibility genes until 2007. However, most of these studies lacked reproducibility due to low power and low density of markers used. Some associations identified by this approach were validated in posterior studies as these reported at *IL2RA* [26] and *IL7R* [27, 28] loci, while others were discarded in well-powered studies as *APOE* [29].

10.5 Genome-Wide Association Studies in MS

The last decade has been very fruitful in identifying loci associated with MS, thanks to the use of the genome-wide association studies (GWASs), a hypothesis-free method that provides almost total coverage of common variants of the genome by tagging the genetic variants through linkage disequilibrium (LD). In 2007, the first GWAS in MS analyzing 334,923 SNPs in 931 family trios was published [30]. Although it is one of the most cited works in genetics of MS and with important posterior repercussion, at first it was a little bit disappointing, since just two modest risk effects at *IL2RA* and *IL7RA* genes were reported, loci that were already known to be associated with MS by candidate gene strategy [26–28]. However, meta-analysis and validations identified a total of 15 associations including the regions of *CD6*, *IRF8*, *TYK2*, *IL12A*, *RGS1*, and *TNFRSF1A* [31–33]. A total of 12 GWASs have been performed to determine the MS susceptibility loci (Table 10.1). Some of these studies were done in very small cohorts but most of them with large populations, finding new MS-associated loci or validating other previously reported. Meta-analysis of several of these GWAS combining 47,351 MS subjects and 68,284

Table 10.1 GWASs and meta-analyses in MS

First author	Year published	Objective of the study	Initial sample size	Replication sample size	Variants reported[a]	Platform [SNPs passing QC]	GWAS catalog study accession
Hafler DA [30]	2007	MS susceptibility	931 European ancestry trios 2431 European ancestry controls	609 European ancestry trios 2322 European ancestry cases 2987 European ancestry controls	6	Affymetrix [334,923]	GCST000062
AulchenkoYS [67]	2008	MS susceptibility	45 European ancestry cases 195 European ancestry controls	1316 European ancestry cases 1423 European ancestry controls 1318 cases and 1507 controls from 756 families	1	Affymetrix [~250,000]	GCST000263
Comabella M [68]	2008	MS susceptibility	242 European ancestry cases 242 European ancestry controls	553 European ancestry cases 1033 European ancestry controls	1	Affymetrix [428,867]	GCST000252
Baranzini ES [69]	2009	MS susceptibility	978 European ancestry cases 883 European ancestry controls	NA	10	Illumina [551,642]	GCST000269
ANZgene [70]	2009	MS susceptibility	1618 European ancestry cases 3413 European ancestry controls	2256 European ancestry cases 2310 European ancestry controls	8	Illumina [302,098]	GCST000425
De Jager PL [31]	2009	Meta-analysis MS susceptibility	2624 European ancestry cases 7220 European ancestry controls	2215 European ancestry cases 2116 European ancestry controls	15	Affymetrix, Illumina [~2,560,000] (imputed)	GCST000424

Baranzini SE [71]	2009	MS age of onset	978 European ancestry cases 883 European ancestry controls	NA	19	Illumina [551,642]	GCST000267
Jakkula E [72]	2010	MS susceptibility	68 Finland founder cases 136 Finland founder controls	83 Finland founder cases 365 Finland founder controls 3285 European ancestry cases 6379 European ancestry controls 1202 cases, 3399 controls	2	Illumina [297,343]	GCST000593
Sanna S [73]	2010	MS susceptibility	882 Sardinian cases 872 Sardinian controls	1775 Sardinian cases 2005 Sardinian controls	2	Affymetrix [6,607,266] (imputed)	GCST000680
Nischwitz S [74]	2010	MS susceptibility	590 European ancestry cases 825 European ancestry controls	NA	4	Illumina [~300,000]	GCST000716
Baranzini SE [75]	2010	MS—brain glutamate levels	382 cases	NA	5	Illumina [~500,000]	GCST000783
Brynedal B [76]	2010	MS severity	1040 European ancestry cases	873 European ancestry cases	1	Affymetrix [105,035]	GCST000577
Sawcer S [18]	2011	MS susceptibility	9772 European ancestry cases 16,849 European ancestry controls	4218 European ancestry cases 7296 European ancestry controls	87	Illumina [465,434]	GCST001198

(continued)

Table 10.1 (continued)

First author	Year published	Objective of the study	Initial sample size	Replication sample size	Variants reported[a]	Platform [SNPs passing QC]	GWAS catalog study accession
Patsopoulos NA [45]	2011	Meta-analysis MS susceptibility	5545 European ancestry cases 12,153 European ancestry controls	NA	19	Affymetrix, Illumina [2,529,394]	GCST001341
IMSGC [77]	2011	MS severity	1470 European ancestry cases	NA	6	Affymetrix [2,110,417] (imputed)	GCST001096
Martinelli-Boneschi F [78]	2012	Progressive MS susceptibility	197 European ancestry cases 234 European ancestry controls	379 European ancestry cases 398 European ancestry controls	1	Affymetrix [277,866]	GCST001459
Matesanz F [79]	2012	MS susceptibility	2127 European ancestry cases 4558 European ancestry controls	2785 European ancestry cases 2940 European ancestry controls	1	Affymetrix, Illumina [130,903]	GCST001505
Leone MA [80]	2013	MS OCB status	49 European ancestry OCB-negative cases 513 European ancestry OCB-positive cases	200 European ancestry OCB-negative cases 1684 European ancestry OCB-positive cases	1	Illumina [504,967]	GCST002072
Gourraud PA [81]	2013	MS brain lesion distribution	284 European ancestry individuals		16	Illumina [208,975]	GCST001860

Mero IL [82]	2013	MS OCB status	1367 European ancestry OCB-positive cases 161 European ancestry OCB-negative cases 428 European ancestry controls	NA	11	Illumina [495,970]	GCST001892
Goris A [39]	2015	Immunoglobulin G index levels in MS	773 European ancestry individuals 165 individuals	2072 individuals	3	NR [485,236]	GCST002757
Goris A [39]	2015	Oligoclonal band status in MS	2232 European ancestry OCB-positive individuals 275 European ancestry OCB-negative individuals 439 OCB-positive individuals, 80 OCB-negative individuals	3026 OCB-positive individuals 452 OCB-negative individuals	3	NR [485,522]	GCST002758
Clarelli F [83]	2015	Response to interferon beta in MS	166 European ancestry responder cases 171 European ancestry non-responder cases	NA	3	Illumina [1,387,466] (imputed)	GCST003193

(continued)

Table 10.1 (continued)

First author	Year published	Objective of the study	Initial sample size	Replication sample size	Variants reported[a]	Platform [SNPs passing QC]	GWAS catalog study accession
Andlauer TF [84]	2016	MS susceptibility	4888 German ancestry cases 10,395 German ancestry controls	2903 Sardinian ancestry cases 3323 Sardinian ancestry controls	1	Illumina [at least 8,143,088] (imputed)	GCST003566
Zhou Y [85]	2016	Epstein Barr virus nuclear antigen 1 IgG levels or MS	3599 individuals 1956 Mexican American individuals 5545 European ancestry multiple sclerosis cases 12,153 European ancestry non-multiple sclerosis controls		4	Illumina [up to 2,529,394] (imputed)	GCST003340
Steri M [56]	2017	MS susceptibility	2273 Sardinian cases 2148 Sardinian controls	6840 European ancestry cases 661 Sardinian cases 3176 cases 6044 European ancestry controls 1244 Sardinian controls, 2958 controls	5	Affymetrix [~12,200,000] (imputed)	GCST004290
Zhou Y [86]	2017	Relapse in MS	268 cases	181 cases	5	Illumina [1,033,813] (imputed)	GCST004752
IMSGC [35]	2017	Meta-analysis MS susceptibility	47,351 MS subjects 68,284 control subjects		200	Affymetrix and Illumina [8,278,136] (imputed)	

[a]Variants reported by the authors. Data obtained from https://www.ebi.ac.uk/gwas/ and from bibliography

control subjects establishes a reference map of the genetic architecture of MS that includes 200 autosomal susceptibility variants outside the MHC, one chromosome X variant, and 32 independent associations within the extended MHC [34, 35]. The effects of the associated variants have odds ratios (ORs) ranging from 1.06 to 2.06 and the allele frequencies of the respective risk allele from 2.1% to 98.4% in the European population. The estimation heritability, including all associations described, ranges between 20 and 30%, most of it assigned to the MHC region [35]. Therefore most of the heritability in MS is still to be revealed, and the focus of attention is being placed on genetic interactions between known variants, rare variants, disease heterogeneity, gene-environment interactions, and epigenetic effects.

Rare variants, unique to specific families or disease conditions, that strongly predispose an individual to MS are a field of intense investigations at this moment. It is being addressed by exome sequencing in families or very large populations, but the results reported until now have not led to the identification of new variants or robust results [36–38].

MS heterogeneity is observed in onset, clinical manifestations, evolution, or treatment response, and these aspects have to be addressed to determine if this phenotypic diversity responds to genetic differences. Most of the GWASs performed in MS susceptibility did not take into consideration this heterogeneity in order to collect large populations to obtain a high statistical power. However, the dilution of the genetic effects due to the mixture of disease forms with different genetic origin could explain the low odds ratio of the variants identified by GWAS as well as being responsible of part of the "missing heritability" of the disease. Some studies have addressed the heterogeneity of the disease stratifying the patients using different criteria as interferon beta (IFNB) response, one of the most common treatments for MS, disease severity, age of onset, or oligoclonal band status (OCBs) (Table 10.1). Using this approach it has been determined that variants associated with immunoglobulin G (IgG) index account for up to two fold differences in the odds of being MS OCB positive [39]. The presence of OCBs and high IgG levels in the CSF of MS patients is considered the principal biomarker of the disease since more than 90% of MS patients exhibit OCBs in the CSF [40].

The next generation of genetic studies in MS will, probably, focus to define the genetic variants' underlying disease heterogeneity to better understand its etiology and use the individual information to approach personalize treatment options and follow-up of the disease.

10.6 Common Genetic Component with Other Autoimmune Diseases

Autoimmune diseases have been observed to coexist within individuals and within families [41], and for many years, it was suspected that they shared etiological similarities. Evidences came from the genetics in which have been demonstrated that most of the recently identified autoimmunity loci are shared among multiple autoimmune diseases. In fact many genetic studies using candidate gene approach have used the criteria of loci associated with other autoimmune disease to select the variants to be analyzed. This is the case of variants at *IRF5* which were firstly associated with systemic lupus erythematosus (SLE) [42] and later with MS [43]. Similarly, *IL2RA* was associated with type 1 diabetes (T1D) [44] and then with MS [26]. However, the more important evidences of the overlap in the genetics underlying susceptibility to autoimmune diseases came from the GWASs in different diseases [18, 45, 46]. A collaborative effort toward the identification of the common genetic bases of the autoimmune diseases was the "Immunochip" project. The Immunochip Consortium developed a 200,000 SNP chip to provide cost-effective genotyping of common and rare variants to fine-map 184 non-MHC loci with genome-wide significant associations to at least one autoimmune disease [47]. A large cohort of 14,498 MS subjects and 24,091 healthy controls were analyzed identifying 48 new susceptibility variants and 49 previously known MS risk loci [48]. Interestingly, some loci associated with two or more diseases revealed heterogeneity of risk variants and alleles. This was the case observed in MS and T1D at the *IL2RA* locus in which one associated variant had a risk effect in one disease and protective in the other, suggesting different roles of IL2RA in these two diseases [49, 50].

10.7 Causal Variants of the MS Associations and Their Functional Effects

Definition of the loci associated with MS is the first step toward the identification of the genes, biological functions and pathways altered in the pathology of MS. However, this is not an easy task; most associated variants do not produce protein-coding changes, suggesting that they must be altering regulatory regions. The signals detected by GWAS are tags representing LD blocks, composed of variable number of SNPs that can be located thousands of bases away from the detected signal; thus assigning the closest gene to the most significant independent effect of a locus as the causative candidate, as was done in the earlier studies, is not a valid approach. In addition, risk variants located in cis-regulatory elements can act at long distances, and their target gene may not be the one closest to the GWAS-detected variant. Fine-mapping through tag-SNP analysis and re-sequencing of the associated loci, together with functional studies of the variants by experimental or in silico analysis, are the approaches used toward the identification of the causal genes of the associations.

Expression quantitative trait loci (eQTL) has been a powerful tool to identify MS risk variants that are associated with changes on expression level of genes [51]. Several MS-associated variants are eQTLs, for example, rs10877013, which alters the enhancer activity of a regulatory element reducing the expression of the *CYP27B1* gene. It encodes the enzyme responsible for the vitamin D activation, affecting the function of vitamin D system [52–55]. Increased levels of TNFSF13B messenger RNA due to its degradation resistance by microRNA have been reported as the mechanism by which an insertion-deletion variant associated with MS alters the function of the BAFF protein encoded by *TNFSF13B* gene [56]. Splicing alteration can also influence gene expression, as it is described for rs28445040. This variant associates with decreased expression of the full-length RNA isoform of *SP140* due to exon 7 skipping [57]. Rs6897932, located within the exon 6 of the *IL7R* gene, disrupts exon splicing silencer altering the amount of soluble and membrane-bound isoforms of the protein [27]. Other variant associated with MS which produces splicing alterations is rs1800693, a SNP located next to the splicing donor of the exon 6 of *TNFRSF1A* which directs the expression of a soluble form of TNFR1 [58]. The truncated soluble isoform of TNFR1 was identified in peripheral blood mononuclear cells (PBMC) from patients carrying the risk allele of rs1800693 variant and is affecting the magnitude of monocyte responses to TNF-α [59, 60].

Several strategies have been developed to determine the gene altered by an associated variant that is located distance away from the causal variant. One of these is the definition of insulator elements bound by CTCF which allowed to determine that the variants associated with MS located within the *EVI5* gene are actually affecting the adjacent gene *GFI1* [61]. However, this seems to be not the only effect associated with MS in this locus. Recently, it was reported that a nonsynonymous variant, strongly associated with MS, induces changes in superficial hydrophobicity patterns of the coiled-coil domain of EVI5 protein, which, in turn, affects the EVI5 interactome [62].

Despite the important advance in the understanding of the genetics of MS, key challenges are ahead of us such as the determination of genes altered by the 200 variants associated with MS, for which we have functional evidence for only some of them, and unravel the missing heritability, not completely detected by GWAS carried out until now. Network analysis of GWAS data addresses these issues [63]. Strategies focused on the overrepresentation of genes at the associated loci in gene ontology (GO) or KEGG pathways [64] or protein–protein and protein–DNA interactions have been used to approach these problems. Network-based pathway analysis of two GWASs in MS, combining data on genetic associations with evidence for protein-protein interactions, obtained overrepresentation of subnetworks of genes from several immunological pathways as well as neural pathways, namely, axon guidance and synaptic potentiation [46]. The IMSGC performed a protein-interaction-network-based pathway analysis (PINBPA) on two large genetic MS studies comprising a total of 15,317 cases and 29,529 controls [65]. The GO analysis of the MS risk genes identified networks of leukocyte activation, apoptosis, and positive regulation of macromolecule metabolic process [66].

10.8 Conclusion

From the first discovery of the HLA-association with MS until now, we have come a long way in the study of the genetics of MS. During this journey, full of successes and failures, we have determined more than 200 loci that independently contribute to disease pathogenesis, we have better defined the HLA variants and their relation with the MS, and we begin to unravel gene-gene and gene-environment interactions underlying MS. However, we have important challenges ahead of us as the contribution of the genetics to MS complexity, evolution, brain atrophy, and treatment response. But, perhaps, the most important challenge that we face is to integrate all these new knowledge into medical practice for a better diagnosis, prognosis, and treatment.

References

1. Murray TJ. The history of multiple sclerosis: the changing frame of the disease over the centuries. J Neurol Sci. 2009;277(Suppl 1):S3–8. https://doi.org/10.1016/S0022-510X(09)70003-6. S0022-510X(09)70003-6 [pii].
2. Ransohoff RM, Hafler DA, Lucchinetti CF. Multiple sclerosis—a quiet revolution. Nat Rev Neurol. 2015;11(3):134–42. https://doi.org/10.1038/nrneurol.2015.14. nrneurol.2015.14 [pii].
3. Disanto G, Berlanga AJ, Handel AE, Para AE, Burrell AM, Fries A, Handunnetthi L, De Luca GC, Morahan JM. Heterogeneity in multiple sclerosis: scratching the surface of a complex disease. Autoimmune Dis. 2010;2011:932351. https://doi.org/10.4061/2011/932351.
4. Browne P, Chandraratna D, Angood C, Tremlett H, Baker C, Taylor BV, Thompson AJ. Atlas of multiple sclerosis 2013: a growing global problem with widespread inequity. Neurology. 2014;83(11):1022–4. https://doi.org/10.1212/WNL.0000000000000768. WNL.0000000000000768 [pii].
5. Multiple Sclerosis International Federation. Atlas of MS, 2013. Mapping multiple sclerosis around the world. 2013. http://www.msif.org/about-us/advocacy/atlas/.
6. Sahraian MA, Sahebkar M, Dehghani R, Derakhshan-Jazari M, Kazami-Moghaddam V, Kouchaki E. Multiple sclerosis—a disease on a dramatically rising trend in Iran: review of possible reasons. Iran J Neurol. 2017;16(1):34–40.
7. Zahoor I, Haq E. Multiple sclerosis in India: iceberg or volcano. J Neuroimmunol. 2017;307:27–30. https://doi.org/10.1016/j.jneuroim.2017.03.015. S0165-5728(17)30058-9 [pii].
8. Midgard R. Incidence and prevalence of multiple sclerosis in Norway. Acta Neurol Scand Suppl. 2012;(195):36–42. https://doi.org/10.1111/ane.12025.
9. Curtius F. Multiple Sklerose und Erbanlage. Leipzig: G. Thieme; 1933.
10. Compston A, Coles A. Multiple sclerosis. Lancet. 2002;359(9313):1221–31. https://doi.org/10.1016/S0140-6736(02)08220-X. S0140-6736(02)08220-X [pii].
11. Compston A. The genetic epidemiology of multiple sclerosis. Philos Trans R Soc Lond Ser B Biol Sci. 1999;354(1390):1623–34. https://doi.org/10.1098/rstb.1999.0507.
12. Kumanovics A, Takada T, Lindahl KF. Genomic organization of the mammalian MHC. Annu Rev Immunol. 2003;21:629–57. https://doi.org/10.1146/annurev.immunol.21.090501.080116. 090501.080116 [pii].
13. Jersild C, Fog T. Histocompatibility (HL-A) antigens associated with multiple sclerosis. Acta Neurol Scand Suppl. 1972;51:377.
14. Naito S, Namerow N, Mickey MR, Terasaki PI. Multiple sclerosis: association with HL-A3. Tissue Antigens. 1972;2(1):1–4.
15. Barcellos LF, Oksenberg JR, Begovich AB, Martin ER, Schmidt S, Vittinghoff E, Goodin DS, Pelletier D, Lincoln RR, Bucher P, Swerdlin A, Pericak-Vance MA, Haines JL, Hauser SL. HLA-DR2 dose effect on susceptibility to multiple sclerosis and influence on disease course. Am J Hum Genet. 2003;72(3):710–6. https://doi.org/10.1086/367781. S0002-9297(07)60586-2 [pii].
16. Dyment DA, Ebers GC, Sadovnick AD. Genetics of multiple sclerosis. Lancet Neurol. 2004;3(2):104–10. S147444220300663X [pii].
17. Marrosu MG, Murru R, Murru MR, Costa G, Zavattari P, Whalen M, Cocco E, Mancosu C, Schirru L, Solla E, Fadda E, Melis C, Porru I, Rolesu M, Cucca F. Dissection of the HLA association with multiple sclerosis in the founder isolated population of Sardinia. Hum Mol Genet. 2001;10(25):2907–16.

18. Sawcer S, Hellenthal G, Pirinen M, Spencer CC, Patsopoulos NA, Moutsianas L, Dilthey A, Su Z, Freeman C, Hunt SE, Edkins S, Gray E, Booth DR, Potter SC, Goris A, Band G, Oturai AB, Strange A, Saarela J, Bellenguez C, Fontaine B, Gillman M, Hemmer B, Gwilliam R, Zipp F, Jayakumar A, Martin R, Leslie S, Hawkins S, Giannoulatou E, D'Alfonso S, Blackburn H, Martinelli Boneschi F, Liddle J, Harbo HF, Perez ML, Spurkland A, Waller MJ, Mycko MP, Ricketts M, Comabella M, Hammond N, Kockum I, McCann OT, Ban M, Whittaker P, Kemppinen A, Weston P, Hawkins C, Widaa S, Zajicek J, Dronov S, Robertson N, Bumpstead SJ, Barcellos LF, Ravindrarajah R, Abraham R, Alfredsson L, Ardlie K, Aubin C, Baker A, Baker K, Baranzini SE, Bergamaschi L, Bergamaschi R, Bernstein A, Berthele A, Boggild M, Bradfield JP, Brassat D, Broadley SA, Buck D, Butzkueven H, Capra R, Carroll WM, Cavalla P, Celius EG, Cepok S, Chiavacci R, Clerget-Darpoux F, Clysters K, Comi G, Cossburn M, Cournu-Rebeix I, Cox MB, Cozen W, Cree BA, Cross AH, Cusi D, Daly MJ, Davis E, de Bakker PI, Debouverie M, D'Hooghe MB, Dixon K, Dobosi R, Dubois B, Ellinghaus D, Elovaara I, Esposito F, Fontenille C, Foote S, Franke A, Galimberti D, Ghezzi A, Glessner J, Gomez R, Gout O, Graham C, Grant SF, Guerini FR, Hakonarson H, Hall P, Hamsten A, Hartung HP, Heard RN, Heath S, Hobart J, Hoshi M, Infante-Duarte C, Ingram G, Ingram W, Islam T, Jagodic M, Kabesch M, Kermode AG, Kilpatrick TJ, Kim C, Klopp N, Koivisto K, Larsson M, Lathrop M, Lechner-Scott JS, Leone MA, Leppa V, Liljedahl U, Bomfim IL, Lincoln RR, Link J, Liu J, Lorentzen AR, Lupoli S, Macciardi F, Mack T, Marriott M, Martinelli V, Mason D, McCauley JL, Mentch F, Mero IL, Mihalova T, Montalban X, Mottershead J, Myhr KM, Naldi P, Ollier W, Page A, Palotie A, Pelletier J, Piccio L, Pickersgill T, Piehl F, Pobywajlo S, Quach HL, Ramsay PP, Reunanen M, Reynolds R, Rioux JD, Rodegher M, Roesner S, Rubio JP, Ruckert IM, Salvetti M, Salvi E, Santaniello A, Schaefer CA, Schreiber S, Schulze C, Scott RJ, Sellebjerg F, Selmaj KW, Sexton D, Shen L, Simms-Acuna B, Skidmore S, Sleiman PM, Smestad C, Sorensen PS, Sondergaard HB, Stankovich J, Strange RC, Sulonen AM, Sundqvist E, Syvanen AC, Taddeo F, Taylor B, Blackwell JM, Tienari P, Bramon E, Tourbah A, Brown MA, Tronczynska E, Casas JP, Tubridy N, Corvin A, Vickery J, Jankowski J, Villoslada P, Markus HS, Wang K, Mathew CG, Wason J, Palmer CN, Wichmann HE, Plomin R, Willoughby E, Rautanen A, Winkelmann J, Wittig M, Trembath RC, Yaouanq J, Viswanathan AC, Zhang H, Wood NW, Zuvich R, Deloukas P, Langford C, Duncanson A, Oksenberg JR, Pericak-Vance MA, Haines JL, Olsson T, Hillert J, Ivinson AJ, De Jager PL, Peltonen L, Stewart GJ, Hafler DA, Hauser SL, McVean G, Donnelly P, Compston A. Genetic risk and a primary role for cell-mediated immune mechanisms in multiple sclerosis. Nature. 2011;476(7359):214–9. https://doi.org/10.1038/nature10251. nature10251 [pii].
19. Moutsianas L, Jostins L, Beecham AH, Dilthey AT, Xifara DK, Ban M, Shah TS, Patsopoulos NA, Alfredsson L, Anderson CA, Attfield KE, Baranzini SE, Barrett J, Binder TMC, Booth D, Buck D, Celius EG, Cotsapas C, D'Alfonso S, Dendrou CA, Donnelly P, Dubois B, Fontaine B, Fugger L, Goris A, Gourraud PA, Graetz C, Hemmer B, Hillert J, Kockum I, Leslie S, Lill CM, Martinelli-Boneschi F, Oksenberg JR, Olsson T, Oturai A, Saarela J, Sondergaard HB, Spurkland A, Taylor B, Winkelmann J, Zipp F, Haines JL, Pericak-Vance MA, Spencer CCA, Stewart G, Hafler DA, Ivinson AJ, Harbo HF, Hauser SL, De Jager PL, Compston A, McCauley JL, Sawcer S, McVean G. Class II HLA interactions modulate genetic risk for multiple sclerosis. Nat Genet. 2015;47(10):1107–13. https://doi.org/10.1038/ng.3395.
20. Patsopoulos NA, Barcellos LF, Hintzen RQ, Schaefer C, van Duijn CM, Noble JA, Raj T, Gourraud PA, Stranger BE, Oksenberg J, Olsson T, Taylor BV, Sawcer S, Hafler DA, Carrington M, De Jager PL, de Bakker PI. Fine-mapping the genetic association of the major histocompatibility complex in multiple sclerosis: HLA and non-HLA effects. PLoS Genet. 2013;9(11):e1003926. https://doi.org/10.1371/journal.pgen.1003926. PGENETICS-D-13-01062 [pii].
21. Ebers GC, Kukay K, Bulman DE, Sadovnick AD, Rice G, Anderson C, Armstrong H, Cousin K, Bell RB, Hader W, Paty DW, Hashimoto S, Oger J, Duquette P, Warren S, Gray T, O'Connor P, Nath A, Auty A, Metz L, Francis G, Paulseth JE, Murray TJ, Pryse-Phillips W, Nelson R, Freedman M, Brunet D, Bouchard JP, Hinds D, Risch N. A full genome search in multiple sclerosis. Nat Genet. 1996;13(4):472–6. https://doi.org/10.1038/ng0896-472.

22. Haines JL, Ter-Minassian M, Bazyk A, Gusella JF, Kim DJ, Terwedow H, Pericak-Vance MA, Rimmler JB, Haynes CS, Roses AD, Lee A, Shaner B, Menold M, Seboun E, Fitoussi RP, Gartioux C, Reyes C, Ribierre F, Gyapay G, Weissenbach J, Hauser SL, Goodkin DE, Lincoln R, Usuku K, Oksenberg JR, et al. A complete genomic screen for multiple sclerosis underscores a role for the major histocompatibility complex. The Multiple Sclerosis Genetics Group. Nat Genet. 1996;13(4):469–71. https://doi.org/10.1038/ng0896-469.
23. Sawcer S, Jones HB, Feakes R, Gray J, Smaldon N, Chataway J, Robertson N, Clayton D, Goodfellow PN, Compston A. A genome screen in multiple sclerosis reveals susceptibility loci on chromosome 6p21 and 17q22. Nat Genet. 1996;13(4):464–8. https://doi.org/10.1038/ng0896-464.
24. GAMES; Transatlantic Multiple Sclerosis Genetics Cooperative. A meta-analysis of whole genome linkage screens in multiple sclerosis. J Neuroimmunol. 2003;143(1–2):39–46. S0165572803003084 [pii].
25. Sawcer S, Ban M, Maranian M, Yeo TW, Compston A, Kirby A, Daly MJ, De Jager PL, Walsh E, Lander ES, Rioux JD, Hafler DA, Ivinson A, Rimmler J, Gregory SG, Schmidt S, Pericak-Vance MA, Akesson E, Hillert J, Datta P, Oturai A, Ryder LP, Harbo HF, Spurkland A, Myhr KM, Laaksonen M, Booth D, Heard R, Stewart G, Lincoln R, Barcellos LF, Hauser SL, Oksenberg JR, Kenealy SJ, Haines JL. A high-density screen for linkage in multiple sclerosis. Am J Hum Genet. 2005;77(3):454–67. https://doi.org/10.1086/444547. S0002-9297(07)63025-0 [pii].
26. Matesanz F, Caro-Maldonado A, Fedetz M, Fernandez O, Milne RL, Guerrero M, Delgado C, Alcina A. IL2RA/CD25 polymorphisms contribute to multiple sclerosis susceptibility. J Neurol. 2007;254(5):682–4. https://doi.org/10.1007/s00415-006-0416-4.
27. Gregory SG, Schmidt S, Seth P, Oksenberg JR, Hart J, Prokop A, Caillier SJ, Ban M, Goris A, Barcellos LF, Lincoln R, McCauley JL, Sawcer SJ, Compston DA, Dubois B, Hauser SL, Garcia-Blanco MA, Pericak-Vance MA, Haines JL. Interleukin 7 receptor alpha chain (IL7R) shows allelic and functional association with multiple sclerosis. Nat Genet. 2007;39(9):1083–91. https://doi.org/10.1038/ng2103. ng2103 [pii].
28. Lundmark F, Duvefelt K, Iacobaeus E, Kockum I, Wallstrom E, Khademi M, Oturai A, Ryder LP, Saarela J, Harbo HF, Celius EG, Salter H, Olsson T, Hillert J. Variation in interleukin 7 receptor alpha chain (IL7R) influences risk of multiple sclerosis. Nat Genet. 2007;39(9):1108–13. https://doi.org/10.1038/ng2106. ng2106 [pii].
29. Lill CM, Liu T, Schjeide BM, Roehr JT, Akkad DA, Damotte V, Alcina A, Ortiz MA, Arroyo R, Lopez de Lapuente A, Blaschke P, Winkelmann A, Gerdes LA, Luessi F, Fernadez O, Izquierdo G, Antiguedad A, Hoffjan S, Cournu-Rebeix I, Gromoller S, Faber H, Liebsch M, Meissner E, Chanvillard C, Touze E, Pico F, Corcia P, Dorner T, Steinhagen-Thiessen E, Baeckman L, Heekeren HR, Li SC, Lindenberger U, Chan A, Hartung HP, Aktas O, Lohse P, Kumpfel T, Kubisch C, Epplen JT, Zettl UK, Fontaine B, Vandenbroeck K, Matesanz F, Urcelay E, Bertram L, Zipp F. Closing the case of APOE in multiple sclerosis: no association with disease risk in over 29 000 subjects. J Med Genet. 2012;49(9):558–62. https://doi.org/10.1136/jmedgenet-2012-101175. jmedgenet-2012-101175 [pii].
30. Hafler DA, Compston A, Sawcer S, Lander ES, Daly MJ, De Jager PL, de Bakker PI, Gabriel SB, Mirel DB, Ivinson AJ, Pericak-Vance MA, Gregory SG, Rioux JD, McCauley JL, Haines JL, Barcellos LF, Cree B, Oksenberg JR, Hauser SL. Risk alleles for multiple sclerosis identified by a genomewide study. N Engl J Med. 2007;357(9):851–62. https://doi.org/10.1056/NEJMoa073493. NEJMoa073493 [pii].
31. De Jager PL, Jia X, Wang J, de Bakker PI, Ottoboni L, Aggarwal NT, Piccio L, Raychaudhuri S, Tran D, Aubin C, Briskin R, Romano S, Baranzini SE, McCauley JL, Pericak-Vance MA, Haines JL, Gibson RA, Naeglin Y, Uitdehaag B, Matthews PM, Kappos L, Polman C, McArdle WL, Strachan DP, Evans D, Cross AH, Daly MJ, Compston A, Sawcer SJ, Weiner HL, Hauser SL, Hafler DA, Oksenberg JR. Meta-analysis of genome scans and replication identify CD6, IRF8 and TNFRSF1A as new multiple sclerosis susceptibility loci. Nat Genet. 2009;41(7):776–82. https://doi.org/10.1038/ng.401. ng.401 [pii].
32. Ban M, Goris A, Lorentzen AR, Baker A, Mihalova T, Ingram G, Booth DR, Heard RN, Stewart GJ, Bogaert E, Dubois B, Harbo HF, Celius EG, Spurkland A, Strange R, Hawkins C,

Robertson NP, Dudbridge F, Wason J, De Jager PL, Hafler D, Rioux JD, Ivinson AJ, McCauley JL, Pericak-Vance M, Oksenberg JR, Hauser SL, Sexton D, Haines J, Sawcer S, Compston A. Replication analysis identifies TYK2 as a multiple sclerosis susceptibility factor. Eur J Hum Genet. 2009;17(10):1309–13. https://doi.org/10.1038/ejhg.2009.41. ejhg200941 [pii].
33. International Multiple Sclerosis Genetics Consortium (IMSGC). IL12A, MPHOSPH9/CDK2AP1 and RGS1 are novel multiple sclerosis susceptibility loci. Genes Immun. 2010;11(5):397–405. https://doi.org/10.1038/gene.2010.28. gene201028 [pii].
34. Baranzini SE, Oksenberg JR. The genetics of multiple sclerosis: from 0 to 200 in 50 years. Trends Genet. 2017;33(12):960–70. https://doi.org/10.1016/j.tig.2017.09.004. S0168-9525(17)30163-4 [pii].
35. International Multiple Sclerosis Genetics Consortium (IMSGC). The Multiple Sclerosis Genomic Map: role of peripheral immune cells and resident microglia in susceptibility. bioRxiv. 2017. https://doi.org/10.1101/143933.
36. Dankowski T, Buck D, Andlauer TF, Antony G, Bayas A, Bechmann L, Berthele A, Bettecken T, Chan A, Franke A, Gold R, Graetz C, Haas J, Hecker M, Herms S, Infante-Duarte C, Jockel KH, Kieseier BC, Knier B, Knop M, Kumpfel T, Lichtner P, Lieb W, Lill CM, Limmroth V, Linker RA, Loleit V, Meuth SG, Moebus S, Muller-Myhsok B, Nischwitz S, Nothen MM, Paul F, Putz M, Ruck T, Salmen A, Stangel M, Stellmann JP, Strauch K, Sturner KH, Tackenberg B, Then Bergh F, Tumani H, Waldenberger M, Weber F, Wiendl H, Wildemann B, Zettl UK, Ziemann U, Zipp F, Hemmer B, Ziegler A. Successful replication of GWAS hits for multiple sclerosis in 10,000 Germans using the exome array. Genet Epidemiol. 2015;39(8):601–8. https://doi.org/10.1002/gepi.21933.
37. Wang Z, Sadovnick AD, Traboulsee AL, Ross JP, Bernales CQ, Encarnacion M, Yee IM, de Lemos M, Greenwood T, Lee JD, Wright G, Ross CJ, Zhang S, Song W, Vilarino-Guell C. Nuclear receptor NR1H3 in familial multiple sclerosis. Neuron. 2016;90(5):948–54. https://doi.org/10.1016/j.neuron.2016.04.039. S0896-6273(16)30126-X [pii].
38. International Multiple Sclerosis Genetics Consortium (IMSGC). NR1H3 p.Arg415Gln is not associated to multiple sclerosis risk. Neuron. 2016;92(4):929. https://doi.org/10.1016/j.neuron.2016.11.010. S0896-6273(16)30848-0 [pii].
39. Goris A, Pauwels I, Gustavsen MW, van Son B, Hilven K, Bos SD, Celius EG, Berg-Hansen P, Aarseth J, Myhr KM, D'Alfonso S, Barizzone N, Leone MA, Martinelli Boneschi F, Sorosina M, Liberatore G, Kockum I, Olsson T, Hillert J, Alfredsson L, Bedri SK, Hemmer B, Buck D, Berthele A, Knier B, Biberacher V, van Pesch V, Sindic C, Bang Oturai A, Sondergaard HB, Sellebjerg F, Jensen PE, Comabella M, Montalban X, Perez-Boza J, Malhotra S, Lechner-Scott J, Broadley S, Slee M, Taylor B, Kermode AG, Gourraud PA, Sawcer SJ, Andreassen BK, Dubois B, Harbo HF. Genetic variants are major determinants of CSF antibody levels in multiple sclerosis. Brain. 2015;138(Pt 3):632–43. https://doi.org/10.1093/brain/awu405. awu405 [pii].
40. Housley WJ, Pitt D, Hafler DA. Biomarkers in multiple sclerosis. Clin Immunol. 2015;161(1):51–8. https://doi.org/10.1016/j.clim.2015.06.015. S1521-6616(15)00219-3 [pii].
41. Somers EC, Thomas SL, Smeeth L, Hall AJ. Autoimmune diseases co-occurring within individuals and within families: a systematic review. Epidemiology. 2006;17(2):202–17. https://doi.org/10.1097/01.ede.0000193605.93416.df. 00001648-200603000-00016 [pii].
42. Sigurdsson S, Nordmark G, Goring HH, Lindroos K, Wiman AC, Sturfelt G, Jonsen A, Rantapaa-Dahlqvist S, Moller B, Kere J, Koskenmies S, Widen E, Eloranta ML, Julkunen H, Kristjansdottir H, Steinsson K, Alm G, Ronnblom L, Syvanen AC. Polymorphisms in the tyrosine kinase 2 and interferon regulatory factor 5 genes are associated with systemic lupus erythematosus. Am J Hum Genet. 2005;76(3):528–37. https://doi.org/10.1086/428480. S0002-9297(07)63349-7 [pii].
43. Kristjansdottir G, Sandling JK, Bonetti A, Roos IM, Milani L, Wang C, Gustafsdottir SM, Sigurdsson S, Lundmark A, Tienari PJ, Koivisto K, Elovaara I, Pirttila T, Reunanen M, Peltonen L, Saarela J, Hillert J, Olsson T, Landegren U, Alcina A, Fernandez O, Leyva L, Guerrero M, Lucas M, Izquierdo G, Matesanz F, Syvanen AC. Interferon regulatory factor 5 (IRF5) gene variants are associated with multiple sclerosis in three distinct populations. J Med Genet. 2008;45(6):362–9. https://doi.org/10.1136/jmg.2007.055012. jmg.2007.055012 [pii].

44. Vella A, Cooper JD, Lowe CE, Walker N, Nutland S, Widmer B, Jones R, Ring SM, McArdle W, Pembrey ME, Strachan DP, Dunger DB, Twells RC, Clayton DG, Todd JA. Localization of a type 1 diabetes locus in the IL2RA/CD25 region by use of tag single-nucleotide polymorphisms. Am J Hum Genet. 2005;76(5):773–9. https://doi.org/10.1086/429843. S0002-9297(07)60724-1 [pii].
45. Patsopoulos NA, Esposito F, Reischl J, Lehr S, Bauer D, Heubach J, Sandbrink R, Pohl C, Edan G, Kappos L, Miller D, Montalban J, Polman CH, Freedman MS, Hartung HP, Arnason BG, Comi G, Cook S, Filippi M, Goodin DS, Jeffery D, O'Connor P, Ebers GC, Langdon D, Reder AT, Traboulsee A, Zipp F, Schimrigk S, Hillert J, Bahlo M, Booth DR, Broadley S, Brown MA, Browning BL, Browning SR, Butzkueven H, Carroll WM, Chapman C, Foote SJ, Griffiths L, Kermode AG, Kilpatrick TJ, Lechner-Scott J, Marriott M, Mason D, Moscato P, Heard RN, Pender MP, Perreau VM, Perera D, Rubio JP, Scott RJ, Slee M, Stankovich J, Stewart GJ, Taylor BV, Tubridy N, Willoughby E, Wiley J, Matthews P, Boneschi FM, Compston A, Haines J, Hauser SL, McCauley J, Ivinson A, Oksenberg JR, Pericak-Vance M, Sawcer SJ, De Jager PL, Hafler DA, de Bakker PI. Genome-wide meta-analysis identifies novel multiple sclerosis susceptibility loci. Ann Neurol. 2011;70(6):897–912. https://doi.org/10.1002/ana.22609.
46. Baranzini SE. The genetics of autoimmune diseases: a networked perspective. Curr Opin Immunol. 2009;21(6):596–605. https://doi.org/10.1016/j.coi.2009.09.014. S0952-7915(09)00210-6 [pii].
47. Cortes A, Brown MA. Promise and pitfalls of the Immunochip. Arthritis Res Ther. 2011;13(1):101. https://doi.org/10.1186/ar3204. ar3204 [pii].
48. Beecham AH, Patsopoulos NA, Xifara DK, Davis MF, Kemppinen A, Cotsapas C, Shah TS, Spencer C, Booth D, Goris A, Oturai A, Saarela J, Fontaine B, Hemmer B, Martin C, Zipp F, D'Alfonso S, Martinelli-Boneschi F, Taylor B, Harbo HF, Kockum I, Hillert J, Olsson T, Ban M, Oksenberg JR, Hintzen R, Barcellos LF, Agliardi C, Alfredsson L, Alizadeh M, Anderson C, Andrews R, Sondergaard HB, Baker A, Band G, Baranzini SE, Barizzone N, Barrett J, Bellenguez C, Bergamaschi L, Bernardinelli L, Berthele A, Biberacher V, Binder TM, Blackburn H, Bomfim IL, Brambilla P, Broadley S, Brochet B, Brundin L, Buck D, Butzkueven H, Caillier SJ, Camu W, Carpentier W, Cavalla P, Celius EG, Coman I, Comi G, Corrado L, Cosemans L, Cournu-Rebeix I, Cree BA, Cusi D, Damotte V, Defer G, Delgado SR, Deloukas P, di Sapio A, Dilthey AT, Donnelly P, Dubois B, Duddy M, Edkins S, Elovaara I, Esposito F, Evangelou N, Fiddes B, Field J, Franke A, Freeman C, Frohlich IY, Galimberti D, Gieger C, Gourraud PA, Graetz C, Graham A, Grummel V, Guaschino C, Hadjixenofontos A, Hakonarson H, Halfpenny C, Hall G, Hall P, Hamsten A, Harley J, Harrower T, Hawkins C, Hellenthal G, Hillier C, Hobart J, Hoshi M, Hunt SE, Jagodic M, Jelcic I, Jochim A, Kendall B, Kermode A, Kilpatrick T, Koivisto K, Konidari I, Korn T, Kronsbein H, Langford C, Larsson M, Lathrop M, Lebrun-Frenay C, Lechner-Scott J, Lee MH, Leone MA, Leppa V, Liberatore G, Lie BA, Lill CM, Linden M, Link J, Luessi F, Lycke J, Macciardi F, Mannisto S, Manrique CP, Martin R, Martinelli V, Mason D, Mazibrada G, McCabe C, Mero IL, Mescheriakova J, Moutsianas L, Myhr KM, Nagels G, Nicholas R, Nilsson P, Piehl F, Pirinen M, Price SE, Quach H, Reunanen M, Robberecht W, Robertson NP, Rodegher M, Rog D, Salvetti M, Schnetz-Boutaud NC, Sellebjerg F, Selter RC, Schaefer C, Shaunak S, Shen L, Shields S, Siffrin V, Slee M, Sorensen PS, Sorosina M, Sospedra M, Spurkland A, Strange A, Sundqvist E, Thijs V, Thorpe J, Ticca A, Tienari P, van Duijn C, Visser EM, Vucic S, Westerlind H, Wiley JS, Wilkins A, Wilson JF, Winkelmann J, Zajicek J, Zindler E, Haines JL, Pericak-Vance MA, Ivinson AJ, Stewart G, Hafler D, Hauser SL, Compston A, McVean G, De Jager P, Sawcer SJ, McCauley JL. Analysis of immune-related loci identifies 48 new susceptibility variants for multiple sclerosis. Nat Genet. 2013;45(11):1353–60. https://doi.org/10.1038/ng.2770. ng.2770 [pii].
49. Maier LM, Lowe CE, Cooper J, Downes K, Anderson DE, Severson C, Clark PM, Healy B, Walker N, Aubin C, Oksenberg JR, Hauser SL, Compston A, Sawcer S, De Jager PL, Wicker LS, Todd JA, Hafler DA. IL2RA genetic heterogeneity in multiple sclerosis and type 1 diabetes susceptibility and soluble interleukin-2 receptor production. PLoS Genet. 2009;5(1):e1000322. https://doi.org/10.1371/journal.pgen.1000322.

50. Alcina A, Fedetz M, Ndagire D, Fernandez O, Leyva L, Guerrero M, Abad-Grau MM, Arnal C, Delgado C, Lucas M, Izquierdo G, Matesanz F. IL2RA/CD25 gene polymorphisms: uneven association with multiple sclerosis (MS) and type 1 diabetes (T1D). PLoS One. 2009;4(1):e4137. https://doi.org/10.1371/journal.pone.0004137.
51. Nica AC, Dermitzakis ET. Expression quantitative trait loci: present and future. Philos Trans R Soc Lond Ser B Biol Sci. 2013;368(1620):20120362. https://doi.org/10.1098/rstb.2012.0362. rstb.2012.0362 [pii].
52. Alcina A, Fedetz M, Fernandez O, Saiz A, Izquierdo G, Lucas M, Leyva L, Garcia-Leon JA, Abad-Grau Mdel M, Alloza I, Antiguedad A, Garcia-Barcina MJ, Vandenbroeck K, Varade J, de la Hera B, Arroyo R, Comabella M, Montalban X, Petit-Marty N, Navarro A, Otaegui D, Olascoaga J, Blanco Y, Urcelay E, Matesanz F. Identification of a functional variant in the KIF5A-CYP27B1-METTL1-FAM119B locus associated with multiple sclerosis. J Med Genet. 2013;50(1):25–33. https://doi.org/10.1136/jmedgenet-2012-101085. jmedgenet-2012-101085 [pii].
53. Karaky M, Alcina A, Fedetz M, Barrionuevo C, Potenciano V, Delgado C, Izquierdo G, Matesanz F. The multiple sclerosis-associated regulatory variant rs10877013 affects expression of CYP27B1 and VDR under inflammatory or vitamin D stimuli. Mult Scler. 2016;22(8):999–1006. https://doi.org/10.1177/1352458515610208. 1352458515610208 [pii].
54. Cortes A, Field J, Glazov EA, Hadler J, Stankovich J, Brown MA. Resequencing and fine-mapping of the chromosome 12q13-14 locus associated with multiple sclerosis refines the number of implicated genes. Hum Mol Genet. 2013;22(11):2283–92. https://doi.org/10.1093/hmg/ddt062. ddt062 [pii].
55. Shahijanian F, Parnell GP, McKay FC, Gatt PN, Shojoei M, O'Connor KS, Schibeci SD, Brilot F, Liddle C, Batten M, Stewart GJ, Booth DR. The CYP27B1 variant associated with an increased risk of autoimmune disease is underexpressed in tolerizing dendritic cells. Hum Mol Genet. 2014;23(6):1425–34. https://doi.org/10.1093/hmg/ddt529. ddt529 [pii].
56. Steri M, Orru V, Idda ML, Pitzalis M, Pala M, Zara I, Sidore C, Faa V, Floris M, Deiana M, Asunis I, Porcu E, Mulas A, Piras MG, Lobina M, Lai S, Marongiu M, Serra V, Sole G, Busonero F, Maschio A, Cusano R, Cuccuru G, Deidda F, Poddie F, Farina G, Dei M, Virdis F, Olla S, Satta MA, Pani M, Delitala A, Cocco E, Frau J, Coghe G, Lorefice L, Fenu G, Ferrigno P, Ban M, Barizzone N, Leone M, Guerini FR, Piga M, Firinu D, Kockum I, Lima Bomfim I, Olsson T, Alfredsson L, Suarez A, Carreira PE, Castillo-Palma MJ, Marcus JH, Congia M, Angius A, Melis M, Gonzalez A, Alarcon Riquelme ME, da Silva BM, Marchini M, Danieli MG, Del Giacco S, Mathieu A, Pani A, Montgomery SB, Rosati G, Hillert J, Sawcer S, D'Alfonso S, Todd JA, Novembre J, Abecasis GR, Whalen MB, Marrosu MG, Meloni A, Sanna S, Gorospe M, Schlessinger D, Fiorillo E, Zoledziewska M, Cucca F. Overexpression of the cytokine BAFF and autoimmunity risk. N Engl J Med. 2017;376(17):1615–26. https://doi.org/10.1056/NEJMoa1610528.
57. Matesanz F, Potenciano V, Fedetz M, Ramos-Mozo P, Abad-Grau Mdel M, Karaky M, Barrionuevo C, Izquierdo G, Ruiz-Pena JL, Garcia-Sanchez MI, Lucas M, Fernandez O, Leyva L, Otaegui D, Munoz-Culla M, Olascoaga J, Vandenbroeck K, Alloza I, Astobiza I, Antiguedad A, Villar LM, Alvarez-Cermeno JC, Malhotra S, Comabella M, Montalban X, Saiz A, Blanco Y, Arroyo R, Varade J, Urcelay E, Alcina A. A functional variant that affects exon-skipping and protein expression of SP140 as genetic mechanism predisposing to multiple sclerosis. Hum Mol Genet. 2015;24(19):5619–27. https://doi.org/10.1093/hmg/ddv256. ddv256 [pii].
58. Gregory AP, Dendrou CA, Attfield KE, Haghikia A, Xifara DK, Butter F, Poschmann G, Kaur G, Lambert L, Leach OA, Promel S, Punwani D, Felce JH, Davis SJ, Gold R, Nielsen FC, Siegel RM, Mann M, Bell JI, McVean G, Fugger L. TNF receptor 1 genetic risk mirrors outcome of anti-TNF therapy in multiple sclerosis. Nature. 2012;488(7412):508–11. https://doi.org/10.1038/nature11307.
59. Comabella M, Caminero AB, Malhotra S, Agullo L, Fernandez O, Reverter F, Vandenbroeck K, Rodriguez-Antiguedad A, Matesanz F, Izquierdo G, Urcelay E, Lopez-Larios A, Sanchez A, Otero S, Tintore M, Montalban X. TNFRSF1A polymorphisms rs1800693 and rs4149584 in

patients with multiple sclerosis. Neurology. 2013;80(22):2010–6. https://doi.org/10.1212/WNL.0b013e318294b2d6. WNL.0b013e318294b2d6 [pii].

60. Ottoboni L, Frohlich IY, Lee M, Healy BC, Keenan BT, Xia Z, Chitnis T, Guttmann CR, Khoury SJ, Weiner HL, Hafler DA, De Jager PL. Clinical relevance and functional consequences of the TNFRSF1A multiple sclerosis locus. Neurology. 2013;81(22):1891–9. https://doi.org/10.1212/01.wnl.0000436612.66328.8a. 01.wnl.0000436612.66328.8a [pii].
61. Martin D, Pantoja C, Fernandez Minan A, Valdes-Quezada C, Molto E, Matesanz F, Bogdanovic O, de la Calle-Mustienes E, Dominguez O, Taher L, Furlan-Magaril M, Alcina A, Canon S, Fedetz M, Blasco MA, Pereira PS, Ovcharenko I, Recillas-Targa F, Montoliu L, Manzanares M, Guigo R, Serrano M, Casares F, Gomez-Skarmeta JL. Genome-wide CTCF distribution in vertebrates defines equivalent sites that aid the identification of disease-associated genes. Nat Struct Mol Biol. 2011;18(6):708–14. https://doi.org/10.1038/nsmb.2059. nsmb.2059 [pii].
62. Didonna A, Isobe N, Caillier SJ, Li KH, Burlingame AL, Hauser SL, Baranzini SE, Patsopoulos NA, Oksenberg JR. A non-synonymous single-nucleotide polymorphism associated with multiple sclerosis risk affects the EVI5 interactome. Hum Mol Genet. 2015;24(24):7151–8. https://doi.org/10.1093/hmg/ddv412. ddv412 [pii].
63. Leiserson MD, Eldridge JV, Ramachandran S, Raphael BJ. Network analysis of GWAS data. Curr Opin Genet Dev. 2013;23(6):602–10. https://doi.org/10.1016/j.gde.2013.09.003. S0959-437X(13)00135-4 [pii].
64. Torkamani A, Topol EJ, Schork NJ. Pathway analysis of seven common diseases assessed by genome-wide association. Genomics. 2008;92(5):265–72. https://doi.org/10.1016/j.ygeno.2008.07.011. S0888-7543(08)00184-5 [pii].
65. International Multiple Sclerosis Genetics Consortium (IMSGC). Network-based multiple sclerosis pathway analysis with GWAS data from 15,000 cases and 30,000 controls. Am J Hum Genet. 2013;92(6):854–65. https://doi.org/10.1016/j.ajhg.2013.04.019. S0002-9297(13)00180-8 [pii].
66. Didonna A, Oksenberg JR. The genetics of multiple sclerosis. 2017. https://doi.org/10.15586/codon.multiplesclerosis.2017.ch1. NBK470155 [bookaccession].
67. Aulchenko YS, Hoppenbrouwers IA, Ramagopalan SV, Broer L, Jafari N, Hillert J, Link J, Lundstrom W, Greiner E, Dessa Sadovnick A, Goossens D, Van Broeckhoven C, Del-Favero J, Ebers GC, Oostra BA, van Duijn CM, Hintzen RQ. Genetic variation in the KIF1B locus influences susceptibility to multiple sclerosis. Nat Genet. 2008;40(12):1402–3. https://doi.org/10.1038/ng.251. ng.251 [pii].
68. Comabella M, Craig DW, Camina-Tato M, Morcillo C, Lopez C, Navarro A, Rio J, Montalban X, Martin R. Identification of a novel risk locus for multiple sclerosis at 13q31.3 by a pooled genome-wide scan of 500,000 single nucleotide polymorphisms. PLoS One. 2008;3(10):e3490. https://doi.org/10.1371/journal.pone.0003490.
69. Baranzini SE, Galwey NW, Wang J, Khankhanian P, Lindberg R, Pelletier D, Wu W, Uitdehaag BM, Kappos L, Polman CH, Matthews PM, Hauser SL, Gibson RA, Oksenberg JR, Barnes MR. Pathway and network-based analysis of genome-wide association studies in multiple sclerosis. Hum Mol Genet. 2009;18(11):2078–90. https://doi.org/10.1093/hmg/ddp120. ddp120 [pii].
70. Australia and New Zealand Multiple Sclerosis Genetics Consortium (ANZgene). Genome-wide association study identifies new multiple sclerosis susceptibility loci on chromosomes 12 and 20. Nat Genet. 2009;41(7):824–8. https://doi.org/10.1038/ng.396. ng.396 [pii].
71. Baranzini SE, Wang J, Gibson RA, Galwey N, Naegelin Y, Barkhof F, Radue EW, Lindberg RL, Uitdehaag BM, Johnson MR, Angelakopoulou A, Hall L, Richardson JC, Prinjha RK, Gass A, Geurts JJ, Kragt J, Sombekke M, Vrenken H, Qualley P, Lincoln RR, Gomez R, Caillier SJ, George MF, Mousavi H, Guerrero R, Okuda DT, Cree BA, Green AJ, Waubant E, Goodin DS, Pelletier D, Matthews PM, Hauser SL, Kappos L, Polman CH, Oksenberg JR. Genome-wide association analysis of susceptibility and clinical phenotype in multiple sclerosis. Hum Mol Genet. 2009;18(4):767–78. https://doi.org/10.1093/hmg/ddn388. ddn388 [pii].

72. Jakkula E, Leppa V, Sulonen AM, Varilo T, Kallio S, Kemppinen A, Purcell S, Koivisto K, Tienari P, Sumelahti ML, Elovaara I, Pirttila T, Reunanen M, Aromaa A, Oturai AB, Sondergaard HB, Harbo HF, Mero IL, Gabriel SB, Mirel DB, Hauser SL, Kappos L, Polman C, De Jager PL, Hafler DA, Daly MJ, Palotie A, Saarela J, Peltonen L. Genome-wide association study in a high-risk isolate for multiple sclerosis reveals associated variants in STAT3 gene. Am J Hum Genet. 2010;86(2):285–91. https://doi.org/10.1016/j.ajhg.2010.01.017. S0002-9297(10)00021-2 [pii].
73. Sanna S, Pitzalis M, Zoledziewska M, Zara I, Sidore C, Murru R, Whalen MB, Busonero F, Maschio A, Costa G, Melis MC, Deidda F, Poddie F, Morelli L, Farina G, Li Y, Dei M, Lai S, Mulas A, Cuccuru G, Porcu E, Liang L, Zavattari P, Moi L, Deriu E, Urru MF, Bajorek M, Satta MA, Cocco E, Ferrigno P, Sotgiu S, Pugliatti M, Traccis S, Angius A, Melis M, Rosati G, Abecasis GR, Uda M, Marrosu MG, Schlessinger D, Cucca F. Variants within the immunoregulatory CBLB gene are associated with multiple sclerosis. Nat Genet. 2010;42(6):495–7. https://doi.org/10.1038/ng.584. ng.584 [pii].
74. Nischwitz S, Cepok S, Kroner A, Wolf C, Knop M, Muller-Sarnowski F, Pfister H, Roeske D, Rieckmann P, Hemmer B, Ising M, Uhr M, Bettecken T, Holsboer F, Muller-Myhsok B, Weber F. Evidence for VAV2 and ZNF433 as susceptibility genes for multiple sclerosis. J Neuroimmunol. 2010;227(1–2):162–6. https://doi.org/10.1016/j.jneuroim.2010.06.003. S0165-5728(10)00258-4 [pii].
75. Baranzini SE, Srinivasan R, Khankhanian P, Okuda DT, Nelson SJ, Matthews PM, Hauser SL, Oksenberg JR, Pelletier D. Genetic variation influences glutamate concentrations in brains of patients with multiple sclerosis. Brain. 2010;133(9):2603–11. https://doi.org/10.1093/brain/awq192. awq192 [pii].
76. Brynedal B, Wojcik J, Esposito F, Debailleul V, Yaouanq J, Martinelli-Boneschi F, Edan G, Comi G, Hillert J, Abderrahim H. MGAT5 alters the severity of multiple sclerosis. J Neuroimmunol. 2010;220(1–2):120–4. https://doi.org/10.1016/j.jneuroim.2010.01.003. S0165-5728(10)00008-1 [pii].
77. International Multiple Sclerosis Genetics Consortium (IMSGC). Genome-wide association study of severity in multiple sclerosis. Genes Immun. 2011;12(8):615–25. https://doi.org/10.1038/gene.2011.34. gene201134 [pii].
78. Martinelli-Boneschi F, Esposito F, Brambilla P, Lindstrom E, Lavorgna G, Stankovich J, Rodegher M, Capra R, Ghezzi A, Coniglio G, Colombo B, Sorosina M, Martinelli V, Booth D, Oturai AB, Stewart G, Harbo HF, Kilpatrick TJ, Hillert J, Rubio JP, Abderrahim H, Wojcik J, Comi G. A genome-wide association study in progressive multiple sclerosis. Mult Scler. 2012;18(10):1384–94. https://doi.org/10.1177/1352458512439118. 1352458512439118 [pii].
79. Matesanz F, Gonzalez-Perez A, Lucas M, Sanna S, Gayan J, Urcelay E, Zara I, Pitzalis M, Cavanillas ML, Arroyo R, Zoledziewska M, Marrosu M, Fernandez O, Leyva L, Alcina A, Fedetz M, Moreno-Rey C, Velasco J, Real LM, Ruiz-Pena JL, Cucca F, Ruiz A, Izquierdo G. Genome-wide association study of multiple sclerosis confirms a novel locus at 5p13.1. PLoS One. 2012;7(5):e36140. https://doi.org/10.1371/journal.pone.0036140. PONE-D-11-24357 [pii].
80. Leone MA, Barizzone N, Esposito F, Lucenti A, Harbo HF, Goris A, Kockum I, Oturai AB, Celius EG, Mero IL, Dubois B, Olsson T, Sondergaard HB, Cusi D, Lupoli S, Andreassen BK, Myhr KM, Guerini FR, Comi G, Martinelli-Boneschi F, D'Alfonso S. Association of genetic markers with CSF oligoclonal bands in multiple sclerosis patients. PLoS One. 2013;8(6):e64408. https://doi.org/10.1371/journal.pone.0064408. PONE-D-12-37153 [pii].
81. Gourraud PA, Sdika M, Khankhanian P, Henry RG, Beheshtian A, Matthews PM, Hauser SL, Oksenberg JR, Pelletier D, Baranzini SE. A genome-wide association study of brain lesion distribution in multiple sclerosis. Brain. 2013;136(Pt 4):1012–24. https://doi.org/10.1093/brain/aws363. aws363 [pii].
82. Mero IL, Gustavsen MW, Saether HS, Flam ST, Berg-Hansen P, Sondergaard HB, Jensen PE, Berge T, Bjolgerud A, Muggerud A, Aarseth JH, Myhr KM, Celius EG, Sellebjerg F, Hillert J, Alfredsson L, Olsson T, Oturai AB, Kockum I, Lie BA, Andreassen BK, Harbo HF. Oligoclonal band status in Scandinavian multiple sclerosis patients is associated with

specific genetic risk alleles. PLoS One. 2013;8(3):e58352. https://doi.org/10.1371/journal.pone.0058352. PONE-D-12-29076 [pii].
83. Clarelli F, Liberatore G, Sorosina M, Osiceanu AM, Esposito F, Mascia E, Santoro S, Pavan G, Colombo B, Moiola L, Martinelli V, Comi G, Martinelli-Boneschi F. Pharmacogenetic study of long-term response to interferon-beta treatment in multiple sclerosis. Pharmacogenomics J. 2017;17(1):84–91. https://doi.org/10.1038/tpj.2015.85. tpj201585 [pii].
84. Andlauer TF, Buck D, Antony G, Bayas A, Bechmann L, Berthele A, Chan A, Gasperi C, Gold R, Graetz C, Haas J, Hecker M, Infante-Duarte C, Knop M, Kumpfel T, Limmroth V, Linker RA, Loleit V, Luessi F, Meuth SG, Muhlau M, Nischwitz S, Paul F, Putz M, Ruck T, Salmen A, Stangel M, Stellmann JP, Sturner KH, Tackenberg B, Then Bergh F, Tumani H, Warnke C, Weber F, Wiendl H, Wildemann B, Zettl UK, Ziemann U, Zipp F, Arloth J, Weber P, Radivojkov-Blagojevic M, Scheinhardt MO, Dankowski T, Bettecken T, Lichtner P, Czamara D, Carrillo-Roa T, Binder EB, Berger K, Bertram L, Franke A, Gieger C, Herms S, Homuth G, Ising M, Jockel KH, Kacprowski T, Kloiber S, Laudes M, Lieb W, Lill CM, Lucae S, Meitinger T, Moebus S, Muller-Nurasyid M, Nothen MM, Petersmann A, Rawal R, Schminke U, Strauch K, Volzke H, Waldenberger M, Wellmann J, Porcu E, Mulas A, Pitzalis M, Sidore C, Zara I, Cucca F, Zoledziewska M, Ziegler A, Hemmer B, Muller-Myhsok B. Novel multiple sclerosis susceptibility loci implicated in epigenetic regulation. Sci Adv. 2016;2(6):e1501678. https://doi.org/10.1126/sciadv.1501678. 1501678 [pii].
85. Zhou Y, Zhu G, Charlesworth JC, Simpson S Jr, Rubicz R, Goring HH, Patsopoulos NA, Laverty C, Wu F, Henders A, Ellis JJ, van der Mei I, Montgomery GW, Blangero J, Curran JE, Johnson MP, Martin NG, Nyholt DR, Taylor BV. Genetic loci for Epstein-Barr virus nuclear antigen-1 are associated with risk of multiple sclerosis. Mult Scler. 2016;22(13):1655–64. https://doi.org/10.1177/1352458515626598. 1352458515626598 [pii].
86. Zhou Y, Graves JS, Simpson S Jr, Charlesworth JC, Mei IV, Waubant E, Barcellos LF, Belman A, Krupp L, Lucas R, Ponsonby AL, Taylor BV. Genetic variation in the gene LRP2 increases relapse risk in multiple sclerosis. J Neurol Neurosurg Psychiatry. 2017;88(10):864–8. https://doi.org/10.1136/jnnp-2017-315971. jnnp-2017-315971 [pii].

Autoimmune Myasthenia Gravis

11

Güher Saruhan-Direskeneli and Amr H. Sawalha

Contents

11.1 Introduction

Myasthenia gravis (MG) is an organ-specific autoimmune disease mediated by autoantibodies against different components, mainly to the nicotinic acetylcholine receptor (AChR), of the neuromuscular junction (NMJ) [1–3]. Patients experience muscular

G. Saruhan-Direskeneli (✉)
Department of Physiology, Istanbul Medical Faculty, Istanbul University, Istanbul, Turkey
e-mail: gsaruhan@istanbul.edu.tr

A. H. Sawalha
Division of Rheumatology, Department of Internal Medicine, University of Michigan, Ann Arbor, MI, USA

Center for Computational Medicine and Bioinformatics, University of Michigan, Ann Arbor, MI, USA
e-mail: asawalha@med.umich.edu

J. Martín, F. D. Carmona (eds.), *Genetics of Rare Autoimmune Diseases*,
Rare Diseases of the Immune System, https://doi.org/10.1007/978-3-030-03934-9_11

fatigability due to the presence of antibodies which inhibit signal transduction across the NMJ. An annual incidence of 8–10 cases and a prevalence of 150–250 cases per one million are reported [4]. Although the disease pathogenesis has been elucidated relatively well, the mechanism of induction of the immune response is not known. Thymic abnormalities are frequently observed, and the involvement of T cells is suggested in the disease pathogenesis [5]. Acquired or autoimmune MG, characterized by autoantibodies, is a heterogeneous disease with respect to age at disease onset, clinical presentation, sex distribution, autoantigens at the NMJ [6, 7], as well as pathogenic mechanisms including genetic risk factors and associated thymic pathologies [8]. Congenital MG and juvenile MG are not covered in this chapter.

11.1.1 MG Associated with Anti-AChR Antibodies (AChR-MG)

The most prevalent MG subtype is due to autoantibodies against the muscle-type AChR [9]. In 80–85% of patients, pathogenic antibodies directed against AChR cause the disease. AChR-MG shows a wide spectrum of clinical findings from pure ocular to generalized MG symptoms. Even AChR-MG is heterogeneous, and subgroups are distinguished [10].

11.1.1.1 Early-Onset (EOMG) and Late-Onset (LOMG) MG with AChR Antibodies

Among patients who have MG with AChR antibodies, the age at onset has a bimodal pattern [11]. Patients with EOMG have onset of their first symptom before age of 50 years. Thymic follicular hyperplasia with lymphoid follicles and germinal centers is the key pathogenic finding and supports an intrathymic initiation of EOMG [12]. Female cases outnumber male cases by three to one [4].

Patients with LOMG have their first onset of symptoms after age of 50 years, and thymic hyperplasia occurs only rarely, whereas thymic atrophy is characteristic of late-onset disease. The disease is slightly more frequently reported in males than females [13].

11.1.2 Thymoma-Associated MG (TAMG)

In about 10–20% of patients, MG is associated with thymoma, typically with generalized muscle involvement in elderly patients with no sex bias. TAMG is commonly accompanied by additional autoimmune diseases [8, 14]. With rare exceptions, TAMG patients have antibodies to the AChR. The spectrum of autoantibody targets in patients with TAMG can be much broader.

11.1.3 Muscle-Specific Kinase (MuSK)-Associated MG (MuSK-MG)

MuSK is a protein expressed in the postsynaptic muscle membrane that is necessary to maintain AChR function. In about ~5% of MG patients, antibodies against MuSK are detected [15–17]. MuSK-positive patients have a severe form of the disease with common muscular atrophy and predominant involvement of cranial and bulbar muscles. No thymus pathological changes are reported [13, 18].

11.1.4 Other Subgroups

MG due to autantibodies against the low-density lipoprotein receptor-related protein 4 (LRP4) [19], agrin [20], and MG without known target autoantigens ("sero-negative MG") [21] have also been described as smaller subgroups. Some other patients have antibodies that can be identified by cell-based methods only [13].

Differences between antibodies in MG subgroups reflect also different pathogenic mechanisms: anti-AChR and anti-LRP4 antibodies are of immunoglobulin (Ig) IgG1 and IgG3 isotypes [19, 22] and exert their effects mainly by the activation of the complement cascade [23, 24], whereas anti-MuSK antibodies are predominantly of the non-complement-fixing IgG4 isotype [16].

11.2 Genetics

Like other complex disorders, genetic susceptibility to MG has been implicated along with environmental factors.

11.2.1 Familial Studies

Neither autosomal nor sex-linked, dominant, or recessive mode of inheritance in MG could be confirmed, although some genetic predisposition to MG seemed to exist [25]. Differences in concordance rates between identical and nonidentical twins in MG (35.5% vs. 4–5%) and some familial occurrence suggested a role of genetic factors in the pathogenesis of the disease [26–28]. In the majority of pairs, the affected twin had an unaffected co-twin, showing that nongenetically determined factors are also critical [29]. However, recent transcriptome and methylome analysis of peripheral blood monocytes (all females) from identical twins also revealed that genetic predisposition may have a strong contribution to the disease [30].

11.2.2 Candidate Genes

11.2.2.1 Human Leukocyte Antigen (HLA)

As in many autoimmune diseases, MG and the subgroups have been examined for HLA associations in different populations at various levels. HLA loci have been reported to be associated with disease development [31–33]. With the first studies, a relation between HL-A8, HL-A2, and MG, mainly in women, was detected in a European population [34]. The association with HLA A1-B8-DR3 haplotype in women with thymus hyperplasia and EOMG was reported consistently [6, 34–38].

In British EOMG patients of European descent, with a strong female bias, HLA-B8 and -DR17 (DR3), and HLA-DR2 in the absence of HLA-DR17, were significantly increased [39, 40]. As *DQB1*0201*, in linkage disequilibrium with HLA-DR3, was found more frequently than HLA-B8 and -DR3 in MG patients with thymus hyperplasia and is negatively associated with thymoma [41–43], DQ was suggested to be the more important locus for disease susceptibility in subgroups of patients. Differential associations of *DQB1* alleles in patients with thymus hyperplasia or with thymoma were reported in EOMG [44] in Norwegian and Swedish cohorts based on the frequencies of HLA-*DQB1*0201* with B8, DR3, and *DQA1*0501* [41, 45]. In many ethnically different and mixed populations, *A*31*, *B*08*, *C*17*, *DRB1*03*, *DQA1*05*, *DQB1*02*, or any single element of the haplotype had increased frequencies among EOMG patients with or without thymic hyperplasia [46–50]. More recently, *HLA-B*08* was mapped to give the strongest contribution to EOMG in Norwegian population [51]. Reflecting the ethnical heterogeneity, a novel haplotype (*DQA1*0401:DQB1*0201*) was the primary factor in the susceptibility to EOMG in a small group of Caucasian-American patients [52].

A protective role of *DRB1*13:01* for both EOMG and LOMG [51] and *DRB1*11 DQA1*0501 DQB1*0301* haplotype was also reported [53]. In some other studies, different immunogenetic backgrounds of ocular and generalized MG were implicated [53, 54].

The studies in less evaluated and smaller MG subgroups and LOMG have revealed different findings. The associations of the HLA-DR7 [33], the *HLA-DRB1*15:01* [51], *HLA-DQB1*05:02 DRB1*16* [55], and *HLA-DRB1*01* [50] were not replicated.

Immunogenetic background in Japanese and Chinese patients has been different from those in Caucasians. Associations of ocular MG with HLA-A2, Bw61, and DRw9, generalized MG with HLA-DRw8 [54], childhood MG with DRw13 and DQw3 [56], and EOMG with HLA-DRw53 [57] and *DPB1*0201* [58] have been reported. In Northern Han Chinese population, *HLA-DRB1*09* was positively and *DRB1*08* negatively associated with MG [59]. In Southern Han Chinese, the association of *HLA-B*4601-DRB1*0901* with MG was demonstrated [60].

Due to the strong linkage disequilibrium across the disease-associated ancestral 8.1 haplotype (*HLA-A*01:01*, *B*08:01*, *DRB1*03:01*, *DQB1*02:01*), the causative locus on this haplotype could not be identified. Another region extending from *HSP70* in class III telomerically into the class I region co-occuring with HLA-B8 showed strongest associations in the patients [40]. The combined analysis of AChR-α-subunit (*CHRNA1*), the α-chain of HLA-DQ, and DR3 haplotype revealed a three-locus association influencing autoantibody titers in a subset of MG patients [61, 62]. The opposing effects of DR3 and DR7 on MG phenotypes according to the presence of thymus hyperplasia or anti-titin antibodies (ATA) have lead to the definition of MYAS1 locus and pathogenetically distinct subsets of MG [33]. MYAS1 locus has been mapped to the class III and proximal class I regions, between the BAT3 and C3-2-11 markers. This region was associated with a marked increase in serum titers of AChR autoantibodies [63]. Other genes contained between C4 and TNF of *DRB1*03* supratype have also been reported for susceptibility to EOMG in women [64].

On the other hand, when genes within the classic major histocompatibility complex (MHC) region are screened by a panel of 1472 single nucleotide polymorphisms (SNP) in 10,576 samples derived from 7 autoimmune disease groups including MG, and complex, multilocus effects were demonstrated [65]. The sequencing of the entire MHC region of patients homozygous for the 8.1 haplotype did not reveal disease-specific variants in EOMG. Inside the HLA region, *HLA-B*08:01* allele has been the unique genetic factor responsible for EOMG. By an intensive screening in the individuals homozygous for *HLA-B*08:01*, *OVCH1* (rs10492374) and *CNYP2* (rs10783780) genes on chromosome 12 were identified as risk factors for MG [66].

11.2.2.2 Subgroup Studies

TAMG

TAMG appeared to have no genetic susceptibility [6]. As the discriminator of thymoma from thymic hyperplasia in MG, HLA-A24 (OR 9.7) and HLA-B8 (OR 0.1) were described as positive and negative predictive factors [37]. The loss of heterozygosity at the HLA locus [67, 68] and a decreased HLA class II expression were demonstrated. The increase of HLA-DR11 [69], *DQB1*0301* [47], and *HLA-DRB1*10* was also reported [50]. A protection associated with *HLA-A*02* in TAMG with a B2-type thymoma emphasized the variation of the histological classification in the genetic study of thymomas [70]. *DRB1*03 DQA1*0501 DQB1*0201* haplotype had negative association with thymomatous MG [53].

MuSK

As a main subgroup of MG, limited number of genetic studies revealed consistent and solid results in MuSK-MG (Table 11.1). In only 23 white Dutch patients with MuSK-MG, a strong association with a relatively rare HLA haplotype (HLA-DR14-DQ5) was detected [71]. In an Italian cohort, *DQB1*05* was associated with *DRB1*16,* not with *DRB1*14,* and an effective role of DQ5 was suggested [72]. Associations of both *DRB1*16* and *DRB1*14* as well as *DQB1∗05* provided support for both loci in susceptibility in Turkish and Serbian [73, 74] as well as Iranian and even in Japanese studies, emphasizing important roles of all these alleles across the races [53, 75]. The genetic association with *DQA1*0104:DQB1*0503* in a group including MuSK-MG patients was interpreted as an indirect evidence for *DRB1*14* haplotype in southern Texas [52].

11.2.2.3 Candidate Genes Associated with Autoimmune Diseases

Protein Tyrosine Phosphatase Type 22 (*PTPN22*)

Protein tyrosine phosphatase type 22 (*PTPN22*) inhibits T-cell activation and interleukin-2 (IL-2) production in lymphoid cells. The PTPN22*R620W variant (*PTPN22* 1858C/T) impaired T-cell activation [76] and is associated with multiple autoimmune diseases [77]. In a French study, *PTPN22* variant 620W allele was increased in nonthymoma EOMG patients without ATA [78], whereas in Hungarian and German patients, the allele was associated with ATA [79]. In the Swedish

Table 11.1 Summary of the HLA association studies in muscle-specific kinase antibody positive MG (MuSK-MG)

HLA	Dutch [71]	Italian [72]	Turkish [73]	Serbian [74]	Japan [75]	Iran [53]
	OR	OR	OR	OR	OR	OR
*DRB1*14*	**18.8 (8.3–42.8)**	1.4 (0.6–3.2)	3.1 (1.5–6.5)	**3.8 (1.9–7.3)**	6.1 (1.9–19.7)	4.0 (1.7–9.2)
*DRB1*16*	6 (1.6–23.4)	**13.5 (6.4–28.9)**	**4.9 (2.4–10.1)**	3.3 (1.9–5.8)	8.2 (1.1–63.4)[a]	**4.3 (1.9–9.4)**
*DQB1*05*	6.3 (2.4–16.6)	3.0 (1.8–5.1)	4.8 (2.4–9.5)	2.2 (1.2–3.9)	**8.5 (2.2–32.9)**	4.1 (2.2–7.5)
*DQB1*0502*		6.7 (3.2–13.7)				
*DQB1*0503*		3.8 (1.4–10.2)				
*DRB1*14-DQB1*05*	**8.5 (3.9–18.7)**	2.2 (0.6–8.3)	2.9 (1.4–6.2)	**3.2 (1.4–7.2)**	5.0 (1.5–16.8)	4.0 (1.7–9.2)
*DRB1*16-DQB1*05*	4.8 (1.1–20.6)	**6.0 (2.1–17.2)**	**4.1 (2.0–8.5)**	2.9 (1.5–5.7)		**4.3 (2.0–9.4)**

Only odds ratios (OR) and 95% confidence intervals (in parentheses) are presented
[a]Not statistically significant

population, the overrepresention of 620W variant was accompanied by higher anti-AChR antibodies and IL-2 production, suggesting a loss-of-function [80]. The *PTPN22* +1858T(+) genotypes were accompanied by decreased intratumorous IL-2 expression in both EOMG and TAMG, implicating *PTPN22* variant as a gain-of-function toward MG [81]. In a Turkish study including disease subgroups, only AChR-MG patients and especially the LOMG group revealed an association [82].

Cytotoxic T Lymphocyte-Associated Antigen-4 (CTLA-4)

Cytotoxic T lymphocyte-associated antigen-4 (CTLA-4) plays a critical role in the downregulation of antigen-activated immune responses. An association of a polymorphism of CTLA-4 gene in a subgroup TAMG [83] has implicated a T cell hyperreactivity via the CD28 pathway [84] and via the effect on the serum levels of sCTLA-4 related to decreased mRNA stability and reduced expression of CTLA-4 [85]. Furthermore, a SNP in the coding region of *CTLA4*, +49 A/G, with functional effect was also associated with TAMG [86]. The CTLA4^{high} genotype (+49A/A), which is protective against several autoimmune diseases, exerted a prominent predisposing effect to TAMG patients supporting the nontolerogenic selection of CD4+ T cells in MG-associated thymomas [87]. In comparison with TAMG, LOMG revealed an association with the CTLA4$^{(low)}$ +49G+ genotypes and decreased low-for-age thymic export of naïve T cells into the blood distinguishing the defects in central thymic or peripheral tolerance induction in TAMG and LOMG [88]. Another SNP in the promoter region and regulating CD152 (*CTLA4*) gene expression was associated with MG and related to elevated levels of sCD152 in the sera [89].

A predisposing effect of SNPs (rs1863800*C, rs733618*C, and rs231775*G) in *CTLA4* was demonstrated, which was likely derived from EOMG and the female patients in Chinese [90]. Following these somehow discordant results, *CTLA4* will be the potential target of further studies (see below).

11.2.2.4 Autoantigen Genes

The main autoantigen of MG, AChR is a pentameric channel that exists in the fetal AChR (α2βδγ) or the adult AChR (α2βδε) composition. The muscle AChR gene encoding the α-subunit of the receptor (*CHRNA1*) was screened extensively. A functional SNP at the promoter conferred a relative risk for MG by disrupting the binding motif of interferon regulatory factor 8 and influencing *CHRNA1* activity in susceptibility [61, 91]. The contribution of the genes encoding the β- (*CHRNB1*) and ε-subunits of the AChR to the susceptibility to MG could not be demonstrated [92, 93]. On the other hand, a microsatellite of *CHRND* encoding the δ-subunit revealed a preferential transmission and an overrepresention in nonthymoma MG patients [94]. In a screening of *PTPN22*, interleukin-10 (*IL10*), *CHRNA1*, autoimmune regulator (*AIRE*), and *CTLA4* genes, the highest association was with SNPs of *CHRNA1* [95].

11.2.2.5 Immunoglubulin (Ig) and T-Cell Receptor Genes

Early studies suggested that the genes predisposing to MG were located within the variable region of the Ig heavy chain loci [96] or T-cell receptor (TCR) variable- and constant-regions [97]. IgG receptor genes (*FCGR2A*, *FCGR3A*, and *FCGR3B*) exhibit functional polymorphisms, which affect efficiency of FcγR-mediated functions. Whereas the frequency of the *FCGR2A* H/H genotype was increased in thymoma MG patients, the distribution of *FCGR3B* alleles did not differ from the controls but was related to the most severe MG [98]. A relative increase of the FCGR2A-R/R131 genotype was suggested as a marker for susceptibility to MG [99]. Among tumor necrosis factor-α and tumor necrosis factor-β (*TNF*, *TNFB*), *FCGR2A*, and *IL10*, susceptibility to MG increased with an increasing number of markers, and *FCGR2A* allelic variants seemed to be the most important determinant of disease [100].

11.2.2.6 Cytokines and Cytokine Receptors

Studies on the effects of cytokine polymorphisms included mainly the genes *TNFB* and *TNF* [101], the lymphotoxin alpha [102, 103], IL-4 and IL-6 [104, 105], *IL1B* [106], *IL1A* [107], *IL10* [108, 109], *IFNG* [110], interleukin-4 receptor alpha [111], *IL17A*, *IL17F*, and MG [112]. Several positive and negative associations are reported with no confirmation in different studies.

11.2.2.7 Other Candidate Genes

The polymorphisms of the β2-adrenergic receptor gene (*ADRB2*) conferred susceptibility to MG probably affecting the density of the receptor on cells [113]. Polymorphisms of the inhibitory receptor, programmed death-1 [114], the MHC class II transactivator (*CIITA*) regulating MHC class II gene expression [115] and interferon regulatory factor 5 (*IRF5*), and TNFα-induced protein 3 (*TNFAIP3*) [116] showed no significant association with the disease.

An association of regulatory region polymorphisms of the galectin-1 (*LGALS1*) was detected in Caucasian MG patients [117]. The association between a SNP in the glucocorticoid receptor (GR) gene was identified as a contributer to drug efficacy in patients [118].

A role of altered expression of decay-accelerating factor (DAF) in the increased prevalence of severe extraocular muscle dysfunction among African MG patients was supported by the association of a regulatory SNP, resulting in inadequate DAF upregulation with consequent complement-mediated damage [119].

The role of epigenetics investigated by examining promoter polymorphisms of the *DNMT3B* gene, coding for the DNA methyltransferase 3B, revealed a contribution to the risk of developing thymoma in MG patients [120]. The functional polymorphism of histamine *N*-methyltransferase (*HNMT*) (A939G) was overrepresented among MG patients with anti-AChR and ATA [121].

Recently, common variants on the IL12/STAT4 and IL10/STAT3 signaling pathways and expression levels of the genes measured in the thymus provided no evidence of functional effects [122]. Thymidylate synthase enhancer region (TSER) polymorphism increased the risk of thymic hyperplasia in AChR-MG patients [123].

In a two-stage association screening of 34 candidate genes, *HLA-DRA*, *CD86*, *AKAP12*, *VAV1*, B-cell activating factor (*BAFF*), and *TNF* were identified as novel loci predisposing to EOMG. Allele frequency difference in female versus male patients at *HLA-DRA* and *TNF* loci was also observed [124].

11.2.3 Genome-Wide Association Studies (GWAS)

MG subgroups have been subject of recent and relatively small GWAS in a few cohorts (Table 11.2). The first GWAS in AChR-MG included only EOMG cases from a North European cohort with a high dominance of women. The discovery and replication analysis as well as meta-analysis in this study confirmed genetic association with variants in the MHC class I as susceptibility markers (rs7750641, $p = 1.2 \times 10^{-92}$; OR, 6.25). *PTPN22* (rs2476601; $p = 8.2 \times 10^{-10}$ OR, 1.71) and TNFAIP3 interacting protein 1 (*TNIP1;* rs4958881; $p = 3.2 \times 10^{-10}$, OR, 1.73) [125]. By imputation and conditional analysis, *HLA-B*08* and *HLA-DRB1*16* (predisposing) and *DRB1*0701* (protective) alleles were suggested as markers in EOMG. The association of *HLA-B*08* was stronger in women compared with men (OR, 6.92 vs. OR, 3.55). In 109 samples from a Korean multicenter and mixed MG cohort, several SNP associations did not pass the threshold for GWAS level of significance [126]. A subsequent GWAS also in AChR-MG patients from two different cohorts (North American and Italian) demonstrated distinct patterns of susceptibility in MHC loci and identified *CTLA4* as another marker for the disease [127]. In the overall case-control cohort with predominantly LOMG patients, association signals at *CTLA4* (rs231770; $p = 3.98 \times 10^{-8}$; OR, 1.37), *HLA-DQA1* (rs9271871; $p = 1.08 \times 10^{-8}$; OR, 2.31), and *TNFRSF11A* (rs4263037; $p = 1.6 \times 10^{-9}$; OR, 1.41)

Table 11.2 Summary of the genome-wide association studies in subgroups of MG

Population	Subgroup	Locus	Marker	*p*	Odds ratio	Reference
649 North European (400 + 249) 2596 HC	ƎOMG	MHC class I	rs7750641	*p* = 1.2 × 10–92	OR, 6.25	Gregersen PK et al. [125]
		HLA-B*08		***p* = 2.9 × 10–113**	**OR, 6.41**	
		PTPN22	rs2476601	*p* = 8.2 × 10–10	OR, 1.71	
		TNIP1	rs4958881	*p* = 3.2 × 10–10	OR, 1.73	
1032 North American 1998 HC and 423 Italian 467 Italian HC	AChR-MG (EOMG and LOMG)	*CTLA4*	rs231770	*p* = 3.98 × 10–8	OR, 1.37	Renton AE et al. [127]
		HLA-DQA1	rs9271871	*p* = 1.08 × 10–8	OR, 2.31	
		TNFRSF11A	rs4263037	*p* = 1.60 × 10–9	OR, 1.41	
		<u>LOMG</u>				
		TNFRSF11A	rs4263037	*p* = 1.32 × 10–12	OR, 1.56	
		HLA-DQA1	rs9271871	*p* = 7.02 × 10–18	OR, 4.27	
		<u>EOMG</u>				
		HLA-DQA1	rs601006	*p* = 2.52 × 10–11	OR, 4.0	
532 European and 2128 HC	LOMG	*TNFRSF11A*	rs4574025	*p* = 3.9 × 10–07	OR, 1.42	Seldin MF et al. [128]
		ZBTB10	rs6998967	*p* = 8.9 × 10–10	OR, 0.53	
		PTPN22	rs2476601	*p* = 6.5 × 10–06	OR, 1.62	
		*DQA1*05:01*		*p* = 5.9 × 10–12	OR, 0.54	
398 Turkish and 541 HC	EOMG, LOMG, and MuSK-MG	<u>EOMG</u>				Saruhan-Direskeneli G et al. [129]
		HLA class I region	rs113519545	*p* = 2.24 × 10–16	OR, 5.71	
		HLA-B*08:01 HLA-C*07:01		***p* = 3.34 × 10–11** ***p* = 2.07 × 10–9**	**OR, 7.04** **OR, 2.74**	
		<u>LOMG</u>				
		HLA class II region	rs111256513	*p* = 2.48 × 10–6	OR, 2.22	
		<u>MuSK-MG</u>				
		HLA-DQB1	rs68081734	*p* = 2.25 × 10–14	OR, 5.86	
		HLA-DQB1*05:02		***p* = 6.88 × 10–13**	**OR, 8.56**	

See [53, 71–75]

were identified and replicated for *CTLA4* and *HLA-DQA1* in an independent cohort of Italian cases. Distinct, but overlapping, disease-associated loci for EOMG and LOMG were described. *TNFRSF11A* (rs4263037; $p = 1.32 \times 10^{-12}$; OR, 1.56) and *HLA-DQA1* (rs9271871; $p = 7.02 \times 10^{-18}$; OR, 4.27) were associated with LOMG, whereas in *HLA-DQA1* (rs601006; $p = 2.52 \times 10^{-11}$; OR, 4.0) was associated with EOMG, although the set of SNP associated was different from that implicated among late-onset cases [127]. In a recent GWAS performed in 532 LOMG cases and 2128 controls matched for sex and population substructure, *TNFRSF11A* association (rs4574025, $p = 3.9 \times 10^{-07}$, OR: 1.42) was confirmed, and a novel candidate gene, *ZBTB10* (rs6998967, $p = 8.9 \times 10^{-10}$, OR, 0.53), was identified. *PTPN22* R620W variant (rs2476601, $p = 6.5 \times 10^{-06}$, OR, 1.62) which was noted in EOMG previously showed suggestive significance. SNPs within the MHC region showing strong associations in LOMG had smaller effect sizes than in EOMG and were in opposite directions (*DQA1*05:01*, $p = 5.9 \times 10^{-12}$, OR, 0.54) [128].

In a smaller study on a single population from Turkey, genetic susceptibility to EOMG, LOMG, and MuSK-MG was investigated at genome-wide level by immunochip [129]. In EOMG, rs113519545 in the HLA class I region ($p = 2.24 \times 10^{-16}$ OR, 5.71), *HLA-B*08:01* ($p = 3.34 \times 10^{-11}$ OR, 7.04), and *HLA-C*07:01* ($p = 2.07 \times 10^{-9}$ OR, 2.74); in LOMG, rs111256513 in the HLA class II region ($p = 2.48 \times 10^{-6}$ OR, 2.22); and in MuSK-MG, an intronic variant within *HLA-DQB1* (rs68081734, $p = 2.25 \times 10^{-14}$ OR, 5.86) and *HLA-DQB1*05:02* ($p = 6.88 \times 10^{-13}$ OR, 8.56) revealed significant associations. Differential genetic susceptibility within the HLA to EOMG, LOMG, and MuSK-MG has been confirmed at a broader level by these data.

11.3 Conclusions

The genetic comparisons of MG subtypes reveal differences between groups implicating variations in pathogenesis. The findings emphasize the value of subgrouping MG patients by clinical and laboratorial criteria for investigations of distinct predisposing mechanisms in MG.

References

1. Drachman DB. Myasthenia gravis. N Engl J Med. 1994;330(25):1797–810.
2. Lindstrom J, Seybold ME, Lennon VA, Whittingham S, Duane DD. Antibody to acetylcholine receptor in myasthenia gravis. Prevalence, clinical correlates, and diagnostic value. Neurology. 1976;26(11):1054–9.
3. Farrugia ME, Vincent A. Autoimmune mediated neuromuscular junction defects. Curr Opin Neurol. 2010;23(5):489–95.
4. Carr AS, Cardwell CR, McCarron PO, McConville J. A systematic review of population based epidemiological studies in Myasthenia Gravis. BMC Neurol. 2010;10:46.
5. Hohlfeld R, Toyka KV, Tzartos SJ, Carson W, Conti-Tronconi BM. Human T-helper lymphocytes in myasthenia gravis recognize the nicotinic receptor alpha subunit. Proc Natl Acad Sci U S A. 1987;84(15):5379–83.

6. Compston D, Vincent A, Newsom-Davis J, et al. Clinical, pathological, HLA antigen and immunological evidence for disease heterogeneity in myasthenia gravis. Brain. 1980;103:579–601.
7. Meriggioli MN, Sanders DB. Autoimmune myasthenia gravis: emerging clinical and biological heterogeneity. Lancet Neurol. 2009;8(5):475–90.
8. Marx A, Willcox N, Leite MI, Chuang WY, Schalke B, Nix W, et al. Thymoma and paraneoplastic myasthenia gravis. Autoimmunity. 2010;43(5–6):413–27.
9. Patrick J, Lindstrom J. Autoimmune response to acetylcholine receptor. Science. 1973;180(4088):871–2.
10. Marx A, Pfister F, Schalke B, Saruhan-Direskeneli G, Melms A, Strobel P. The different roles of the thymus in the pathogenesis of the various myasthenia gravis subtypes. Autoimmun Rev. 2013;12(9):875–84.
11. Heldal AT, Owe JF, Gilhus NE, Romi F. Seropositive myasthenia gravis: a nationwide epidemiologic study. Neurology. 2009;73(2):150–1.
12. Wekerle H, Ketelsen UP. Intrathymic pathogenesis and dual genetic control of myasthenia gravis. Lancet. 1977;1(8013):678–80.
13. Gilhus NE, Verschuuren JJ. Myasthenia gravis: subgroup classification and therapeutic strategies. Lancet Neurol. 2015;14(10):1023–36.
14. Kisand K, Lilic D, Casanova JL, Peterson P, Meager A, Willcox N. Mucocutaneous candidiasis and autoimmunity against cytokines in APECED and thymoma patients: clinical and pathogenetic implications. Eur J Immunol. 2011;41(6):1517–27.
15. Hoch W, McConville J, Helms S, Newsom-Davis J, Melms A, Vincent A. Auto-antibodies to the receptor tyrosine kinase MuSK in patients with myasthenia gravis without acetylcholine receptor antibodies. Nat Med. 2001;7(3):365–8.
16. Verschuuren JJ, Huijbers MG, Plomp JJ, Niks EH, Molenaar PC, Martinez-Martinez P, et al. Pathophysiology of myasthenia gravis with antibodies to the acetylcholine receptor, muscle-specific kinase and low-density lipoprotein receptor-related protein 4. Autoimmun Rev. 2013;12(9):918–23.
17. Deymeer F, Gungor-Tuncer O, Yilmaz V, Parman Y, Serdaroglu P, Ozdemir C, et al. Clinical comparison of anti-MuSK- vs anti-AChR-positive and seronegative myasthenia gravis. Neurology. 2007;68(8):609–11.
18. Berrih-Aknin S, Frenkian-Cuvelier M, Eymard B. Diagnostic and clinical classification of autoimmune myasthenia gravis. J Autoimmun. 2014;48–49:143–8.
19. Higuchi O, Hamuro J, Motomura M, Yamanashi Y. Autoantibodies to low-density lipoprotein receptor-related protein 4 in myasthenia gravis. Ann Neurol. 2012;69(2):418–22.
20. Zhang B, Shen C, Bealmear B, Ragheb S, Xiong W-C, Lewis RA, et al. Autoantibodies to agrin in myasthenia gravis patients. PLoS One. 2014;9(3):e91816.
21. Zisimopoulou P, Brenner T, Trakas N, Tzartos SJ. Serological diagnostics in myasthenia gravis based on novel assays and recently identified antigens. Autoimmun Rev. 2013;12(9):924–30.
22. Rodgaard A, Nielsen F, Djurup R, Somnier F, Gammeltoft S. Acetylcholine receptor antibody in myasthenia gravis: predominance of IgG subclasses 1 and 3. Clin Exp Immunol. 1987;67:82–8.
23. Drachman DB. Myasthenia gravis (first of two parts). N Engl J Med. 1978;298(3):136–42.
24. Engel AG, Sahashi K, Fumagalli G. The immunopathology of acquired myasthenia gravis. Ann N Y Acad Sci. 1981;377:158–74.
25. Pirskanen R. Genetic aspects in myasthenia gravis. A family study of 264 Finnish patients. Acta Neurol Scand. 1977;56(5):365–88.
26. Namba T, Shapiro MS, Brunner NG, Grob D. Myasthenia gravis occurring in twins. J Neurol Neurosurg Psychiatry. 1971;34(5):531–4.
27. Seybold ME, Lindstrom JM. Antiacetylcholine receptor antibody and its relationship to HLA type in asymptomatic siblings of a patient with myasthenia gravis. Neurology. 1981;31(6):778–80.
28. Leslie RD, Hawa M. Twin studies in auto-immune disease. Acta Genet Med Gemellol (Roma). 1994;43(1–2):71–81.

29. Ramanujam R, Pirskanen R, Ramanujam S, Hammarstrom L. Utilizing twins concordance rates to infer the predisposition to myasthenia gravis. Twin Res Hum Genet. 2011;14(2):129–36.
30. Mamrut S, Avidan N, Truffault F, Staun-Ram E, Sharshar T, Eymard B, et al. Methylome and transcriptome profiling in Myasthenia Gravis monozygotic twins. J Autoimmun. 2017;82:62–73.
31. Pirskanen R, Tiilikainen A, Hokkanen E. Histocompatibility (HL-A) antigens associated with myasthenia gravis. A preliminary report. Ann Clin Res. 1972;4(5):304–6.
32. Fritze D, Herrman C Jr, Naeim F, Smith GS, Walford RL. HL-A antigens in myasthenia gravis. Lancet. 1974;1(7851):240–2.
33. Giraud M, Beaurain G, Yamamoto AM, Eymard B, Tranchant C, Gajdos P, et al. Linkage of HLA to myasthenia gravis and genetic heterogeneity depending on anti-titin antibodies. Neurology. 2001;57(9):1555–60.
34. Feltkamp TE, van den Berg-Loonen PM, Nijenhuis LE, Engelfriet CP, van Rossum AL, van Loghem JJ, et al. Myasthenia gravis, autoantibodies, and HL-A antigens. Br Med J. 1974;1(5899):131–3.
35. Carlsson B, Wallin J, Pirskanen R, Matell G, Smith CI. Different HLA DR-DQ associations in subgroups of idiopathic myasthenia gravis. Immunogenetics. 1990;31(5–6):285–90.
36. Kaul R, Shenoy M, Goluszko E, Christadoss P. Major histocompatibility complex class II gene disruption prevents experimental autoimmune myasthenia gravis. J Immunol. 1994;152(6):3152–7.
37. Machens A, Loliger C, Pichlmeier U, Emskotter T, Busch C, Izbicki JR. Correlation of thymic pathology with HLA in myasthenia gravis. Clin Immunol. 1999;91(3):296–301.
38. Pirskanen R. Genetic associations between myasthenia gravis and the HL-A system. J Neurol Neurosurg Psychiatry. 1976;39(1):23–33.
39. Ratanachaiyavong S, Fleming D, Janer M, Demaine AG, Willcox N, Newsom-Davis J, et al. HLA-DPB1 polymorphisms in patients with hyperthyroid Graves' disease and early onset myasthenia gravis. Autoimmunity. 1994;17(2):99–104.
40. Janer M, Cowland A, Picard J, Campbell D, Pontarotti P, Newsom-Davis J, et al. A susceptibility region for myasthenia gravis extending into the HLA-class I sector telomeric to HLA-C. Hum Immunol. 1999;60(9):909–17.
41. Spurkland A, Gilhus NE, Ronningen KS, Aarli JA, Vartdal F. Myasthenia gravis patients with thymus hyperplasia and myasthenia gravis patients with thymoma display different HLA associations. Tissue Antigens. 1991;37(2):90–3.
42. Vieira M, Caillat- Zuchman S, Gajdos P, et al. Identification by genomic typing of non-DR3 HLA class II genes associated with myasthenia gravis. J Neuroimmunol. 1993;47:115–22.
43. Bell J, Rassenti L, Smoot S, Smith K, Newby C, Hohlfeld R, et al. HLA-DQ beta-chain polymorphism linked to myasthenia gravis. Lancet. 1986;1(8489):1058–60.
44. Hjelmstrom P, Giscombe R, Lefvert AK, Pirskanen R, Kockum I, Landin-Olsson M, et al. Different HLA-DQ are positively and negatively associated in Swedish patients with myasthenia gravis. Autoimmunity. 1995;22(1):59–65.
45. Hjelmstrom P, Giscombe R, Lefvert AK, Pirskanen R, Kockum I, Landin-Olsson M, et al. Polymorphic amino acid domains of the HLA-DQ molecule are associated with disease heterogeneity in myasthenia gravis. J Neuroimmunol. 1996;65(2):125–31.
46. Hajeer AH, Sawidan FA, Bohlega S, Saleh S, Sutton P, Shubaili A, et al. HLA class I and class II polymorphisms in Saudi patients with myasthenia gravis. Int J Immunogenet. 2009;36(3):169–72.
47. Saruhan-Direskeneli G, Kilic A, Parman Y, Serdaroglu P, Deymeer F. HLA-DQ polymorphism in Turkish patients with myasthenia gravis. Hum Immunol. 2006;67(4–5):352–8.
48. Donmez B, Ozakbas S, Oktem MA, Gedizlioglu M, Coker I, Genc A, et al. HLA genotypes in Turkish patients with myasthenia gravis: comparison with multiple sclerosis patients on the basis of clinical subtypes and demographic features. Hum Immunol. 2004;65(7):752–7.
49. Fernandez-Mestre MT, Vargas V, Montagnani S, Cotua M, Ogando V, Layrisse Z. HLA class II and class I polymorphism in Venezuelan patients with myasthenia gravis. Hum Immunol. 2004;65(1):54–9.

50. Santos E, Bettencourt A, da Silva AM, Boleixa D, Lopes D, Brás S, et al. HLA and age of onset in myasthenia gravis. Neuromuscul Disord. 2017;27(7):650–4.
51. Maniaol AH, Elsais A, Lorentzen AR, Owe JF, Viken MK, Saether H, et al. Late onset myasthenia gravis is associated with HLA DRB1*15:01 in the Norwegian population. PLoS One. 2012;7(5):e36603.
52. Deitiker PR, Oshima M, Smith RG, Mosier D, Atassi MZ. Association with HLA DQ of early onset myasthenia gravis in Southeast Texas region of the United States. Int J Immunogenet. 2011;38(1):55–62.
53. Ehsan S, Amirzargar A, Yekaninejad MS, Mahmoudi M, Mehravar S, Moradi B, Nafissi S. Association of HLA class II (DRB1, DQA1, DQB1) alleles and haplotypes with myasthenia gravis and its subgroups in the Iranian population. J Neurol Sci. 2015;359(1):335–42. https://doi.org/10.1016/j.jns.2015.11.021.
54. Kida K, Hayashi M, Yamada I, Matsuda H, Yoshinaga J, Takami S, et al. Heterogeneity in myasthenia gravis: HLA phenotypes and autoantibody responses in ocular and generalized types. Ann Neurol. 1987;21(3):274–8.
55. Testi M, Terracciano C, Guagnano A, Testa G, Marfia GA, Pompeo E, et al. Association of HLA-DQB1 *05:02 and DRB1 *16 alleles with late-onset, nonthymomatous, AChR-Ab-positive myasthenia gravis. Autoimmune Dis. 2012;2012:541760.
56. Matsuki K, Juji T, Tokunaga K, Takamizawa M, Maeda H, Soda M, et al. HLA antigens in Japanese patients with myasthenia gravis. J Clin Invest. 1990;86(2):392–9.
57. Morita K, Moriuchi J, Inoko H, Tsuji K, Arimori S. HLA class II antigens and DNA restriction fragment length polymorphism in myasthenia gravis in Japan. Ann Neurol. 1991;29(2):168–74.
58. Horiki T, Inoko H, Moriuchi J, Ichikawa Y, Arimori S. Combinations of HLA-DPB1 and HLA-DQB1 alleles determine susceptibility to early-onset myasthenia gravis in Japan. Autoimmunity. 1994;19(1):49–54.
59. Xie YC, Qu Y, Sun L, Li HF, Zhang H, Shi HJ, et al. Association between HLA-DRB1 and myasthenia gravis in a northern Han Chinese population. J Clin Neurosci. 2011;18(11):1524–7.
60. Feng HY, Yang LX, Liu WB, Huang X, Qiu L, Li Y. The HLA-B*4601-DRB1*0901 haplotype is positively correlated with juvenile ocular myasthenia gravis in a southern Chinese Han population. Neurol Sci. 2015;36(7):1135–40.
61. Giraud M, Beaurain G, Eymard B, Tranchant C, Gajdos P, Garchon HJ. Genetic control of autoantibody expression in autoimmune myasthenia gravis: role of the self-antigen and of HLA-linked loci. Genes Immun. 2004;5(5):398–404.
62. Djabiri F, Caillat-Zucman S, Gajdos P, Jais JP, Gomez L, Khalil I, et al. Association of the AChRalpha-subunit gene (CHRNA), DQA1*0101, and the DR3 haplotype in myasthenia gravis. Evidence for a three-gene disease model in a subgroup of patients. J Autoimmun. 1997;10(4):407–13.
63. Vandiedonck C, Beaurain G, Giraud M, Hue-Beauvais C, Eymard B, Tranchant C, et al. Pleiotropic effects of the 8.1 HLA haplotype in patients with autoimmune myasthenia gravis and thymus hyperplasia. Proc Natl Acad Sci U S A. 2004;101(43):15464–9.
64. Franciotta D, Cuccia M, Dondi E, Piccolo G, Cosi V. Polymorphic markers in MHC class II/III region: a study on Italian patients with myasthenia gravis. J Neurol Sci. 2001;190(1–2):11–6.
65. International MHC and Autoimmunity Genetics Network, Rioux JD, Goyette P, Vyse TJ, Hammarstrom L, et al. Mapping of multiple susceptibility variants within the MHC region for 7 immune-mediated diseases. Proc Natl Acad Sci U S A. 2009;106(44):18680–5.
66. Varade J, Wang N, Lim CK, Zhang T, Zhang Y, Liu X, et al. Novel genetic loci associated HLA-B*08:01 positive myasthenia gravis. J Autoimmun. 2018;88:43–9.
67. Strobel P, Chuang WY, Chuvpilo S, Zettl A, Katzenberger T, Kalbacher H, et al. Common cellular and diverse genetic basis of thymoma-associated myasthenia gravis: role of MHC class II and AIRE genes and genetic polymorphisms. Ann N Y Acad Sci. 2008;1132:143–56.
68. Zettl A, Strobel P, Wagner K, Katzenberger T, Ott G, Rosenwald A, et al. Recurrent genetic aberrations in thymoma and thymic carcinoma. Am J Pathol. 2000;157(1):257–66.
69. Garcia-Ramos G, Tellez-Zenteno JF, Zapata-Zuniga M, Yamamoto-Furusho JK, Ruiz-Morales JA, Villarreal-Garza C, et al. HLA class II genotypes in Mexican Mestizo patients with myasthenia gravis. Eur J Neurol. 2003;10(6):707–10.

70. Vandiedonck C, Raffoux C, Eymard B, Tranchant C, Dulmet E, Krumeich S, et al. Association of HLA-A in autoimmune myasthenia gravis with thymoma. J Neuroimmunol. 2009;210(1–2):120–3.
71. Niks EH, Kuks JB, Roep BO, Haasnoot GW, Verduijn W, Ballieux BE, et al. Strong association of MuSK antibody-positive myasthenia gravis and HLA-DR14-DQ5. Neurology. 2006;66(11):1772–4.
72. Bartoccioni E, Scuderi F, Augugliaro A, Chiatamone Ranieri S, Sauchelli D, Alboino P, et al. HLA class II allele analysis in MuSK-positive myasthenia gravis suggests a role for DQ5. Neurology. 2009;72(2):195–7.
73. Alahgholi-Hajibehzad M, Yilmaz V, Gulsen-Parman Y, Aysal F, Oflazer P, Deymeer F, Saruhan-Direskeneli G. Association of HLA-DRB1 *14, -DRB1 *16 and -DQB1 *05 with MuSK-myasthenia gravis in patients from Turkey. Hum Immunol. 2013;74(12):1633–5. https://doi.org/10.1016/j.humimm.2013.08.271.
74. Nikolic AV, Andric ZP, Simonovic RB, Rakocevic Stojanovic VM, Basta IZ, Bojic SD, Lavrnic DV. High frequency of DQB1*05 and absolute absence of DRB1*13 in muscle-specific tyrosine kinase positive myasthenia gravis. Eur J Neurol. 2015;22(1):59–63. https://doi.org/10.1111/ene.12525.
75. Kanai T, Uzawa A, Kawaguchi N, Sakamaki T, Yoshiyama Y, Himuro K, et al. HLA-DRB1*14 and DQB1*05 are associated with Japanese anti-MuSK antibody-positive myasthenia gravis patients. J Neurol Sci. 2016;363:116–8. https://doi.org/10.1016/j.jns.2016.02.031.
76. Bottini N, Musumeci L, Alonso A, Rahmouni S, Nika K, Rostamkhani M, et al. A functional variant of lymphoid tyrosine phosphatase is associated with type I diabetes. Nat Genet. 2004;36(4):337–8.
77. Burn GL, Svensson L, Sanchez-Blanco C, Saini M, Cope AP. Why is PTPN22 a good candidate susceptibility gene for autoimmune disease? FEBS Lett. 2011;585(23):3689–98.
78. Vandiedonck C, Capdevielle C, Giraud M, Krumeich S, Jais JP, Eymard B, et al. Association of the PTPN22*R620W polymorphism with autoimmune myasthenia gravis. Ann Neurol. 2006;59(2):404–7.
79. Greve B, Hoffmann P, Illes Z, Rozsa C, Berger K, Weissert R, et al. The autoimmunity-related polymorphism PTPN22 1858C/T is associated with anti-titin antibody-positive myasthenia gravis. Hum Immunol. 2009;70(7):540–2.
80. Lefvert AK, Zhao Y, Ramanujam R, Yu S, Pirskanen R, Hammarstrom L. PTPN22 R620W promotes production of anti-AChR autoantibodies and IL-2 in myasthenia gravis. J Neuroimmunol. 2008;197(2):110–3.
81. Chuang WY, Strobel P, Belharazem D, Rieckmann P, Toyka KV, Nix W, et al. The PTPN22gain-of-function+1858T(+) genotypes correlate with low IL-2 expression in thymomas and predispose to myasthenia gravis. Genes Immun. 2009;10(8):667–72.
82. Kaya GA, Coskun AN, Yilmaz V, Oflazer P, Gulsen-Parman Y, Aysal F, et al. The association of PTPN22 R620W polymorphism is stronger with late-onset AChR-myasthenia gravis in Turkey. PLoS One. 2014;9(8):e104760.
83. Huang D, Liu L, Noren K, Xia SQ, Trifunovic J, Pirskanen R, et al. Genetic association of CTLA-4 to myasthenia gravis with thymoma. J Neuroimmunol. 1998;88(1–2):192–8.
84. Huang D, Giscombe R, Zhou Y, Pirskanen R, Lefvert AK. Dinucleotide repeat expansion in the CTLA-4 gene leads to T cell hyper-reactivity via the CD28 pathway in myasthenia gravis. J Neuroimmunol. 2000;105(1):69–77.
85. Wang XB, Kakoulidou M, Giscombe R, Qiu Q, Huang D, Pirskanen R, et al. Abnormal expression of CTLA-4 by T cells from patients with myasthenia gravis: effect of an AT-rich gene sequence. J Neuroimmunol. 2002;130(1–2):224–32.
86. Wang XB, Kakoulidou M, Qiu Q, Giscombe R, Huang D, Pirskanen R, et al. CDS1 and promoter single nucleotide polymorphisms of the CTLA-4 gene in human myasthenia gravis. Genes Immun. 2002;3(1):46–9.
87. Chuang WY, Strobel P, Gold R, Nix W, Schalke B, Kiefer R, et al. A CTLA4high genotype is associated with myasthenia gravis in thymoma patients. Ann Neurol. 2005;58(4):644–8.

88. Chuang WY, Strobel P, Bohlender-Willke AL, Rieckmann P, Nix W, Schalke B, et al. Late-onset myasthenia gravis—CTLA4(low) genotype association and low-for-age thymic output of naive T cells. J Autoimmun. 2014;52:122–9.
89. Wang XB, Pirskanen R, Giscombe R, Lefvert AK. Two SNPs in the promoter region of the CTLA-4 gene affect binding of transcription factors and are associated with human myasthenia gravis. J Intern Med. 2008;263(1):61–9.
90. Sun L, Meng Y, Xie Y, Zhang H, Zhang Z, Wang X, et al. CTLA4 variants and haplotype contribute genetic susceptibility to myasthenia gravis in northern Chinese population. PLoS One. 2014;9(7):e101986.
91. Garchon HJ, Djabiri F, Viard JP, Gajdos P, Bach JF. Involvement of human muscle acetylcholine receptor alpha-subunit gene (CHRNA) in susceptibility to myasthenia gravis. Proc Natl Acad Sci U S A. 1994;91(11):4668–72.
92. Djabiri F, Gajdos P, Eymard B, Gomez L, Bach JF, Garchon HJ. No evidence for an association of AChR beta-subunit gene (CHRNB1) with myasthenia gravis. J Neuroimmunol. 1997;78(1–2):86–9.
93. Bonifati DM, Willcox N, Vincent A, Beeson D. Lack of association between acetylcholine receptor epsilon polymorphisms and early-onset myasthenia gravis. Muscle Nerve. 2004;29(3):436–9.
94. Giraud M, Eymard B, Tranchant C, Gajdos P, Garchon HJ. Association of the gene encoding the delta-subunit of the muscle acetylcholine receptor (CHRND) with acquired autoimmune myasthenia gravis. Genes Immun. 2004;5(1):80–3.
95. Li HF, Hong Y, Zhang X, Xie Y, Skeie GO, Hao HJ, et al. Gene polymorphisms for both auto-antigen and immune-modulating proteins are associated with the susceptibility of autoimmune myasthenia gravis. Mol Neurobiol. 2017;54(6):4771–80.
96. Demaine A, Willcox N, Janer M, Welsh K, Newsom-Davis J. Immunoglobulin heavy chain gene associations in myasthenia gravis: new evidence for disease heterogeneity. J Neurol. 1992;239(1):53–6.
97. Oksenberg JR, Sherritt M, Begovich AB, Erlich HA, Bernard CC, Cavalli-Sforza LL, et al. T-cell receptor V alpha and C alpha alleles associated with multiple and myasthenia gravis. Proc Natl Acad Sci U S A. 1989;86(3):988–92.
98. Raknes G, Skeie GO, Gilhus NE, Aadland S, Vedeler C. FcgammaRIIA and FcgammaRIIIB polymorphisms in myasthenia gravis. J Neuroimmunol. 1998;81(1–2):173–6.
99. van der Pol WL, Jansen MD, Kuks JB, de Baets M, Leppers-van de Straat FG, Wokke JH, et al. Association of the Fc gamma receptor IIA-R/R131 genotype with myasthenia gravis in Dutch patients. J Neuroimmunol. 2003;144(1–2):143–7.
100. Amdahl C, Alseth EH, Gilhus NE, Nakkestad HL, Skeie GO. Polygenic disease associations in thymomatous myasthenia gravis. Arch Neurol. 2007;64(12):1729–33.
101. Zelano G, Lino MM, Evoli A, Settesoldi D, Batocchi AP, Torrente I, et al. Tumour necrosis factor beta gene polymorphisms in myasthenia gravis. Eur J Immunogenet. 1998;25(6):403–8.
102. Hjelmstrom P, Peacock CS, Giscombe R, Pirskanen R, Lefvert AK, Blackwell JM, et al. Polymorphism in tumor necrosis factor genes associated with myasthenia gravis. J Neuroimmunol. 1998;88(1–2):137–43.
103. Skeie GO, Pandey JP, Aarli JA, Gilhus NE. TNFA and TNFB polymorphisms in myasthenia gravis. Arch Neurol. 1999;56(4):457–61.
104. Huang D, Xia S, Zhou Y, Pirskanen R, Liu L, Lefvert AK. No evidence for interleukin-4 gene conferring susceptibility to myasthenia gravis. J Neuroimmunol. 1998;92(1–2):208–11.
105. Huang D, Zheng C, Giscombe R, Matell G, Pirskanen R, Kari Lefvert A. Polymorphisms at -174 and in the 3′-flanking region of interleukin-6 (IL-6) gene in patients with myasthenia gravis. J Neuroimmunol. 1999;101(2):197–200.
106. Huang D, Pirskanen R, Hjelmstrom P, Lefvert AK. Polymorphisms in IL-1beta and IL-1 receptor antagonist genes are associated with myasthenia gravis. J Neuroimmunol. 1998;81(1–2):76–81.

107. Sciacca FL, Ferri C, Veglia F, Andreetta F, Mantegazza R, Cornelio F, et al. IL-1 genes in myasthenia gravis: IL-1A -889 polymorphism associated with sex and age of disease onset. J Neuroimmunol. 2002;122(1–2):94–9.
108. Huang DR, Zhou YH, Xia SQ, Liu L, Pirskanen R, Lefvert AK. Markers in the promoter region of interleukin-10 (IL-10) gene in myasthenia gravis: implications of diverse effects of IL-10 in the pathogenesis of the disease. J Neuroimmunol. 1999;94(1–2):82–7.
109. Alseth EH, Nakkestad HL, Aarseth J, Gilhus NE, Skeie GO. Interleukin-10 promoter polymorphisms in myasthenia gravis. J Neuroimmunol. 2009;210(1–2):63–6.
110. Yilmaz V, Demirbilek V, Gurses C, Yentur SP, Uysal S, Yapici Z, et al. Interleukin (IL)-12, IL-2, interferon-gamma gene polymorphisms in subacute sclerosing panencephalitis patients. J Neurovirol. 2007;13(5):410–5.
111. Pal Z, Varga Z, Semsei A, Remenyi V, Rozsa C, Falus A, et al. Interleukin-4 receptor alpha polymorphisms in autoimmune myasthenia gravis in a Caucasian population. Hum Immunol. 2012;73(2):193–5.
112. Yue YX, Hong Y, Xie Y, Hao HJ, Sui Y, Gu CK, et al. Association study between IL-17A and IL-17F gene polymorphism and myasthenia gravis in Chinese patients. Neurol Sci. 2016;37(1):123–30.
113. Xu BY, Huang D, Pirskanen R, Lefvert AK. beta2-adrenergic receptor gene polymorphisms in myasthenia gravis (MG). Clin Exp Immunol. 2000;119(1):156–60.
114. Sakthivel P, Ramanujam R, Wang XB, Pirskanen R, Lefvert AK. Programmed Death-1: from gene to protein in autoimmune human myasthenia gravis. J Neuroimmunol. 2008;193(1–2):149–55.
115. Ramanujam R, Zhao Y, Pirskanen R, Hammarstrom L. Lack of association of the CIITA -168A-->G promoter SNP with myasthenia gravis and its role in autoimmunity. BMC Med Genet. 2010;11:147.
116. Zagoriti Z, Georgitsi M, Giannakopoulou O, Ntellos F, Tzartos SJ, Patrinos GP, et al. Genetics of myasthenia gravis: a case-control association study in the Hellenic population. Clin Dev Immunol. 2012;2012:484919.
117. Pal Z, Antal P, Millinghoffer A, Hullam G, Paloczi K, Toth S, et al. A novel galectin-1 and interleukin 2 receptor beta haplotype is associated with autoimmune myasthenia gravis. J Neuroimmunol. 2010;229(1–2):107–11.
118. Xie Y, Meng Y, Li HF, Hong Y, Sun L, Zhu X, et al. GR gene polymorphism is associated with inter-subject variability in response to glucocorticoids in patients with myasthenia gravis. Eur J Neurol. 2016;23(8):1372–9.
119. Heckmann JM, Uwimpuhwe H, Ballo R, Kaur M, Bajic VB, Prince S. A functional SNP in the regulatory region of the decay-accelerating factor gene associates with extraocular muscle pareses in myasthenia gravis. Genes Immun. 2010;11(1):1–10.
120. Coppedè F, Ricciardi R, Denaro M, De Rosa A, Provenzano C, Bartoccioni E, et al. Association of the DNMT3B -579G>T polymorphism with risk of thymomas in patients with myasthenia gravis. PLoS One. 2013;8(11):e80846.
121. Kellermayer B, Polgar N, Pal J, Banati M, Maasz A, Kisfali P, et al. Association of myasthenia gravis with polymorphisms in the gene of histamine N-methyltransferase. Hum Immunol. 2013;74(12):1701–4.
122. Zagoriti Z, Lagoumintzis G, Perroni G, Papathanasiou G, Papadakis A, Ambrogi V, et al. Evidence for association of STAT4 and IL12RB2 variants with Myasthenia gravis susceptibility: what is the effect on gene expression in thymus? J Neuroimmunol. 2018;319:93–9.
123. Lopomo A, Ricciardi R, De Rosa A, Guida M, Maestri M, Lucchi M, et al. The thymidylate synthase enhancer region (TSER) polymorphism increases the risk of thymic lymphoid hyperplasia in patients with Myasthenia Gravis. Gene. 2018;642:376–80.
124. Avidan N, Le Panse R, Harbo HF, Bernasconi P, Poulas K, Ginzburg E, et al. VAV1 and BAFF, via NFkappaB pathway, are genetic risk factors for myasthenia gravis. Ann Clin Transl Neurol. 2014;1(5):329–39.

125. Gregersen PK, Kosoy R, Lee AT, Lamb J, Sussman J, McKee D, et al. Risk for myasthenia gravis maps to a (151) Pro-->Ala change in TNIP1 and to human leukocyte antigen-B*08. Ann Neurol. 2012;72(6):927–35.
126. Na SJ, Lee JH, Kim SW, Kim DS, Shon EH, Park HJ, et al. Whole-genome analysis in Korean patients with autoimmune myasthenia gravis. Yonsei Med J. 2014;55(3):660–8.
127. Renton AE, Pliner HA, Provenzano C, Evoli A, Ricciardi R, Nalls MA, et al. A genome-wide association study of myasthenia gravis. JAMA Neurol. 2015;72(4):396–404.
128. Seldin MF, Alkhairy OK, Lee AT, Lamb JA, Sussman J, Pirskanen-Matell R, et al. Genome-wide association study of late-onset myasthenia gravis: confirmation of TNFRSF11A, and identification of ZBTB10 and three distinct HLA associations. Mol Med. 2015;21:769–81.
129. Saruhan-Direskeneli G, Hughes T, Yilmaz V, Durmus H, Adler A, Alahgholi-Hajibehzad M, et al. Genetic heterogeneity within the HLA region in three distinct clinical subgroups of myasthenia gravis. Clin Immunol. 2016;166–167:81–8.

Common Genetic Component in Autoimmunity

12

Gisela Orozco and Blanca Rueda

Contents

12.1 Introduction

Autoimmune diseases (ADs) comprise a heterogeneous group of disorders characterized by an altered immune response that results in a serious damage of diverse organ and tissues. Worldwide, 7.9–9.4% of the population is estimated to be affected by an AD such as rheumatoid arthritis (RA), systemic lupus erythematosus (SLE),

G. Orozco (✉)
Faculty of Biology, Medicine and Health, The University of Manchester, Manchester, UK
e-mail: Gisela.orozco@manchester.ac.uk

B. Rueda
Faculty of Health Sciences, University of Granada, Granada, Spain

J. Martín, F. D. Carmona (eds.), *Genetics of Rare Autoimmune Diseases*,
Rare Diseases of the Immune System, https://doi.org/10.1007/978-3-030-03934-9_12

type 1 diabetes (T1D), or inflammatory bowel disease (IBD) among others [1]. Knowledge of etiology and pathogenic mechanisms causing AD remain limited, but it is well stablished that the alteration of the immune response results from a complex interplay between environmental factors and genetic susceptibility.

Since long time ago, it was suggested that ADs would share a genetic component on the basis of the important overlap of clinical and immunological characteristics, the familial aggregation for autoimmunity and the co-occurrence of two or more AD in the same individual. During the past 10 years, the development of powerful genotyping and technical and analytical tools has allowed for a great advance in the characterization of the shared genetic background for autoimmunity. The major advance happened with the expansion of genome-wide association studies (GWASs). With this approach, common variants, typically single nucleotide polymorphisms (SNPs), across the whole genome are examined in case-control groups including thousands of individuals. Over the past decade, more than 100 GWASs have been conducted in different ADs uncovering hundreds of risk loci predisposing for ADs, of which almost half overlap between diseases [2, 3] (Fig. 12.1). In addition, a specific immune-genetic genotyping array (Immunochip) was designed for the replication and fine mapping of established GWAS loci for autoimmune and inflammatory diseases [4]. Several novel autoimmunity loci that were not detected in GWAS studies have been identified with the Immunochip studies conducted in different ADs [5–8]. On the other hand, recently cross-disease studies analyzing data set coming from GWASs of different ADs have also contributed to expand the known genetic susceptibility loci for autoimmunity [9–13].

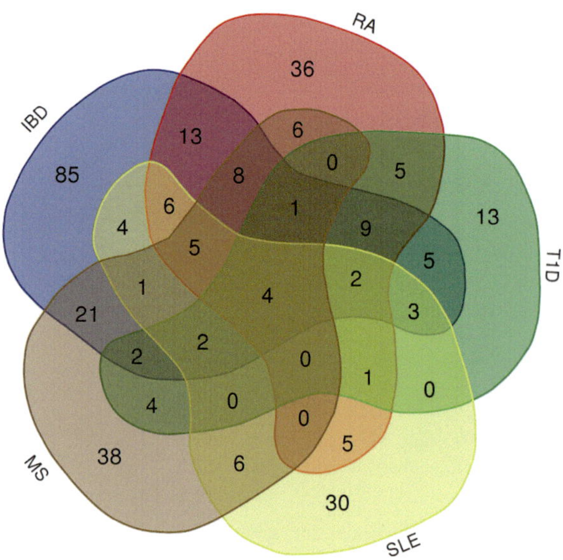

Fig. 12.1 A number of overlapping genetic risk loci for five of the most common and best studied autoimmune diseases: RA, T1D, SLE, MS, and IBD. All risk loci listed in the NHGRI GWAS Catalog (https://www.ebi.ac.uk/gwas/) showing an association p value $<10^{-5}$ were included. *RA* rheumatoid arthritis, *T1D* type 1 diabetes, *SLE* systemic lupus erythematosus, *MS* multiple sclerosis, *IBD* inflammatory bowel disease

Thus, at present a huge number of AD-shared risk loci have been identified convincingly. Nevertheless, this overlap is complicated and could comprise different scenarios, with the same SNP/haplotype accounting for the risk of different ADs, discordant associations in which the same SNP exerts a protective role in one disease and confer risk for another, and shared loci for which a different haplotype is associated in each disease. To add more complexity, the genes implicated frequently present differential expression patterns and could exert pleiotropic immune functions.

In this chapter we will highlight the most relevant shared pathways involved in the development of ADs discovered from recent advances in genetic studies, including antigen presentation, cytokine profile, or lymphocyte activity modulation.

12.2 Antigen Presentation

The major histocompatibility complex (MHC) is a genomic region including hundreds of genes with immune functions, including antigen presentation. This region is characterized by wide allelic variation and linkage disequilibrium. For most autoimmune conditions, the first reported genetic association was with MHC loci, previous to the GWAS era, and still remains as the strongest genetic effect [14]. Usually, ADs with the presence of autoantibodies such as RA, T1D, SLE, systemic sclerosis (SSc), or celiac disease (CD) are associated with HLA class II alleles, whereas HLA class I alleles confer risk for ADs in which autoantibodies are not a common feature (i. e., Behçet's disease, ankylosing spondylitis (AS), or psoriasis) [15–19]. Notably, Crohn's disease is an exception since although it is associated with SNPs in the MHC region, classical HLA alleles do not associate with this condition [20].

Recent studies including large data sets, high-throughput genotyping techniques, and novel analysis tools, such as imputation of alleles, have characterized independent non-HLA associations within the region for some ADs. In RA, an extensive study using imputation of classical HLA alleles as well as SNPs across the MCH identified independent association with *HLA-B* and *HLA-DPβ1* and refined the classical shared epitope association to three amino acid positions of the peptide-binding groove [21]. Similarly, an independent signal at *HLA-A**0201 was defined for ankylosing spondylitis through the imputation analysis of Immunochip data [7].

For T1D and multiple sclerosis, association at *HLA-A/HLA-B* and *HLA-DPB1*, respectively, was described as independent of the classical HLA susceptibility signals [22, 23].

In spite of the robust and largely characterized contribution of MHC genes to autoimmunity, for the majority of risk loci, causal alleles remain undiscovered. This is a difficult issue due to the extensive variability and the strong linkage disequilibrium in this region. Probably, causal alleles would be different for each disease conditioning distinctive patterns of antigen recognition starting the altered immune response. On the other hand, considering that the MHC region contains a dense number of genes, it is likely that non-HLA genes contribute to the genetic risk of ADs. Thus, another challenge for researches is to identify independent genetic variants outside the common classical HLA haplotypes that would help to the characterization of novel pathways involved in the autoimmune process. In this line, for SLE a role of non-HLA alleles in the multiple MHC association with the disease has been described [24].

Together with the implication of MHC genes, there are interesting findings about the role of different aminopeptidase genes in antigen presentation. Variants in endoplasmic reticulum aminopeptidase 1 (*ERAP1*) gene located at chromosome 5 are associated with AS, psoriasis, and Behçet's disease. This gene encodes for an endoplasmic reticulum aminopeptidase involved, among other functions, in the preparation of peptides for HLA class I presentation. Interestingly, data from GWAS studies revealed a gene-gene interaction between *ERAP1* and *HLA-B*27* in AS, *ERAP1* and *HLA-Cw6* in psoriasis, and *ERAP1* with *HLA-B*51* with Behçet's disease that reinforces the importance of antigen presentation in the pathogenesis of these diseases [25–27]. Likewise, a SNP in the *ERAP2* gene was associated with a protective effect in AS and Crohn's disease. The variant associated causes a splice site variation that leads to a decay of ERAP2 expression and to the deficiency of the translated protein [28, 29].

12.3 Cytokines Pathways

Cytokines play an important role in autoimmunity and inflammation in general, since they mediate the recruitment, activation, and intercellular communication of inflammatory cells in the site of inflammation. A dysregulated expression of cytokines is a common feature of autoimmune lesions, and therefore, substantial efforts have been made to elucidate their potential role as genetic risk factors for autoimmune disease. GWASs have further highlighted the importance of genetic polymorphism in cytokine genes, as many associations have been found with multiple autoimmune diseases. A summary of the most important ones is described below.

12.3.1 TNF Superfamily

There are 18 ligands (TNFSF) and 29 receptors (TNFRSF) in the tumor necrosis factor (TNF) cytokine and receptor superfamilies, respectively. These molecules are involved in the modulation of immunological responses via co-stimulation, maturation, and cell death signaling pathways [30]. Mutations in genes of this TNF superfamily are responsible for the development of Mendelian autoimmune diseases like autoimmune lymphoproliferative syndrome (ALPS) and TNF receptor-associated periodic syndrome (TRAPS), which are caused by mutations in FAS and TNFRSF1A, respectively [31–33].

For complex autoimmune diseases, GWASs have identified associations with genetic variants close to around a quarter of the 88 autosomal genes encoding TNFSF cytokines, their receptors, and downstream signaling molecules. In addition, a number of these genetic variants are associated with multiple diseases, and several diseases are associated with several variants in TNFSF network genes [34].

Diseases showing association with genes in these pathways include ankylosing spondylitis, celiac disease, Crohn's disease, multiple sclerosis, primary biliary cirrhosis, psoriasis, rheumatoid arthritis, Sjögren's syndrome, SLE, ulcerative colitis, and vitiligo [35]. Some of these SNPs associated with autoimmunity have also been shown to be correlated with the expression levels of nearby TNFSF and TNFRSF members, for example, *TNFSF4* [36, 37], *TNFRSF1A* [38], *TNFSF14* [39], *CD40* [40], *TNFRSF6B* [41], and *TNFSF15* [42–45].

Further evidence supporting a key role of TNFSF and TNFRSF genes in autoimmunity is (a) increased expression of these genes in the serum and/or at the site of inflammation in patients, including RA [46–48], inflammatory bowel disease (IBD) [49–53], and SLE [54–56]; (b) amelioration of autoimmune disease in mouse models by blockade of several TNFRSF signaling pathways [57]; and (c) successful treatment of disease in humans by targeting TNF [58] and TNFSF13B (BAFF) [59].

12.3.2 IL23R

One of the strongest genetic associations in Crohn's disease and ulcerative colitis is with *IL23R* [60], which is also associated with psoriasis [61] and ankylosing spondylitis [62]. *IL23R* encodes for one of the subunits of the interleukin-23 (IL-23) receptor. IL-23 is known to play a crucial role in the development and maintenance of T helper 17 cells. The missense variant R381Q in *IL23R*, encoding the receptor molecule for IL-23, is perhaps one of the best studied of SNPs associated with autoimmunity. Functional studies have shown that human CD4+ T cells carrying the *IL23R* R381Q protective allele display reduced phosphorylation of signal transducer and activator of transcription 3 (STAT3) upon stimulation with IL-23 and decreased production of IL-17, which suggests that reduced responsiveness in Th17 cells protects against those ADs [63]. In addition to the R381Q variant, several other independent association signals have been found in a haplotype block encompassing the C-terminal seven exons of *IL23R* and the intergenic region between *IL23R* and its close homolog, *IL12RB2*.

The association of genes in the IL-23 pathway illustrates how GWAS findings have sparked the successful repositioning of drugs; biologic drugs targeting components of this pathway are now used routinely for psoriasis and psoriatic arthritis and have been shown to be effective in the treatment of ankylosing spondylitis and inflammatory bowel disease [64–66]. It has been proposed that the annual sales of these medications alone are likely to be greater than the total amount spent on GWASs in the past decade [67].

12.3.3 IL2RA

GWASs have implicated multiple, distinct noncoding variants in the *IL2RA* locus as risk factors for eight autoimmune diseases, including juvenile idiopathic arthritis, type 1 diabetes, autoimmune thyroiditis, multiple sclerosis (MS), primary sclerosing cholangitis, vitiligo, Crohn's disease, and alopecia areata [68]. *IL2RA* encodes a subunit of the high-affinity interleukin-2 (IL-2) receptor (IL-2Ra, also known as CD25) and plays an important role in T-cell stimulation and Treg function [69]. These variants map to regulatory rather than coding sequences, and several studies have aimed to understand how they affect *IL2RA*. For example, it has been shown that the rs2104286 risk allele, associated with both MS and T1D, is correlated with increased expression of IL-2Ra on effector T cells and Tregs [70–72], and it is also associated with decreased STAT5 signaling downstream of IL-2 [71]. Investigation of SNPs mapping to the 5′ flanking region and the first intron of *IL2RA* showed that the minor allele is associated with lower transcript levels and altered transcription factor binding [73]. The implication of rs61839660, which has been shown to be responsible for the risk of IBD at the *IL2RA* locus in a fine-mapping study [74], in the regulation of *IL2RA* expression was later confirmed in a high-throughput CRISPR activation study; it was also found that this SNP delayed the timing of *IL2RA* activation in response to stimulation and the deletion of the enhancer containing the variant skewed polarization of naive T cells toward a pro-inflammatory TH17 cell state [75]. Interestingly, the identification of multiple T1D susceptibility genes in the IL-2 pathway (*IL2RA*, *IL2*, *IL21*, *BACH2*, *PTPN2*, *IL10*) through GWAS [76, 77] promoted the use of aldesleukin (Proleukin; recombinant human IL-2) at low doses to treat this condition [78].

12.4 Interferon Signature

A dysregulation of the adaptive immune system is considered a principal disease mechanism in autoimmunity, but multiple lines of evidence suggest that the innate immune system also plays an important role in such conditions. Type I interferons (IFNs) are key signaling cytokines involved in the activation of the innate immune response and recruitment of adaptive immune mediators [79] and are implicated in the pathogenesis of some autoimmune diseases, especially SLE [80]. Multiple genes involved in interferon signaling have been associated with autoimmune diseases [81]. In SLE, GWASs have identified multiple loci associated with type I interferon signaling pathways, including *TLR7*, *IRAK1*, *IRF5*, *TYK2*, *IRF7*, and *IFIH1* [82]. Some of these genes also are shared with other autoimmune diseases: *IRF5* is associated with rheumatoid arthritis, inflammatory bowel diseases, and primary biliary cirrhosis; *IFIH1* is associated with type 1 diabetes, psoriasis, and inflammatory diseases.

STAT4 is also an important gene in the IFN signaling pathway that has been shown to be associated with RA, SLE, Sjögren's syndrome, and psoriasis, among other diseases [81]. *STAT4* is activated by type I interferons and is essential for the production of IFN-γ in T cells and natural killer cells [83].

Strong and independently replicated associations have been detected between polymorphic variants within or near IRF8 gene for systemic lupus erythematosus [84], ulcerative colitis [85], Crohn's disease [86, 87], RA [88], and MS [89, 90]. The MS-associated SNP rs17445836, mapping 61 kb downstream of *IRF8*, is also associated with higher peripheral blood mononuclear cell IRF8 mRNA levels [89].

2006;314(5804):1461–3. http://www.ncbi.nlm.nih.gov/pubmed/17068223%5Cn; http://www.pubmedcentral.nih.gov/articlerender.fcgi?artid=PMC4410764.
61. Cargill M, Schrodi SJ, Chang M, Garcia VE, Brandon R, Callis KP, et al. A large-scale genetic association study confirms IL12B and leads to the identification of IL23R as psoriasis-risk genes. Am J Hum Genet [Internet]. 2007;80(2):273–90. http://linkinghub.elsevier.com/retrieve/pii/S0002929707626858.
62. Burton PR, Clayton DG, Cardon LR, Craddock N, Deloukas P, Duncanson A, et al. Association scan of 14,500 nonsynonymous SNPs in four diseases identifies autoimmunity variants. Nat Genet [Internet]. 2007;39(11):1329–37. [cited 2013 Oct 24]. http://www.pubmedcentral.nih.gov/articlerender.fcgi?artid=2680141&tool=pmcentrez&rendertype=abstract.
63. Sarin R, Wu X, Abraham C. Inflammatory disease protective R381Q IL23 receptor polymorphism results in decreased primary CD4+ and CD8+ human T-cell functional responses. Proc Natl Acad Sci U S A [Internet]. 2011;108(23):9560–5. http://www.pnas.org/cgi/doi/10.1073/pnas.1017854108.
64. McInnes IB, Sieper J, Braun J, Emery P, van der Heijde D, Isaacs JD, et al. Efficacy and safety of secukinumab, a fully human anti-interleukin-17A monoclonal antibody, in patients with moderate-to-severe psoriatic arthritis: a 24-week, randomised, double-blind, placebo-controlled, phase II proof-of-concept trial. Ann Rheum Dis [Internet]. 2014;73(2):349–56. [cited 2018 Mar 7]. http://www.ncbi.nlm.nih.gov/pubmed/23361084.
65. Hueber W, Patel DD, Dryja T, Wright AM, Koroleva I, Bruin G, et al. Effects of AIN457, a fully human antibody to interleukin-17A, on psoriasis, rheumatoid arthritis, and uveitis. Sci Transl Med [Internet]. 2010;2(52):52ra72. [cited 2018 Mar 7]. http://www.ncbi.nlm.nih.gov/pubmed/20926833.
66. Sieper J, Deodhar A, Marzo-Ortega H, Aelion JA, Blanco R, Jui-Cheng T, et al. Secukinumab efficacy in anti-TNF-naive and anti-TNF-experienced subjects with active ankylosing spondylitis: results from the MEASURE 2 Study. Ann Rheum Dis [Internet]. 2017;76(3):571–92. [cited 2018 Mar 7]. http://www.ncbi.nlm.nih.gov/pubmed/27582421.
67. Visscher PM, Wray NR, Zhang Q, Sklar P, McCarthy MI, Brown MA, et al. 10 years of GWAS discovery: biology, function, and translation [Internet]. Am J Hum Genet. 2017;101:5–22. Cell Press; [cited 2018 Mar 7]. https://www.sciencedirect.com/science/article/pii/S0002929717302409?via%3Dihub.
68. Farh KKH, Marson A, Zhu J, Kleinewietfeld M, Housley WJ, Beik S, et al. Genetic and epigenetic fine mapping of causal autoimmune disease variants. Nature. 2015;518(7539):337–43.
69. Parkes M, Cortes A, van Heel DA, Brown MA. Genetic insights into common pathways and complex relationships among immune-mediated diseases. Nat Rev Genet [Internet]. 2013;14(9):661–73. [cited 2013 Oct 18]. http://www.ncbi.nlm.nih.gov/pubmed/23917628.
70. Hartmann FJ, Khademi M, Aram J, Ammann S, Kockum I, Constantinescu C, et al. Multiple sclerosis-associated IL2RA polymorphism controls GM-CSF production in human THcells. Nat Commun. 2014;5:5056.
71. Cerosaletti K, Schneider A, Schwedhelm K, Frank I, Tatum M, Wei S, et al. Multiple autoimmune-associated variants confer decreased IL-2R signaling in CD4+CD25hiT cells of type 1 diabetic and multiple sclerosis patients. PLoS One. 2013;8(12):e83811.
72. Dendrou CA, Plagnol V, Fung E, Yang JHM, Downes K, Cooper JD, et al. Cell-specific protein phenotypes for the autoimmune locus IL2RA using a genotype-selectable human bioresource. Nat Genet [Internet]. 2009;41(9):1011–5. [cited 2013 Oct 24]. http://www.pubmedcentral.nih.gov/articlerender.fcgi?artid=2749506&tool=pmcentrez&rendertype=abstract.
73. Ye CJ, Feng T, Kwon H-K, Raj T, Wilson MT, Asinovski N, et al. Intersection of population variation and autoimmunity genetics in human T cell activation. Science. 2014;345(6202):1254665. http://www.sciencemag.org/cgi/doi/10.1126/science.1254665.
74. Huang H, Fang M, Jostins L, Umićević Mirkov M, Boucher G, Anderson CA, et al. Fine-mapping inflammatory bowel disease loci to single-variant resolution. Nature. 2017;547(7662):173–8.

75. Simeonov DR, Gowen BG, Boontanrart M, Roth TL, Gagnon JD, Mumbach MR, et al. Discovery of stimulation-responsive immune enhancers with CRISPR activation. Nature. 2017;549:111–5.
76. Lowe CE, Cooper JD, Brusko T, Walker NM, Smyth DJ, Bailey R, et al. Large-scale genetic fine mapping and genotype-phenotype associations implicate polymorphism in the IL2RA region in type 1 diabetes. Nat Genet [Internet]. 2007;39(9):1074–82. [cited 2013 Oct 24]. http://www.ncbi.nlm.nih.gov/pubmed/17676041.
77. Todd JA, Walker NM, Cooper JD, Smyth DJ, Downes K, Plagnol V, et al. Robust associations of four new chromosome regions from genome-wide analyses of type 1 diabetes. Nat Genet [Internet]. 2007;39(7):857–64. [cited 2013 Oct 24]. http://www.pubmedcentral.nih.gov/articlerender.fcgi?artid=2492393&tool=pmcentrez&rendertype=abstract.
78. Todd JA, Evangelou M, Cutler AJ, Pekalski ML, Walker NM, Stevens HE, et al. Regulatory T cell responses in participants with type 1 diabetes after a single dose of interleukin-2: a non-randomised, open label, adaptive dose-finding trial. PLoS Med. 2016;13(10):e1002139.
79. Forster S. Interferon signatures in immune disorders and disease. Immunol Cell Biol. 2012;90:520–7.
80. López de Padilla CM, Niewold TB. The type I interferons: basic concepts and clinical relevance in immune-mediated inflammatory diseases. Gene. 2016;576:14–21.
81. Delgado-Vega AM, Alarcón-Riquelme ME, Kozyrev SV. Genetic associations in type I interferon related pathways with autoimmunity. Arthritis Res Ther. 2010;12:S2.
82. Niewold TB. Advances in lupus genetics. Curr Opin Rheumatol. 2015;27:440–7.
83. Liang Y, Pan H-F, Ye D-Q. Therapeutic potential of STAT4 in autoimmunity. Expert Opin Ther Targets [Internet]. 2014;18(8):945–60. http://www.tandfonline.com/doi/full/10.1517/14728222.2014.920325.
84. Graham DS, Morris DL, Bhangale TR, Criswell LA, Syvänen AC, Rönnblom L, et al. Association of NCF2, IKZF1, IRF8, IFIH1, and TYK2 with systemic lupus erythematosus. PLoS Genet. 2011;7(10):e1002341.
85. Anderson CA, Boucher G, Lees CW, Franke A, D'Amato M, Taylor KD, et al. Meta-analysis identifies 29 additional ulcerative colitis risk loci, increasing the number of confirmed associations to 47. Nat Genet. 2011;43:246–52.
86. Barrett JC, Hansoul S, Nicolae DL, Cho JH, Duerr RH, Rioux JD, et al. Genome-wide association defines more than 30 distinct susceptibility loci for Crohn's disease. Nat Genet [Internet]. 2008;40(8):955–62. [cited 2013 Oct 24]. http://www.pubmedcentral.nih.gov/articlerender.fcgi?artid=2574810&tool=pmcentrez&rendertype=abstract.
87. Elding H, Lau W, Swallow DM, Maniatis N. Dissecting the genetics of complex inheritance: linkage disequilibrium mapping provides insight into Crohn disease. Am J Hum Genet [Internet]. 2011;89(6):798–805. [cited 2013 Oct 24]. http://www.pubmedcentral.nih.gov/articlerender.fcgi?artid=3234369&tool=pmcentrez&rendertype=abstract.
88. Okada Y, Wu D, Trynka G, Raj T, Terao C, Ikari K, et al. Genetics of rheumatoid arthritis contributes to biology and drug discovery. Nature [Internet]. 2014;506(7488):376–81. [cited 2018 Mar 26]. http://www.nature.com/articles/nature12873.
89. De Jager PL, Jia X, Wang J, De Bakker PIW, Ottoboni L, Aggarwal NT, et al. Meta-analysis of genome scans and replication identify CD6, IRF8 and TNFRSF1A as new multiple sclerosis susceptibility loci. Nat Genet [Internet]. 2009;41(7):776–82. https://doi.org/10.1038/ng.401.
90. Leppä V, Surakka I, Tienari PJ, Elovaara I, Compston A, Sawcer S, et al. The genetic association of variants in CD6, TNFRSF1A and IRF8 to multiple sclerosis: a multicenter case-control study. PLoS One. 2011;6(4):e18813.
91. Bottini N, Musumeci L, Alonso A, Rahmouni S, Nika K, Rostamkhani M, et al. A functional variant of lymphoid tyrosine phosphatase is associated with type I diabetes. Nat Genet [Internet]. 2004;36(4):337–8. [cited 2013 Oct 24]. http://www.ncbi.nlm.nih.gov/pubmed/15004560.
92. Lee YH, Rho YH, Choi SJ, Ji JD, Song GG, Nath SK, et al. The PTPN22 C1858T functional polymorphism and autoimmune diseases—a meta-analysis. Rheumatology. 2007;46(1):49–56.

93. Gourh P, Tan FK, Assassi S, Ahn CW, McNearney TA, Fischbach M, et al. Association of the PTPN22 R620W polymorphism with anti-topoisomerase I- and anticentromere antibody-positive systemic sclerosis. Arthritis Rheum. 2006;54(12):3945–53.
94. Hedjoudje A, Cheurfa C, Briquez C, Zhang A, Koch S, Vuitton L. Rs2476601 polymorphism in PTPN22 is associated with Crohn's disease but not with ulcerative colitis: a meta-analysis of 16,838 cases and 13,356 controls. Ann Gastroenterol. 2017;30(2):197–208.
95. Zhang J, Zahir N, Jiang Q, Miliotis H, Heyraud S, Meng X, et al. The autoimmune disease-associated PTPN22 variant promotes calpain-mediated Lyp/Pep degradation associated with lymphocyte and dendritic cell hyperresponsiveness. Nat Genet [Internet]. 2011;43(9):902–7. https://doi.org/10.1038/ng.904.
96. Stanford SM, Bottini N. PTPN22: the archetypal non-HLA autoimmunity gene. Nat Rev Rheumatol. 2014;10:602–11.
97. Ma A, Malynn BA. A20: linking a complex regulator of ubiquitylation to immunity and human disease. Nat Rev Immunol. 2012;12:774–85.
98. Musone SL, Taylor KE, Lu TT, Nititham J, Ferreira RC, Ortmann W, et al. Multiple polymorphisms in the TNFAIP3 region are independently associated with systemic lupus erythematosus. Nat Genet [Internet]. 2008;40(9):1062–4. [cited 2013 Oct 24]. http://www.ncbi.nlm.nih.gov/pubmed/19165919.
99. Martin JE, Broen JC, Carmona FD, Teruel M, Simeon CP, Vonk MC, et al. Identification of CSK as a systemic sclerosis genetic risk factor through Genome Wide Association Study follow-up. Hum Mol Genet. 2012;21(12):2825–35.
100. Adrianto I, Wen F, Templeton A, Wiley G, King JB, Lessard CJ, et al. Association of a functional variant downstream of TNFAIP3 with systemic lupus erythematosus. Nat Genet. 2011;43:253–8.
101. Elsby LM, Orozco G, Denton J, Worthington J, Ray DW, Donn RP. Functional evaluation of TNFAIP3 (A20) in rheumatoid arthritis. Clin Exp Rheumatol. 2010;28(5):708–14. http://www.scopus.com/inward/record.url?eid=2-s2.0-78650560490&partnerID=MN8TOARS.
102. McGovern A, Schoenfelder S, Martin P, Massey J, Duffus K, Plant D, et al. Capture Hi-C identifies a novel causal gene, IL20RA, in the pan-autoimmune genetic susceptibility region 6q23. Genome Biol. 2016;17(1):212. http://europepmc.org/abstract/med/27799070.
103. Gateva V, Sandling JK, Hom G, Taylor KE, Chung SA, Sun X, et al. A large-scale replication study identifies TNIP1, PRDM1, JAZF1, UHRF1BP1 and IL10 as risk loci for systemic lupus erythematosus. Nat Genet. 2009;41(11):1228–33.
104. Harden JL, Krueger JG, Bowcock AM. The immunogenetics of psoriasis: a comprehensive review. J Autoimmun. 2015;64:66–73.
105. Bossini-Castillo L, López-Isac E, Martín J. Immunogenetics of systemic sclerosis: defining heritability, functional variants and shared-autoimmunity pathways. J Autoimmun. 2015;64:53–65.
106. Alpi AF, Chaugule V, Walden H. Mechanism and disease association of E2-conjugating enzymes: lessons from UBE2T and UBE2L3. Biochem J. 2016;473(20):3401–19.
107. Järvinen TM, Hellquist A, Zucchelli M, Koskenmies S, Panelius J, Hasan T, et al. Replication of GWAS-identified systemic lupus erythematosus susceptibility genes affirms B-cell receptor pathway signalling and strengthens the role of IRF5 in disease susceptibility in a Northern European population. Rheumatology. 2012;51(1):87–92.
108. Génin E, Coustet B, Allanore Y, Ito I, Teruel M, Constantin A, et al. Epistatic interaction between BANK1 and BLK in rheumatoid arthritis: results from a large trans-ethnic meta-analysis. PLoS One. 2013;8(4):e61044.
109. Rueda B, Gourh P, Broen J, Agarwal SK, Simeon C, Ortego-Centeno N, et al. BANK1 functional variants are associated with susceptibility to diffuse systemic sclerosis in Caucasians. Ann Rheum Dis. 2010;69(4):700–5.
110. Gourh P, Agarwal SK, Martin E, Divecha D, Rueda B, Bunting H, et al. Association of the C8orf13-BLK region with systemic sclerosis in North-American and European populations. J Autoimmun. 2010;34(2):155–62.

111. Yokoyama K, Su IH, Tezuka T, Yasuda T, Mikoshiba K, Tarakhovsky A, et al. BANK regulates BCR-induced calcium mobilization by promoting tyrosine phosphorylation of IP3receptor. EMBO J. 2002;21(1–2):83–92.
112. Kozyrev SV, Abelson AK, Wojcik J, Zaghlool A, Linga Reddy MVP, Sanchez E, et al. Functional variants in the B-cell gene BANK1 are associated with systemic lupus erythematosus. Nat Genet. 2008;40(2):211–6.
113. Tretter T, Ross AE, Dordai DI, Desiderio S. Mimicry of pre–B cell receptor signaling by activation of the tyrosine kinase Blk. J Exp Med. 2003;198(12):1863–73.
114. Hom G, Graham RR, Modrek B, Taylor KE, Ortmann W, Garnier S, et al. Association of systemic lupus erythematosus with C8orf13-BLK and ITGAM-ITGAX. N Engl J Med. 2008;358(9):900–9.
115. Castillejo-López C, Delgado-Vega AM, Wojcik J, Kozyrev SV, Thavathiru E, Wu YY, et al. Genetic and physical interaction of the B-cell systemic lupus erythematosus-associated genes BANK1 and BLK. Ann Rheum Dis. 2012;71(1):136–42.
116. Subramanian V, Knight JS, Parelkar S, Anguish L, Coonrod SA, Kaplan MJ, et al. Design, synthesis, and biological evaluation of tetrazole analogs of Cl-amidine as protein arginine deiminase inhibitors. J Med Chem. 2015;58(3):1337–44.
117. Kawalkowska J, Quirke AM, Ghari F, Davis S, Subramanian V, Thompson PR, et al. Abrogation of collagen-induced arthritis by a peptidyl arginine deiminase inhibitor is associated with modulation of T cell-mediated immune responses. Sci Rep. 2016;6:26430.
118. Maurano MT, Humbert R, Rynes E, Thurman RE, Haugen E, Wang H, et al. Systematic localization of common disease-associated variation in regulatory DNA. Science. 2012;337(6099):1190–5.
119. Schaub MA, Boyle AP, Kundaje A, Batzoglou S, Snyder M. Linking disease associations with regulatory information in the human genome. Genome Res. 2012;22(9):1748–59.
120. Freedman ML, Monteiro AN, Gayther SA, Coetzee GA, Risch A, Plass C, et al. Principles for the post-GWAS functional characterization of cancer risk loci. Nat Genet [Internet]. 2011;43(6):513–8. [cited 2013 Oct 18]. http://www.pubmedcentral.nih.gov/articlerender.fcgi?artid=3325768&tool=pmcentrez&rendertype=abstract.
121. Ward LD, Kellis M. Interpreting noncoding genetic variation in complex traits and human disease. Nat Biotechnol. 2012;30:1095–106.
122. Krijger PHL, de Laat W. Regulation of disease-associated gene expression in the 3D genome. Nat Rev Mol Cell Biol [Internet]. 2016;17(12):771–82. [cited 2018 Mar 26]. http://www.nature.com/articles/nrm.2016.138.
123. Lieberman-Aiden E, van Berkum NL, Williams L, Imakaev M, Ragoczy T, Telling A, et al. Comprehensive mapping of long-range interactions reveals folding principles of the human genome. Science [Internet]. 2009;326(5950):289–93. [cited 2013 Oct 17]. http://www.pubmedcentral.nih.gov/articlerender.fcgi?artid=2858594&tool=pmcentrez&rendertype=abstract.
124. Dryden NH, Broome LR, Dudbridge F, Johnson N, Orr N, Schoenfelder S, et al. Unbiased analysis of potential targets of breast cancer susceptibility loci by Capture Hi-C. Genome Res. 2014;24(11):1854–68.
125. Jäger R, Migliorini G, Henrion M, Kandaswamy R, Speedy HE, Heindl A, et al. Capture Hi-C identifies the chromatin interactome of colorectal cancer risk loci. Nat Commun. 2015;6:6178.
126. Javierre BM, Sewitz S, Cairns J, Wingett SW, Várnai C, Thiecke MJ, et al. Lineage-specific genome architecture links enhancers and non-coding disease variants to target gene promoters. Cell. 2016;167(5):1369–84.e19.
127. Martin P, McGovern A, Orozco G, Duffus K, Yarwood A, Schoenfelder S, et al. Capture Hi-C reveals novel candidate genes and complex long-range interactions with related autoimmune risk loci. Nat Commun. 2015;6:10069. http://europepmc.org/abstract/med/26616563.
128. Gallagher MD, Chen-Plotkin AS. The post-GWAS era: from association to function. Am J Hum Genet [Internet]. 2018;102(5):717–30. [cited 2018 May 11]. http://www.ncbi.nlm.nih.gov/pubmed/29727686.

Index

J. Martin, F. D. Carmona (eds.), *Genetics of Rare Autoimmune Diseases*, Rare Diseases of the Immune System, https://doi.org/10.1007/978-3-030-03934-9

Printed by Printforce, the Netherlands